Palliative Care Nursing of Children and Young People

Rita Pfund

Lecturer (Child Health)
University of Nottingham School of Nursing

Foreword by

Professor Susan Fowler-Kerry PhD

College of Nursing
University of Saskatchewan, Canada

Radcliffe Publishing
Oxford • Seattle

Radcliffe Publishing Ltd
18 Marcham Road
Abingdon
Oxon OX14 1AA
United Kingdom

www.radcliffe-oxford.com
Electronic catalogue and worldwide online ordering facility.

———————————————

British Library Cataloguing in Publication Data

A catalogue record for this book is available from the British Library.

ISBN-10: 1 84619 019 3
ISBN-13: 978 1 84619 019 3

Typeset by Wordspace, Lewes, East Sussex
Printed and bound by TJ International Ltd, Padstow, Cornwall

Contents

Group 4: Conditions with severe neurological disability which may cause weakness and susceptibility to health complications, and may deteriorate unpredictably, but are not usually considered progressive. Examples: severe multiple disabilities such as following brain or spinal cord injuries including some children with severe cerebral palsy

Foreword

Every year, the unthinkable still happens and children continue to die from trauma, lethal congenital conditions, extreme prematurity, heritable disorders, or acquired illness. With every medical breakthrough reported, every child saved creates a burden of expectation that the next child can also be saved. Aggressive treatment in our death denying society has become synonymous with buying time and holds out the possibility of a cure. When a child's life is at stake, many in our society believe there is no such thing as going too far, a philosophical position misunderstood in relation to what palliative care truly is.

To assist with the necessary cognitive lane change, Rita begins her text by making a cogent point that it is no longer acceptable practice to utilize adult models of palliative care with children and youth, where the underlying assumption exists that palliative care begins when curative fails, thereby eliminating the option of cure. This assumption is not true in the pediatric context, where there may still be curative options available. She succinctly points out that pediatric definitions of palliative care reflect a broader, holistic dimension to children's health care that most health professionals would agree is applicable to all children and their families, regardless of their diagnosis. Within these definitions is a strong emphasis towards an integrated model of care which is evidence based. This emphasis is a logical outcome, where health care professionals are forced to think of an integrated approach to care due to the diagnostic diversity, protracted nature of many of the illness trajectories, as well as the developmental needs of the child and their family.

Implicit within the text is the belief that palliative care programs must be regarded as a right of children globally. Several international statutes including the Universal Declaration of Human Rights and Convention on the Rights of the Child have recognized children as citizens in their own right and as independent bearers of rights. These manifestos articulate worldwide moral standards for the treatment of children. Within this context, it is no longer acceptable not to provide comprehensive, evidence based palliative care to all children and families who require these services. The development of new models in different locales, nationally and internationally, must receive government funding to create a sustainable subsidiary.

Rita's passion and commitment as an advocate for improving the quality of life of children with life-limiting and life-threatening illness and their families is clearly evident throughout every page of this book, a text that she herself asserts was never intended to be the definitive source of palliative care for children and young people. Rather, as nurse educator, she approaches the subject from an applied clinical perspective, examining the current state of practice. Children's palliative care is an evolving speciality and as such our knowledge base cannot remain static. Rita constantly challenges the reader to critically analyze their own practices and beliefs within an evidence-based framework and as such makes a valuable contribution to the growing body of knowledge on this important subject.

Childhood is an enigma. The home of all the great questions about life and death, reality and dreams. Recognizing the uniqueness of childhood, Rita has provided the reader with a new lens to view the changing and individualized palliative care needs of children and their families.

Professor Susan Fowler-Kerry PhD
College of Nursing
University of Saskatchewan, Canada
September 2006

Preface

The original intention of this book was to examine the evidence base within palliative care for children and young people. The time of writing coincided with a huge number of publications resulting from the implementation of and further developments around 'Every Child Matters' and the National Service Framework for Children. The book resulting from this captures not just the rapidly evolving evidence base but also as many current developments as possible and applies them in a meaningful way to the care of infants, children and young people living with life-limiting illness, and their families. However, it can only provide a snapshot at a time when children's services in general, and children's and young people's palliative care services in particular, are undergoing rapid changes.

My hope is that this book will offer an overview of contemporary issues to readers and will help to stimulate the type of dialogue that can bring about the actions that will make a real difference for the children, young people and families in our care.

Rita Pfund
September 2006

About the author

Rita Pfund is a lecturer in child health at the University of Nottingham, with a professional interest in palliative care for children and young people. This developed following considerable experience of caring for children and young people with life-limiting illnesses and their families, in both regional and district general hospitals as well as a children's hospice.

Acknowledgements

I would like to thank the following individuals and institutions for their help and constructive criticism:

- Dr Mike Miller, Paediatric Palliative Care Consultant, Martin House Hospice
- Lizzie Chambers, Chief Executive, Association for Children with Life-Threatening or Terminal Conditions and their Families (ACT)
- Erica Brown, Head of Research and Development, Acorns Children's Hospice
- Dr Richard Hain, Senior Lecturer in Paediatric Palliative Medicine, Children's Hospital of Wales, Cardiff
- Jackie Browne and Gillian Bishop, Paediatric Bereavement Services, University Hospitals Nottingham
- Jo Rooney, Kite–Team Co-ordinator, Children's Services, Derby City General Hospital
- Di Melvin, Consultant Clinical Psychologist, Department of Psychological Medicine, Great Ormond Street Hospital
- David Widdas, Nurse Consultant for Children with Complex Needs, North and South Warwickshire, Coventry and Rugby Primary Care Trusts
- Janneke van Wageningen, Psychologist, and Riet Niezen, Bartimeus, NCL Expertise Centre, Netherlands
- Royal College of Paediatrics and Child Health, for permission to reproduce a large section of *Withholding and Withdrawing Life-Saving Treatment in Children: a framework of practice* (published in 2004)
- Dr Sasha Scambler, King's College London
- Brother Francis, Clinical Nurse Specialist in Paediatric Oncology and Related Palliative Care
- Jonathan Perks, Charge Nurse, Transitional Care Unit, Great Ormond Street Hospital
- all the staff on Dolphin Unit, Derby City General Hospital Children's Unit
- Maureen Gambles, Research Team, Liverpool Pathway for the Dying Child
- The Reverend Julian Hemstock, Chaplaincy Services, University Hospitals Nottingham
- Wes Magee, children's author
- My colleagues: Dr Carol Hall, Prof Davina Porrock, Paula Dawson, Sally Melling, Dawn Ritchie, School of Nursing, University of Nottingham.

This book is for all the boys and girls whose mums and dads
just wanted them to be ordinary kids.

The hardest part of living is giving up what has been given. And you know no one could love you more. Whatever the future has in store I want you to remember that we laughed.

We Laughed, **by Billy Bragg and**
Maxine Edgington
From the CD *Rosetta Requiem* **(2005)**
produced by Rosetta Life, London.

How this book works

This book is about working with life-limited children and young people and their families, and it uses scenarios throughout. Although care is needed when generalising from these scenarios, they are useful for highlighting themes that affect families. They provide an opportunity to look at how a multi-disciplinary team might organise care for a family and what the outcomes could be.

Recently there have been a number of new initiatives, such as the ACT Care Pathways published by the Association for Children with Life-Threatening or Terminal Conditions and their Families (ACT),[1] and the National Service Framework for Children, Young People and Maternity Services (the NSF).[2,3] This book shows how working with them in a reflective way and giving evidence-based care helps to improve the lives of life-limited children and young people and their families.

The book emphasises the application of key skills, particularly communication, working with others, problem solving, improving one's own learning, and information technology.

Working with the key documents

'Every Child Matters'[4] and the Children Act 2004[5] provide the legislative backbone. There is also a new Children's Bill.[6]

The NSF provides the guidelines, and the Knowledge and Skills Framework (KSF),[7] as its name suggests, is a framework for the knowledge and skills required for the job.

The ACT Care Pathway represents the application of these.

This book shows how the contents of these documents can be applied in practice.

Aynsley-Green[8] has predicted that the processes, debate, discussion and awareness generated around the NSF will create an unstoppable movement which will deliver real change for children's services irrespective of political agendas and governments. The child's journey might take them to an Accident and Emergency department in a district general hospital (DGH), and might then involve transfer to a regional centre, transfer back to the DGH and then back to society to face the next milestone. Aynsley-Green has mapped the needs of the child and their family at each of these milestones, and alongside these are mapped the competencies required to deliver them in the context of giving an explanation to families so that they know:

- what is going to happen to their child
- what they are going to be faced with
- how they are going to support their child as he or she moves through different circumstances.

According to Aynsley-Green, the NSF provides much detail, but nothing will happen unless there is local action driven by practitioners as agents for change for children. To seize this momentum, this book challenges some views, practices and attitudes, and is sometimes provocative. It integrates theory and practice and provides a wealth of evidence-based literature for the reader to follow up. Although on the surface it might appear to be repetitive in parts, this is not the case, but it does require the reader to transfer skills and thought processes from one situation to another.

What this book does not do is provide all the answers, because it is assumed that these need to be sought and implemented in the reader's own working environment. The intention is not to provide comprehensive information about disease processes and corresponding care, as it is assumed that the reader has access to information about the actual illnesses portrayed in the scenarios.

Format of the book

The book has three parts.

1. Part One defines palliative care for children and young people and goes on to explore the emotional safety needs of children and young people who are experiencing adverse events.
2. Part Two explores factors that affect children and young people with life-limiting illness and their families, and considers how their needs can be met. The chapters in this section follow the same format, with a scenario setting the scene and the reader then reflecting on the emotions generated by this. A brief SWOT (strengths, weaknesses, opportunities and threats) analysis encourages the reader to explore their existing knowledge as well as their attitudes and learning needs resulting from the scenario.
3. Part Three explores safe practice in expanding boundaries and exploring personal issues and attitudes, as well as professional, legal and ethical issues that guide professional practice.

An enquiry-based learning style is used throughout the book. This means that the reader decides to what extent suggested material is followed up in terms of both theoretical knowledge and practice. However, it is strongly suggested that the reader familiarises himor herself with the key documents discussed in the Appendix. These not only underpin practitioners' work in all areas of child health, but also provide the tools and ammunition necessary to advocate effectively for the children and young people and their families in our care.

The scenarios

There are nine scenarios in the book, structured around the four groups of life-limited illness as identified by ACT and the Royal College of Paediatrics and Child Health:[9,10]

- a neonatal death
- a young child with a sudden serious illness
- an adolescent with cancer
- a young adult who has 'outgrown' paediatric services
- a family affected by HIV
- a young child with a neurological degenerative illness
- a cognate school-age child with a degenerative illness
- a technology-dependent child
- a child with complex needs.

Each scenario identifies biopsychosocial and spiritual issues that require fact finding and considering all aspects of the family's life.

Personal reflection

After each scenario, the reader is encouraged to reflect on their personal feelings and responses, and the memories that the scenario evokes of similar situations. Whittle[11] describes the emotions experienced by nurses when caring for dying children as stressful and rewarding feelings, as well as feelings of guilt, intense sorrow and sadness, with a need to give meaning to these experiences. Benner[12] offers a poignant account of such a reflection:

> The significance of this event in my life is multi-faceted. First it made me examine myself and the way I deal with others, particularly the quiet parent....Often that reserve is a façade over their inner terror. Although they appear to be coping, a few non-threatening questions...some trivial chit-chat can open them up and allow them to express their fears, thoughts and questions.

This process is described by White and Epstein[13] as 'externalisation.' Manley *et al.*[14] consider reflective ability (reflexivity) to be important not only in the ability to uncover expertise, but also in a person's ability to further analyse and synthesise insightfulness to others in a meaningful way.

This book acknowledges the difficulties that are faced by practitioners working in this field. Not only do they have to deal with the death of young people, but they also have to cope with the expectations of families and colleagues. By working through the chapters, the reader is helped to understand the roles of the different members of the multi-disciplinary team.

SWOT analysis

Below is an example of a SWOT analysis. Some suggestions are made to help the reader to get started. What are your learning needs when considering this chapter? They could look similar to the following:

Strengths	*Weaknesses*
• Having a range of documents to guide practice. • There is an increasing research base and I am becoming more confident about accessing it.	• On the surface it all sounds rather vague.
Opportunities	*Threats*
• This very vagueness offers plenty of scope for imaginative interpretation. • A lot of work is being done to improve care for life-limited children and young people and their families. • There is plenty of opportunity for networking.	• The sheer volume of guiding literature – do I really need to know all this? • Imaginative interpretation can be viewed in terms of providing best practice or be interpreted differently to protect the budget.

Throughout the book the reader is encouraged to examine their personal thoughts and needs. For example, their initial response might be 'I really do not want to deal with this.' After reflection and relating the situation to their own working practices and environment, this could become 'What are my responsibilities in this situation?'

The final part of the book considers safe practice in expanding boundaries, and a coping exercise that examines personal resources and demands made on individuals is suggested. However, the reader might wish to examine their personal coping mechanisms as part of each chapter.

Guiding questions

These offer some questions and model answers to prompt the reader to think further about the subject. The family's situation is explored by following the ACT Care Pathways. It is recommended that readers use a marker pen to identify where on the pathways they might find themselves at any one time.

The relevant sections of the NSF are highlighted and skills required are mapped against the Knowledge and Skills Framework (KSF).[7]

Enquiry-based learning

Enquiry-based learning (EBL) is an educational method which uses real-life scenarios that allow readers to learn from them. Clinical skills as required by the KSF[7] are explored. McSherry and Proctor-Childs[15] highlight the importance of integrating theory and practice, as this encourages the practice of evidence-based nursing.

Contemporary issues

Most chapters contain additional information, including recent research, that is relevant to the chapter topic. There is also cross-referencing between chapters (indicated at the beginning of each chapter).

Clinical governance and suggestions for work-based learning and networking

According to Scally and Donaldson,[16] clinical governance is:

> A framework through which NHS organisations are accountable for continually improving the quality of their services and safeguarding high standards of care by creating an environment in which excellence in clinical care will flourish.

Clinical governance and suggestions for work-based learning and networking encourage the reader to explore issues that are particularly relevant to their own practice, and they are asked to 'play through' all three sections of the ACT Care Pathway in their own working environment. Resources for this are suggested. A further SWOT analysis points the reader towards formulating an action plan for further learning.

References

1. Elston S (2004) *Integrated Multi-Agency Care Pathways for Children with Life-Threatening and Life-Limiting Conditions.* Association for Children with Life-Threatening or Terminal Conditions and their Families, Bristol.
2. Department of Health (2003) *Getting the Right Start: National Service Framework for chil-*

dren. Standard for hospital services. Department of Health, London; www.doh.uk/nsf/children/gettingtherightstart

3. Department of Health (2004) National Service Framework for Children, Young People and Maternity Services: core standards. Department of Health, London.

4. Department for Education and Skills (2003) *Every Child Matters.* DfES Publications, Nottingham; www.everychildmatters.gov.uk/publications/

5. Children Act 2004; www.opsi.gov.uk/acts/acts2004/20040031.htm

6. Children's Bill 2004; http://image.guardian.co.uk/sys-files/Society/documents/2004/03/04/bill.pdf

7. Department of Health (2004) The NHS Knowledge and Skills Framework (NHS KSF) and the Development Review Process. Department of Health, London.

8. Aynsley-Green A (2003) *Practical implications of the emerging NSF for children.* Conference presentation, January 2003.

9. Association for Children with Life-Threatening or Terminal Conditions and their Families (ACT) and the Royal College of Paediatrics and Child Health (1997) *A Guide to the Development of Children's Palliative Care Services.* ACT, Bristol.

10. Association for Children with Life-Threatening or Terminal Conditions and their Families (ACT) and the Royal College of Paediatrics and Child Health (2003) *A Guide to the Development of Children's Palliative Care Services.* ACT, Bristol.

11. Whittle M (2002) Death education: what should student children's nurses be taught? *J Child Health Care.* **6:** 189–201.

12. Benner P (1991) The role of experience, narrative and community in skilled ethical comportment. *Adv Nurs Sci.* **14:** 1–21.

13. White M and Epstein D (1990) *Narrative Means to Therapeutic Ends.* WW Norton, London.

14. Manley K, Hardy S, Titchen A *et al.* (2005) *Changing Patients' Worlds Through Nursing Practice Expertise.* Royal College of Nursing, London.

15. McSherry R and Proctor-Childs T (2001) Promoting evidence-based practice through an integrated model of care: patient case studies as a teaching method. *Nurse Educ Pract.* **1:** 19–26.

16. Scally G and Donaldson L (1998) Clinical governance and the drive for quality improvement in the new NHS in England. *BMJ.* **317:** 61–5; www.cgsupport.nhs.uk/About_CGST/Clinical_Governance_defined.asp

DIAGNOSIS OR RECOGNITION

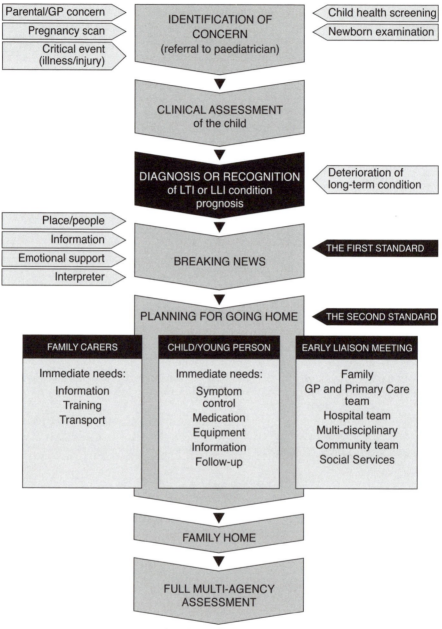

Parental/GP concern

Pregnancy scan

Critical event (illness/injury)

Child health screening

Newborn examination

IDENTIFICATION OF CONCERN
(referral to paediatrician)

▼

CLINICAL ASSESSMENT
of the child

▼

DIAGNOSIS OR RECOGNITION
of LTI or LLI condition
prognosis

Deterioration of long-term condition

▼

Place/people

Information

Emotional support

Interpreter

BREAKING NEWS

THE FIRST STANDARD

▼

PLANNING FOR GOING HOME

THE SECOND STANDARD

FAMILY CARERS	CHILD/YOUNG PERSON	EARLY LIAISON MEETING
Immediate needs: Information Training Transport	Immediate needs: Symptom control Medication Equipment Information Follow-up	Family GP and Primary Care team Hospital team Multi-disciplinary Community team Social Services

▼

FAMILY HOME

▼

FULL MULTI-AGENCY ASSESSMENT

(continues Pathway 2)

LIVING WITH A LIFE-THREATENING OR LIFE-LIMITING CONDITION

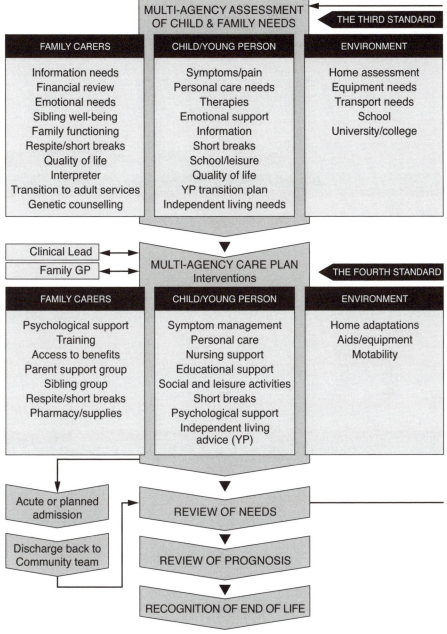

MULTI-AGENCY ASSESSMENT OF CHILD & FAMILY NEEDS

THE THIRD STANDARD

FAMILY CARERS	CHILD/YOUNG PERSON	ENVIRONMENT
Information needs	Symptoms/pain	Home assessment
Financial review	Personal care needs	Equipment needs
Emotional needs	Therapies	Transport needs
Sibling well-being	Emotional support	School
Family functioning	Information	University/college
Respite/short breaks	Short breaks	
Quality of life	School/leisure	
Interpreter	Quality of life	
Transition to adult services	YP transition plan	
Genetic counselling	Independent living needs	

Clinical Lead

Family GP

MULTI-AGENCY CARE PLAN
Interventions

THE FOURTH STANDARD

FAMILY CARERS	CHILD/YOUNG PERSON	ENVIRONMENT
Psychological support	Symptom management	Home adaptations
Training	Personal care	Aids/equipment
Access to benefits	Nursing support	Motability
Parent support group	Educational support	
Sibling group	Social and leisure activities	
Respite/short breaks	Short breaks	
Pharmacy/supplies	Psychological support	
	Independent living advice (YP)	

Acute or planned admission

Discharge back to Community team

REVIEW OF NEEDS

REVIEW OF PROGNOSIS

RECOGNITION OF END OF LIFE

(continues Pathway 3)

END OF LIFE AND BEREAVEMENT

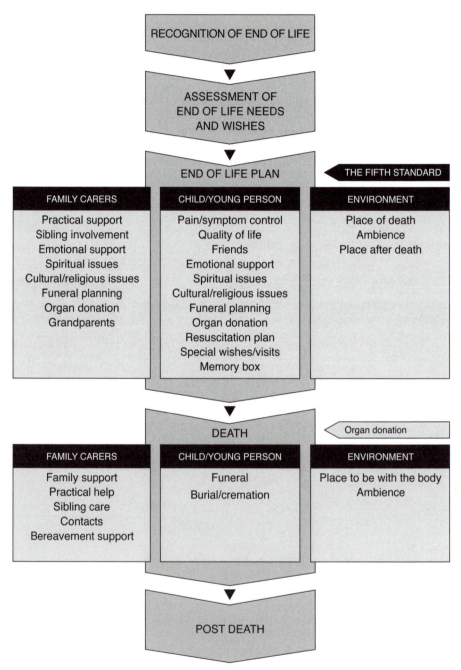

RECOGNITION OF END OF LIFE

ASSESSMENT OF
END OF LIFE NEEDS
AND WISHES

END OF LIFE PLAN   THE FIFTH STANDARD

FAMILY CARERS	CHILD/YOUNG PERSON	ENVIRONMENT
Practical support	Pain/symptom control	Place of death
Sibling involvement	Quality of life	Ambience
Emotional support	Friends	Place after death
Spiritual issues	Emotional support	
Cultural/religious issues	Spiritual issues	
Funeral planning	Cultural/religious issues	
Organ donation	Funeral planning	
Grandparents	Organ donation	
	Resuscitation plan	
	Special wishes/visits	
	Memory box	

DEATH   Organ donation

FAMILY CARERS	CHILD/YOUNG PERSON	ENVIRONMENT
Family support	Funeral	Place to be with the body
Practical help	Burial/cremation	Ambience
Sibling care		
Contacts		
Bereavement support		

POST DEATH

Introduction

Palliative care for children and young people has been recognised as a specialist field within paediatrics for around 25 years. During this time many advances have been made in the care of life-limited and life-threatened children, and particularly in recent months rapid changes have taken place, mainly prompted by the introduction of the National Service Framework for Children.[1,2] Concern is frequently expressed that, as a specialty in its own right, palliative care for children and young people has only a limited evidence base.

Examining the evidence base

In an attempt to examine the evidence base for palliative care for children and young people, I aimed to contextualise the following:

- what we understand by children's and young people's palliative care
- the scope and range of situations in which families might benefit from palliative care
- whether a distinction between a child being 'palliative' or not is relevant or justified
- the frameworks in which palliative care for children and young people can be delivered
- contemporary issues within palliative care for children and young people
- how we translate palliative care for children and young people into practice.

I found a wealth of information, including examples of research on almost every topic I examined, and an almost overwhelming number of relevant documents published in rapid succession, which proved a considerable challenge to keep up with. To present this information I therefore had to be selective about which topics I was going to discuss. I had to make some choices, and I opted for the topics that on balance I considered to be particularly relevant.

This is not a definitive text on palliative care for children and young people, and it makes the assumption that the reader has access to information on the diseases discussed in the book as well as an opportunity to follow up suggested links and documents.

Focusing on just one section of the World Health Organization model of palliative care,[3] on the subject of 'dying care', Porock[4] examined the role of the nurse in the outcome of 'dying care.' She made the sobering point that if a dying person was left alone in a room, without a friend or relative and without a nurse, the outcome for that person would be the same – they would die. This does not seem a good way to enthuse readers about working with families facing life-limiting illness!

The difference we as professionals make is not in the outcome, but in the process – how the child and the family live, often for many years, how the child dies and how the family continues to live.

The special case for palliative care for children and young people – unlike the adult model, which tends to focus on the terminal stages of the disease – is that it aims to accompany the whole family from the child's diagnosis right through to end-of-life care and bereavement.

Because children and families might be living with the child's condition for many years, this book is about living. For the children and young people whose life is limited, life is about living, and about a peaceful death. For the people who are left behind, life is about living, too, and having the support necessary to give them strength at the time of diagnosis, throughout the child's illness and following the death, so that they come through this with their physical and mental health intact.

So where is this 'evidence' in a specialty that has been around for about 25 years? And how can children's palliative care generate evidence? What kind of research are we talking about? It is easy to conjure up images of researchers conducting double-blind controlled trials, and immediately this raises questions of whether it is 'moral' or morally acceptable to undertake research on children and their families during their distress, at a time when every day and every moment is at a premium. Who would undertake this research and generate this evidence?

It can be argued that there is now a considerable body of knowledge, and it is high time that professionals working in the field of children's nursing take ownership of their achievement. With ownership comes a new kind of responsibility, namely preserving the evidence. In palliative care for children and young people this can be disjointed, with little awareness that it is there.

In the wake of a number of high-profile reports,[5,6] new frameworks are being provided to guide and ensure safe care, largely adapted from adult or related disciplines. Accountability and advocacy, clinical governance and benchmarking are all high on the agenda and, importantly when it comes to preserving evidence, the Data Protection Act[7] dictates the minimum time for which records must be kept, although it does not state a maximum time limit. While some areas of 'research' on patients and/or their families would be neither feasible nor ethically acceptable, these early records might provide a wealth of information for retrospective studies, ranging from shedding light on some of the extremely rare conditions that are encountered to evaluating approaches to care.

Looking back: a personal view

Perhaps we need to take a step back and reflect on what it is we are looking at. When I started working in children's palliative care, I thought I was a well-trained all-rounder. I had worked in various settings, ranging from district general hospitals to tertiary referral units. I had seen, or so I believed, a good range of problems with which children presented, and a good proportion of these were very unusual problems. How naive I had been! I soon met children and their families in situations I most certainly had not encountered before. Some conditions were so rare that there were only a handful of cases known in Europe or even worldwide. Some families had the tragedy of having a life-limited child suffering from a rare disease repeated several times over. I shall never forget the family with four children all with Sanfilipo syndrome. Three of the children were profoundly hyperactive, while the fourth had reached the stage of final decline. I had previously met a child with Sanfilipo syndrome as a day case on a neurology ward. I realise now that at the time I had no idea what this meant to the family, all day, every day, every year – in the knowledge that their child would never grow up.

Some children had no diagnosis, and one family in which there were three children affected by the same disease, which had no name, had the syndrome named after them.

The problems and needs of the families I cared for varied tremendously, encompassing every specialty represented in paediatrics. On one day a knowledge base pertaining mainly to neurology, but also to cardiology, might be needed. The next day there might be a child requiring ventilator support and another one needing peritoneal dialysis, while the child coming in the following day was worked up for his third liver transplant. These children and their families all needed respite and competent down-to-earth practical support.

Children's palliative care is constantly evolving, and we cannot pretend that there can ever be one knowledge base capable of covering all eventualities. Similarly, there will never be one decisive text on palliative care. Twenty-five years down the line there still seems to be unease and a degree of confusion about the type of children who fall into this category, and indeed about what 'palliative care' in the context of children and young people actually means.

The changing face of palliative care for children and young people

There have been tremendous changes and challenges in this field. It started with one children's hospice, Helen House, created in 1982 by Mother Frances Dominica, who had the vision and determination to help families with life-limited children. When Martin House opened in 1987 in Boston Spa, many professionals felt that perhaps one more children's hospice could satisfy the demand for such a facility across the country.

The Association for Children with Life-Threatening or Terminal Conditions and their Families (ACT)[8] was established in the late 1980s to advocate actively for children with life-limiting conditions and their families, and it was registered as a national charity in 1992. Starting with the ACT charter for children with life-threatening or terminal conditions and their families in 1993, the research conducted and published through ACT has had a significant impact both on the understanding and acknowledgement of needs, and on the improvement and development of care.

Research conducted through ACT[9] revealed the extent of unmet needs and the staggering numbers of families affected. There are now 36 hospices, and a further 29 are being planned.[10] Different models of support for life-limited children and their families were developed and are still developing, reflecting and responding to identified needs. Community (Diana) teams were set up next, to meet the needs of children who are best cared for in their own environment. The New Opportunities Fund has enabled a massive expansion of this. At the time of going to press, government funding for the children's hospices of £27 million over the next three years has been announced. Funding for children's palliative care services over the longer term is under discussion. There are now three paediatric palliative care consultants working in a range of settings, and we are seeing the first nurse consultant posts developing. Many more models of child and adolescent care practitioners are evolving to suit different local settings. All of these developments are contributing to better cohesion of a service that has historically been driven by the independent sector.

The face of children's palliative care itself is changing. This in part pertains to the age groups catered for. Back in the 1980s it was well recognised that a transition age to adult services of 16 years was not workable, as for many young people this coincided with the time of greatest need. There was virtually no transitional care provided by adult services, and adult hospices, which were mainly geared to caring for adult cancer sufferers, were not an option. Young people frequently and informally continued to be supported by children's services. There are currently two models in operation. One aims for the transfer of young people to adult services. The other operates by keeping young people within one umbrella organisation, with a children's hospice and a separate young people's hospice that caters for young people up to the age of 40 years. Other models of transitional care are being developed.

The range of conditions that present themselves to children's palliative care services has also changed in nature. This challenges the original philosophy, which was based on treatment and prognosis in the classification used in the 1980s. Increasingly there appears to be a dilemma as to whether some children and young people are 'palliative', as well as whether there can be a distinction between 'palliative care' and 'complex needs'.

A framework for palliative care for children and young people

Something else has changed – we now have a clearer framework in which to work. There is evidence of the scope of palliative care for children and young people, thanks to a range of reports published over the last few years. The ACT Care Pathways[11] guide the care that families require on the journey. The National Service Framework[1,2] drives care provision and requires strategic planning at all levels by those providing care. Evidence guides the choices and best care for children, young people and their families. Last but not least, the Knowledge and Skills Framework (KSF)[12] stipulates clear care dimensions for practitioners to follow, supported by a developmental review process that puts practitioners in the driving seat so that they can identify their own learning needs.

Going global

Chambers[13] has observed that many children's palliative care services worldwide work in isolation and find themselves reinventing what has been developed elsewhere, when there could have been opportunity for mutual learning. A virtual global network to facilitate future working and information sharing was set up as the International Children's Palliative Care Network.[14] This is a collaborative partnership between ACT, Help the Hospices and the Association of Children's Hospices (ACH), with the common objectives of information sharing and advocacy for children's hospice and palliative care globally, as well as education and training support.

This is an exciting time for children's palliative care. There are so many strengths to build on. There are also weaknesses that need to be addressed, and there are threats, of course. But more than anything else there are opportunities to be seized. These are what this book is about.

References

1   All the documents for the National Service Framework for Children can be accessed via the Department of Health website; www.dh.gov.uk/PolicyAndGuidance/ HealthAndSocialCareTopics/ChildrenServices/ChildrenServicesInformation/Children ServicesInformationArticle/fs/en?CONTENT_ID=4089111&chk=U8Ecln

2   Department of Health (2004) *National Service Framework for Children, Young People and Maternity Services: core standards*. Department of Health, London.

3   Davies R and Higginson IJ (2004) *Better Palliative Care for Older People*; www.euro.who.int/document/E82933.pdf

4   Porock D (2005) *Dying for Survival: theoretical imperatives for palliative care*. Inaugural lecture, University of Nottingham, Nottingham, 18 October 2005.

5   Laming, WH, Lord (2003) *The Victoria Climbie Inquiry*; www.victoria-climbie-inquiry.org.uk/finreport/report.pdf

6   Kennedy I (2001) *Learning Lessons from Bristol. The Report of the Public Inquiry into Children's Heart Surgery at the Bristol Royal Infirmary 1984–1995*; www.bristol-inquiry.org.uk

7   Data Protection Act 1998; www.opsi.gov.uk/acts/acts1998/19980029.htm

8   Association for Children with Life-Threatening or Terminal Conditions and their Families (ACT); www.act.org.uk

9   Association for Children with Life-Threatening or Terminal Conditions and their Families (ACT) and the Royal College of Paediatrics and Child Health (2003) *A Guide to the Development of Children's Palliative Care Services*. ACT, Bristol.

10 Joy I (2005) *Valuing Short Lives: children with terminal conditions*. New Philanthropy Capital, London.

11 Elston S (ed.) (2004) *Integrated Multi-Agency Care Pathways for Children with Life-Threatening and Life-Limiting Conditions*. ACT, Bristol.

12 Department of Health (2004) *The NHS Knowledge and Skills Framework (NHS KSF) and the Development Review Process*. Department of Health, London.

13 Chambers L (2005) 'A global children's hospice and palliative care website'. *Int J Palliat Nurs*. 11: 292–3.

14 International Children's Palliative Care Network; www.ICPCN.org

Part One

The concept of palliative care for children and young people

Chapter 1

From resistance to resilience: revisiting the concept of palliative care for children and young people

This chapter covers

Content	Relevant to other areas of palliative care for children and young people
• What does the term 'palliative' mean? • Definition of palliative care for children and young people • Definition of life-limiting conditions • Four broad groups • The special case of palliative care for children • Difficulties encountered in provision • Meeting the needs of children, young people and their families • Key outcomes for children • The emotional cost • Common core of skills and knowledge for the children's workforce • High hopes for the NSF • Disability/complex needs/palliative care needs and early referral • Difficulty with the terminology • Principles for assessment work • Principles for effective multi-disciplinary working • Summary	• The concept of palliative care for children and young people is relevant to all other chapters

Why do we need a definition? What does the term 'palliative' mean?

One issue that repeatedly proved to be a stumbling block when researching pertinent aspects of issues to be included in this book was the response 'Our children are not palliative.' It appears that the 'label' matters whether a child gets referred for relevant services or not. Langerman and Worrall[1] quote a service manager: 'We can take only the tip of the iceberg. Many children don't meet our criteria, and they might have quite complex needs but they don't have palliative care needs or degenerative conditions, so they get nothing.' Therefore the first contemporary issue to be explored is the challenge of identifying children and young people who might benefit from palliative care.

Three themes emerged:

1. difficulty with the terminology
2. the need for dissemination of knowledge
3. funding issues.

The last two items will be discussed in detail in individual chapters to highlight how on a day-to-day basis these issues directly affect children and their families. This chapter attempts to clarify what is meant by palliative care for children and young people.

So what does the term 'palliative care' mean in the context of care for children and young people? Are the definition and the perceptions realistic and can the 'progress' seen in paediatrics over the last 25 years justify a demarcation between 'life-limited' and 'chronically ill' children when the common denominator often means that both groups have 'complex' needs, but have very different philosophies and access to funding in the approach to their care?

Definition of palliative care for children and young people

According to the *Concise Oxford Dictionary*,[2] the term 'palliate' means 'to alleviate without curing.'

> Palliative care for children and young people with life-limiting conditions is an active and total approach to care, embracing physical, emotional, social and spiritual elements.
>
> It focuses on enhancement of quality of life for the child and support for the family, and includes the management of distressing symptoms, provision of respite, and care through death and bereavement. It is provided for children for whom curative treatment is no longer the main focus of care, and may extend over many years.
>
> ACT and Royal College of Paediatrics and Child Health[3]

Definition of life-limiting conditions

Life-limiting conditions have been defined as:

> Those for which there is no reasonable hope of cure and from which children will die. Many of these conditions cause progressive deterioration, rendering the child increasingly dependent on parents and carers.
>
> ACT and Royal College of Paediatrics and Child Health[4]

Knebel and Hudgings[5] stress that the healthcare community needs to find a way to talk about end-of-life issues earlier in the course of a disease, so that unnecessary conflict between palliative care and life-prolonging treatments can be avoided. Social, cultural and environmental contexts all influence end-of-life issues.

Four broad groups

The Association for Children with Life-Threatening or Terminal Conditions and their Families (ACT) has identified four broad groups.[3] These have been used to structure the different chapters involving scenarios in this book. The value of these categories soon becomes obvious, as given the long-term nature of palliative care for children and young people, they identify the times when families are most likely to require services. This can assist in the planning and commissioning of services such as respite care provision.

Group 1

- Life-threatening conditions for which curative treatment may be feasible but can fail.
- Palliative care may be necessary during periods of prognostic uncertainty and when treatment fails.
- Children in long-term remission are not included.
- Examples include cancer, and irreversible organ failure of the heart, liver or kidneys.

Group 2

- Conditions for which there may be long periods of intensive treatment aimed at prolonging life and allowing participation in normal childhood activities, although premature death is still possible.
- Examples include cystic fibrosis, muscular dystrophy and HIV.

Group 3

- Progressive conditions without curative treatment options, where treatment is exclusively palliative and may commonly extend over many years.
- Examples include Batten's disease and mucopolysaccharidosis.

Group 4

- Conditions characterised by severe neurological disability which may cause weakness and susceptibility to health complications. Such conditions may deteriorate unpredictably, but are not usually considered to be progressive.
- Examples include severe multiple disabilities (e.g. following brain or spinal cord injuries) and children with severe cerebral palsy.

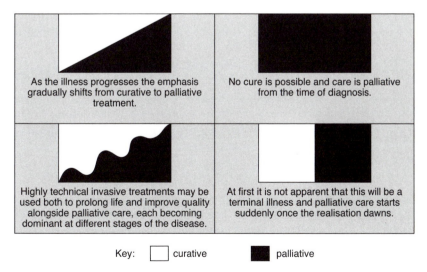

As the illness progresses the emphasis gradually shifts from curative to palliative treatment.

No cure is possible and care is palliative from the time of diagnosis.

Highly technical invasive treatments may be used both to prolong life and improve quality alongside palliative care, each becoming dominant at different stages of the disease.

At first it is not apparent that this will be a terminal illness and palliative care starts suddenly once the realisation dawns.

Key: ☐ curative ■ palliative

Figure 1.1. Curative and palliative care relationship (adapted from ACT and RCPCH[4]).

The special case of palliative care for children[4]

- Small numbers of individuals are involved compared with adults.
- Many of the conditions are extremely rare. Diagnosis is often specific to paediatrics, although the child might survive into early adulthood.
- There is a different timescale to that for adults. The condition may last for only a few days or months, or may extend over several years.
- Many illnesses are familial, and there may be more than one affected child. Genetic counselling should be offered.
- Care embraces the whole family. Parents and siblings are especially vulnerable, and parents bear a heavy responsibility for personal and nursing care.
- A unique characteristic of childhood is the continuing physical, emotional and cognitive development, which is reflected in the child's communication skills and affects their understanding of disease and death.
- Provision of education is essential and is a legal requirement. It also adds an additional professional intervention which increases the complexity of care provision.

Difficulties encountered in provision

- This area is largely unrecognised and underdeveloped, and there is a need for research and evidence-based practice.
- There are limited epidemiological data. In a district with 50,000 children, five are likely to die of progressive illness that requires palliative care, and 50 are likely to have life-limiting illness with some palliative care needs (for half of whom the needs will be substantial).
- This was not previously recognised as a unified group.
- The most comprehensive model at present is cancer nursing, based on outreach nurses working from tertiary centres, district hospitals or community units enabling supportive care by primary healthcare teams. Provision for children with other life-limiting conditions is patchy.
- The needs of families are likely to be complex.
- There is a need for close collaboration between members of a multi-disciplinary team.
- Day-to-day care should be provided in the community.
- Often the components for provision that are needed are already available; there is a need for the support of schools.
- There is considerable psychological stress for the ill child, their siblings, their parents and the staff who are working closely with the family. There is a need for mental healthcare professionals to be available to support families and staff.
- At present most funding is from the voluntary sector. There is a need for integration of funding into overall planning (e.g. Diana nurses).

Meeting the needs of children, young people and their families[3]

Every child and family should expect to:

1. receive a flexible service according to a care plan which is based on individual assessment of their needs, with reviews at appropriate intervals; children and families should be included in the process of care planning
2. be provided with appropriate and timely information
3. have their own named key worker to coordinate their holistic care and provide access to appropriate professionals across the network
4. have access to a local paediatrician in their home area and have access to a local

multi-disciplinary children's palliative care team with a knowledge of the whole range of relevant services

5. be in the care of an identified lead consultant paediatrician who is an expert on the child's condition

6. be supported in the day-by-day management of the child's physical and emotional symptoms and have access to 24-hour care in the terminal stage

7. receive help in meeting the needs of parents and siblings, both during the child's illness and during death and bereavement

8. be offered a range of regular respite, both in the home and away from home and over varying periods of time; this should include nursing care and symptom management

9. have available appropriate supplies of medications, oxygen and specialised feeds, and have all disposable items such as feeding tubes, suction catheters and stoma products supplied regularly, effectively and preferably through a single source

10. have access to housing adaptations and specialised equipment for use at home and at school, in an efficient and timely manner without recourse to several agencies

11. be given assistance in procuring benefits, grants and other financial help.

These are the key elements that are integral to the ACT Care Pathways.[6]

Key outcomes for children

The UK has recently seen a major review of the legal framework governing all children in the form of the Children Act 2004,[7] driven forward by 'Every Child Matters.'[8] There are five key outcomes:

- being healthy
- staying safe
- enjoying and achieving
- making a positive contribution
- economic well-being.

For 'the child in need'[7] there is now a clear duty on local authorities to promote cooperation between agencies (through children's trusts bringing together health, education and social services within a single agency). This will enable professionals from different agencies working together as one team to benefit children and families. Compared with 'Every Child Matters',[8] the National Service Framework for Children does not appear to enjoy such a high profile, but could be viewed as the implementation of the former. Two years into the 10-year plan of the NSF[9,10] large gaps in provision can still be identified, although anecdotal evidence points towards 'first glimpses of changes', such as combining home occupational therapists' assessments for social services and health, thus speeding up assessment and reducing the number of different assessments that need to be undertaken. However, many organisational problems result from care being subject to different policies. For example, the discharge home of a technology-dependent child can still be delayed by up to 3 years if the family needs to be found alternative accommodation appropriate for the additional equipment and carers necessary.

The emotional cost

The emotional cost of having a life-limited child is high for the child him- or herself, the parents and the siblings. This cost will be explored in different contexts in the various chapters of this book. The cost in terms of the physical and mental health of the carers is discussed in Chapters 6 and 9. Various other chapters, notably Chapters 8 and 11, also put this into a financial perspective.

Common core of skills and knowledge for the children's workforce

The common core of skills and knowledge for the children's workforce[11] is discussed in the Appendix (*see* p. 245), and indicates an expectation that there is a knowledge of the services available, and the skills for multi-agency working and information sharing.

High hopes for the NSF

Two years into the NSF there is still much to do. One practical problem with the layout of a complex framework such as the children's NSF in distinct sections is the temptation to compartmentalise the various standards. Although different sections cross-reference to each other, it is difficult to see how they integrate. The ACT Care Pathway[6] is a companion document for Standard 8, Disabled Children and Young People,[12] and those with complex health needs, which is implicitly applicable to different care settings and allows for application to neonatal or critical care, but requires the appropriate knowledge and motivation for this. As the care of children and young people has to be dynamic, perhaps it requires an explicit 'hopping off' point for youngsters whose prognosis improves dramatically. This is not as far-fetched as it sounds. For example, a young person with Duchenne muscular dystrophy (DMD) who was born in the late 1970s or early 1980s could expect to survive to their early or mid teens. However, as treatment has become more sophisticated, especially with ventilatory support, the outlook has changed dramatically and will continue to improve, as it is likely that for younger patients with DMD supportive treatment will be started earlier in the course of the disease in order to delay the onset of pulmonary and cardiac complications.

Similarly, in the case of children receiving transplants, there is a real chance that despite an often protracted period of palliative care needs, many of these children will eventually 'hop off' the palliative care pathway.

Although many areas of care are pushing forward and achieving spectacular successes, for some families the reality looks rather different, and there is no clearly recognised pathway.

An inherent problem for pathways may be that practitioners become overly reliant on them and expect patients to follow an exact pattern (e.g. the diabetes pathway published as part of the NSF). Yet for each child with complex needs and their family the situation is completely different, and this cannot be easily projected on to a standard path.

Pathways do serve as a useful framework that enables professionals to collaborate and to ensure that no major omissions are made, and they can be useful tools for the commissioning of services. An attempt is made in this book to utilise the ACT Care Pathways[6] for the care planning process. Needs that are identified will be very specific to individual families, requiring individual attention within the constraints of very individual local adaptability.

A major issue is the inter-professional collaboration required within the NSF,[9,10,12] the ACT Care Pathways[6] and the Knowledge and Skills Framework (KSF).[13] Palliative care for children and young people is not exclusive to a group of staff who specialise in this area. It is necessary for there to be a wide understanding of what palliative care for children and young people actually is, as opposed to palliative care for adults, which historically refers to end-of-life care (*see* Chapter 6). Only then will practitioners feel comfortable applying the principles appropriately to all who can benefit from such care. It is therefore necessary for practitioners working in both general and critical care, who are usually the first points of contact for these children and their families, to have a sound understanding of palliative care and a robust approach to referral.

There is also a need for adult services to reach out to the paediatric services at the point of transfer to the adult services, allowing for reciprocation of the process, rather than the paediatric services invariably taking the lead. According to the Department of Health,[10] this process should commence when the young person has reached the age of 14 years. The Ellenor Foundation is a hospice-at-home service which, according to Joy,[14] is piloting a pathway for adolescents and young adults, based on persuading professionals in adult services to develop relationships with young people who will come into their care, from the age of 16 years, two years before their transfer at the age of 18 years. During this time the young person might still be completing several loops of the second ACT pathway before reaching the third (end-of-life) pathway.

Having a distinct specialty within child health called 'palliative care' might prove to be less dynamic than a system whereby each specialty identifies the palliative care needs of their patient group, develops the expertise necessary to meet those needs and takes ownership of them. The remit of each specialty is then to appropriately collaborate with the multi-disciplinary team involved with palliative care for children and young people.

Disability/complex needs/palliative care needs and early referral

Hampshire and Polney[15] highlight early identification and intervention as one of the key themes of the NSF, and explain that this means that when potential problems are identified, children should be referred without delay.

But what should they be referred for? Taking as an example the very premature baby whose parents are informed that he or she has a 50% chance of survival, every effort goes into keeping the baby alive. Whether this is the most appropriate care for all such babies is part of an ongoing ethical debate, and it is the right choice for the 50% who come through and consequently enjoy a good quality of life. However, this also means that there is a 50% chance that such a baby might not survive, or would have a poor quality of life if it did. The interpretation of seamless care means that a pathway needs to be in place that allows for the best possible care for both eventualities. This view is not unduly pessimistic. It does not preclude the possibility that the baby will receive the best possible care, but it avoids the situation where there is a feeling that we are 'giving up' on this baby. It also avoids a situation where the parents only gradually over a period of months or years become aware of the full impact of their child's situation, with little coordination of support for them.

Langerman and Worrall[1] describe disability as the interaction between impairment and social, attitudinal, economic or physical barriers. They conclude that if society chooses to spend large amounts of money keeping very premature babies alive, then it must guarantee that adequate services and financial support are available to meet the lifetime care needs of these children. This group of children represents a proportion of disabled children.

Langerman and Worrall[1] highlight the following statistics.

- According to the 2001 General Household Survey,[16] 789,000 children under the age of 16 years are disabled (given that different reports produce different statistics, this is nearly 10% of all children).
- In total, 25,000 children under the age of 19 years suffer from a life-limiting condition.
- In total, 241 children under the age of 16 years were registered as technology dependent. This represented an increase of 77% (from 136) in just three years.

The above figures refer to ventilator-dependent children. However, there are no clear statistics on the total number of children who are in some way 'technology dependent.'

Wang[17] states that the US Congress Office of Technology considers children to be technology dependent if they use 'a medical device to compensate for the loss of a vital bodily function and substantial and ongoing nursing care to avert death or further disability.' According to Wang,[17] discharging these children into the community involves a number of unprecedented social implications that warrant policy consideration, beginning with an understanding of the phenomenon of caring for technology-dependent children who are living at home.

According to the definition put forward by Wang,[17] children who are living with gastrostomies, or who are having daily interventions such as peritoneal dialysis administered by parents, etc., are 'technology dependent.' The extent of the challenges that are created will vary from one child to another. For example, a child with a gastrostomy might superficially appear easy to look after in the community. However, taking into consideration the fact that, unlike pre-gastrostomy management of children with swallowing difficulties, this child will now be normal weight for their age and will live longer, the real challenge might be in providing appropriate equipment, moving and handling aids, appropriate housing and regular reassessment of what Wang[17] summarises as physical, mental, social and financial stress, particularly when dependent children require an ongoing supply of expensive equipment, continuous nursing care and home help.

Difficulty with the terminology

Professional and voluntary groups working with children with life-limiting conditions do not always recognise that they are already providing palliative care, due to the complexity of the definition.[18] The emotive terminology relating to hospices and palliative care can also prevent uptake of services.[19] With regard to the meaning of the term 'palliation', Hain[20] suggests that it may have very different meanings to different people. On the one hand, it could be viewed as the embodiment of compassion – rescuing dying children from the talons of technology and the turmoil of modern medicine. On the other hand, it could be interpreted as the antithesis of good healthcare – denying a child the hope of cure and the chance of life. Yet according to Hain,[20] technology (e.g. the use of ventilation or gastrostomies) and palliation are no longer opposites. In fact, in his call for papers for the third international conference on paediatric palliative care, Hain[20] suggested that the pendulum may have swung too far in allowing palliation to become increasingly invasive.

The discussion therefore seems to have come full circle. Laypeople and professionals alike might have an understanding of adult palliative care anchored in its origins of cancer care, although also expanding towards a wider definition of life-limiting illnesses.

The definition of palliative care for children and young people which has developed over the past 25 years has encompassed the range of needs of the families. Different concepts have evolved in parallel to palliative care for children and young people during this time, including terms such as 'complex needs' and 'technology dependent.' Technology has not just impacted on how it can be used successfully in the palliation of children and young people. Concurrently, technology has been used increasingly not only in groups of children and young people with disabilities, but also for a growing number of children of all ages who have become ventilator dependent for a variety of reasons. Some of these, such as young people with muscular dystrophy, will eventually succumb to their illness. However, for many ventilated children the expectation is that they will 'outgrow' their medical problem by mid-childhood. An optimistic approach is utilised here and the 'label' of 'palliative care' is firmly rejected. All of these families present the same needs for support and care as children in the traditional 'palliative care' categories, because:

> The needs of these families are likely to be many and complex. A proportion have long-term needs with elements in common with severe disability. The parents often carry out much of the care themselves, but they need effective support, help with complex nursing care in the home and the opportunity for short-term breaks which include health provision. Above all they need a named key worker to ensure that provision is planned, coordinated and appropriate.[3]

Principles for assessment work

Planning and coordination need to be based on sound assessment. The Association for Children with Life-Threatening or Terminal Conditions and their Families (ACT)[21] suggests the following principles for assessment work.

- Assessment should be a process, not a single event. Action and services may be provided in parallel.
- A holistic and multi-disciplinary approach should be used.
- Assessment should be in partnership with the family.
- The child or young person should be kept in focus and involved in the process.
- Care should be taken to include fathers, siblings and significant others identified by the child and their family.
- Individuality and ethnicity should be respected.
- Information should be systematically gathered and recorded to ensure consistency and equal opportunities.
- Straightforward, jargon-free language should be used with families.
- The issues of confidentiality and consent should be appropriately addressed.
- Assessment information and action plans should be shared with the family.
- There should be clarity of roles, responsibilities and lines of communication, both for the family and between the different professionals involved.
- Needs should be reviewed and reassessed as an ongoing activity.
- Those undertaking assessments should have appropriate skills and local knowledge.

Principles for effective multi-disciplinary working

Planning and implementing effective care requires effective multi-disciplinary working, the principles of which are set out by ACT[21] as follows:

- clarity with regard to lead role/responsibility
- early joint planning
- cooperation between disciplines and agencies
- clear channels of communication
- shared information
- shared protocols with regard to consent and confidentiality
- understanding each others' roles and terminology.

Summary

This chapter has examined the use of the term 'palliative care' in the context of children and young people experiencing life-limiting illness, and their families. Some children have a label such as 'complex needs' or 'technology dependent', and it is the assessment of the needs of each child and their family that should result in the activation of relevant services to meet the needs that have been identified. The implementation of the Children Act 2004,[7] 'Every Child Matters'[8] and the NSF[9,10] should facilitate and clarify the entitlement to services for 'the child in need.' Care can then be planned, implemented and evaluated using the ACT Care Pathway.[6]

References

1. Langerman C and Worrall E (2005) *Ordinary Lives: disabled children and their families.* New Philanthropy Capital, London.
2. Fowler H and Fowler F (eds) (1992) *Concise Oxford Dictionary.* Clarendon Press, Oxford.
3. Association for Children with Life-Threatening or Terminal Conditions and their

Families (ACT) and the Royal College of Paediatrics and Child Health (2003) *A Guide to the Development of Children's Palliative Care Services*. ACT, Bristol.

4. Association for Children with Life-Threatening or Terminal Conditions and their Families (ACT) and the Royal College of Paediatrics and Child Health (1997) *A Guide to the Development of Children's Palliative Care Services*. ACT, Bristol.

5. Knebel A and Hudgings C (2002) End-of-life issues in genetic disorders: literature and research directions. *Genet Med.* **4:** 366–72.

6. Elston S (ed.) (2004) *Integrated Multi-Agency Care Pathways for Children with Life-Threatening and Life-Limiting Conditions*. ACT, Bristol.

7. Children Act 2004; www.opsi.gov.uk/acts/acts2004/20040031.htm

8. Department for Education and Skills (2003) *Every Child Matters*. DfES Publications, Nottingham.

9. Department of Health (2003) *Getting the Right Start: National Service Framework for children. Standard for hospital services*. Department of Health, London; www.doh.uk/nsf/children/gettingtherightstart

10. Department of Health (2004) *National Service Framework for Children, Young People and Maternity Services: core standards*. Department of Health, London.

11. Department for Education and Skills (2005) *Common Core of Skills and Knowledge for the Children's Workforce. Every child matters*. DfES Publications, Nottingham.

12. Department of Health (2004) *National Service Framework for Children, Young People and Maternity Services: disabled child*. Department of Health, London.

13. Department of Health (2004) *The NHS Knowledge and Skills Framework (NHS KSF) and the Development Review Process*. Department of Health, London.

14. Joy I (2005) *Valuing Short Lives: children with terminal conditions*. New Philanthropy Capital, London.

15. Hampshire A and Polnay L (2005) Referring to others from primary care. In: R Chambers and K Licence (eds) *Looking After Children in Primary Care*. Radcliffe Publishing, Oxford.

16. Walker A, O'Brien M, Traynor J *et al.* (2002) *Living in Britain: results from the 2001 General Household Survey*. Office of National Statistics, Colchester.

17. Wang (2004) Technology-dependent children and their families: a review. *J Adv Nurs.* **45:** 36–46.

18. Irish Department of Health and Children and the Irish Hospice Foundation (2005) *Design and Guidelines for Specialist Palliative Care Settings*. Irish Department of Health and Children, Dublin.

19. Sharman S (2005) *Palliative Care: year two evaluation findings*. The Big Lottery Fund Research Issue 18; www.biglotteryfund.org.uk

20. Hain R (2005) *Call for papers to Third International Conference on Paediatric Palliative Care*, University of Cardiff, 21–23 June 2006; www.cf.ac.uk/medicine/study/child_health/research/palliative_care

21. Association for Children with Life-Threatening or Terminal Conditions and their Families (ACT) and the Royal College of Paediatrics and Child Health (2003) *Assessment of Children with Life-Limiting Conditions and their Families: a guide to effective care planning*. ACT, Bristol.

Chapter 2

Emotional safety in adverse events

This chapter covers

Content

- The NSF standard
- The ACT Care Pathway
- The National Curriculum
- The media
- Grief in children: how bereavements affect children
- Religious, cultural and spiritual context
- Therapeutic work with children
- Books for children
- Books for adolescents
- A book with a cautionary note
- Children who need specialised professional support
- Post-traumatic stress disorder (PTSD)
- Suicide-bereaved children
- Refugee children and victims of public disaster and terrorism
- Clinical governance and suggestions for work-based learning and networking
- Summary

Relevant to other areas of palliative care for children and young people

- Many issues will be relevant to other areas of palliative care for children and young people

Relevant topics in other chapters

- Chapter 4: children with sudden serious illness
- Chapter 5: communication with young people
- Chapter 8: information needs for children with learning disability
- Chapter 9: cognate children who are terminally ill, with a sibling suffering from the same illness
- Chapter 10: information needs for children with acquired learning disability

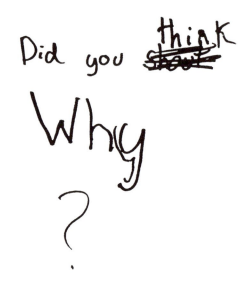

Figure 2.1. Reproduced with permission from Brown.[13]

The day after[1]

I went to school
The day after dad died.
Teacher knew all about it.
She put a hand on my shoulder
And sighed.

In class things seemed much the same
Although I felt strangely subdued.
Breaktime was the same too,
And at lunchtime the usual crew
Played up the dinner supervisors.
Fraggle was downright rude.

I joined in the football game
But volunteered to go in goal.
That meant I was left almost alone,
Could think things over on my own.
For once I let the others shout
And race and roll.

First thing that afternoon,
Everyone in his and her place
For silent reading,
I suddenly felt hot tears streaming
Down my face.
Salty tears slashed down
And soaked into my book's page.
Sobs heaved in my chest.

Teacher peered over her half specs
And said quietly, 'Ben come here.'
I stood at her desk, crying. At my age!
I felt like an idiot, a clown.

'Don't feel ashamed,' teacher said.
'It's only right to weep.
Here have these tissues to keep.'
I dabbed my eyes, then looked around.
Bowed into books, every head.

'Have a cold drink.
Go with James. He'll understand.'
In the boys' cloaks I drank deeply
Then slowly wiped my mouth
On the back of my hand.
Sheepishly I said, 'my dad died.'
'I know,' said James.
'We'd best get back to class. Come on.'
Walking down the corridor I thought of dad...gone.
In class no one sniggered,
They were busy getting changed for games.
No one noticed I'd cried.

All day I felt sad.
After school I reached my street,
Clutching the tissues, dragging my feet.
Mum was there in our house
But no dad,

No dad.

For any family, any of the scenarios discussed in this book may represent their own very personal tragedy. There are also situations where children are affected by public tragedies. In recent years there have been some very public and violent attacks, such as the Dunblane school shootings in 1996, the hostage taking and subsequent killing of children and parents in Beslan, Russia in 2004, the attacks of 9/11 in New York in 2001, and the terrorist attacks in London in July 2005, as well as natural disasters such as the Boxing Day tsunami along the coasts of the Pacific in 2004, and the South Asian earthquake in October 2005. All of these events will quickly evoke images in our minds, illustrating just how well known they are.

There are also increasing numbers of refugee children entering the UK, all with their own experiences of loss and violence, which they are often unable to verbalise due to their age, language difficulties and/or the trauma they have experienced. They are also often unable to access services for evaluation of their physical or mental health needs.

This chapter will explore how children learn about loss and bereavement, and will suggest some simple steps that we can all take to keep the communication channels open and assist children with this learning process. It then moves on to examine the child's perspective when experiencing death that is complicated by the manner in which it occurred (e.g. through suicide, natural disaster or violence).

SWOT

Where are you in this context with regard to your personal learning needs? They could look similar to the following:

Strengths	*Weaknesses*
• I work in a supportive environment within a multi-skilled team. • I have greatly enjoyed reading books with my own children. Often minor incidents have led to us making up silly little stories that are now precious to us as a family.	• I have had little exposure to families from different cultures and am worried that I won't know how to deal with them or that I might offend them.
Opportunities	*Threats*
• I can follow up the suggestions in this chapter.	• I lack the confidence to initiate 'therapeutic work' with children.

The NSF standard[2]

Standard 9: The mental health and psychological well-being of children and young people

- Page 36 Inter-agency commitment.
- Page 52 Clinical governance arrangements should ensure that all staff are trained, supported and able to deliver sound, ethical and safe services.
- Page 14 Families who are refugees or who are seeking asylum.

Standard 8: Disabled child

- Page 13 Refers to Standard 9.
- Page 16 Refers to the Children Act: framework for the assessment of children in need and their families.
- Page 34 Refers to the death of a child: 'death in childhood may be sudden and unexpected, for example as a result of a road traffic accident, or may occur at the end of a long-term illness. Whatever their circumstances, it is very important that families receive care which is sensitive, and appropriate to their individual needs.'

Skills and knowledge[3]

The following are implied in the clinical governance statement of Standard 9:

1. communication

2. personal and people development
3. health, safety and security
4. service improvement
5. quality
6. equality and diversity.

The ACT Care Pathway[4]

This serves as a companion to the NSF, but little can be drawn from the latter to guide how the needs should be assessed and then duly met. The pathway allows for sibling care (Diagram 3: end of life and bereavement) but is unlikely to extend to all of the situations discussed in this chapter. It will be up to individual organisations whether they offer advice and support when approached. However, it would be hoped that, if approached, they would refer families on to organisations such as 'Winston's Wish' (see below). The concern is that there is no clear path indicating how families and professionals can access this information easily.

The National Curriculum

The Government response to the House of Commons Health Committee Report on Palliative Care[5] discusses opportunities that are provided within the national curriculum to deal with issues surrounding death and bereavement, a topic specifically covered in Personal, Social and Health Education (PSHE). According to the above report, effective PSHE provision helps pupils to cope with and understand a wider range of issues as they mature:

> younger pupils will be taught about the process of growing from young to old and how people's needs change. They will also have opportunities to reflect on spiritual, moral, social and cultural issues, using imagination to understand other people's experiences. Older pupils should be taught to recognise the stages of emotions associated with loss and change caused by death and bereavement, and how to deal positively with the strength of their feelings in different situations. They should also be taught about the impact of bereavement on families and how to adapt to changing circumstances.

The media

Natural disasters and terrorist attacks are very public affairs, and consideration needs to be given by the media to their responsibility to vulnerable children and young people. Children are bombarded by the media in a manner that cannot be easily controlled by adults. A TV set can be switched off so that children are not exposed to news coverage during waking hours. However, curiosity often prevails, and particularly when public disasters or terrorist attacks are unfolding there is usually round-the-clock coverage. Newspapers also pay little attention to the effect of their news coverage on young minds. Many parents reported that their children had nightmares following the September 11th attack in New York. The possibility of aircraft flying into houses can be a very real threat to a young mind, especially if their house is on a flight path of the local airport, or even if they are just aware of planes flying overhead.

Impressively, 'Newsround' on CBBC carefully explains world affairs to young listeners. This is backed up by a well-edited website[6] that offers links to other web pages should a child be worried about a particular item ('advice on what to do if the news upsets you'). For example, at the time of the London terrorist attacks, children were reassured about their own personal safety and the safety in their school, and were given some general advice on how to keep safe. Suggestions were made that children who were particularly worried should confide in a trusted adult, such as a parent or a teacher. Links were offered to organisations such as the National Society for the Prevention of Cruelty to Children (NSPCC). These web pages are a permanent feature and are cross-referenced with each potentially upsetting report, such as the report on the anniversary of the Beslan school siege.

Grief in children: how bereavements affect children

Most children gradually learn about the life cycle – for example, by realising that leaves fall off trees to make way for new leaves to grow the following spring.[7] Often a first bereavement is that of a pet. The pet has probably been much loved, but if the situation is handled well the child learns about feelings of sadness, missing the pet, the permanence of the loss of the pet, and maybe rituals surrounding death if the pet has a funeral in the garden.

The grief response is commonly linked to a child's cognitive development,[8–11] as described below.

0–2 years

Children in this age group are very sensitive to separation (for a discussion of attachment and loss theory, the reader is referred to a developmental text[12]). A young child might search for a parent, call out, and respond with protests, sadness and despair. Young children tend to experience loss in a playful context, such as 'Peek-a-Boo' and 'All gone.'

The child in the picture above assumed that when she died, mummy would come with her and still care for her. As there is no grasp of permanence, it's not really tough on mummy…

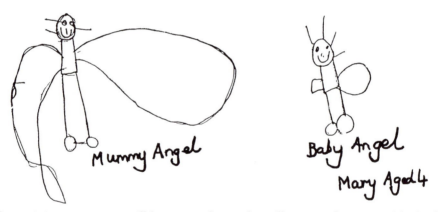

Figure 2.2. 'My mummy will be an angel too. She will come to heaven and look after me.' Reproduced with permission from Brown.[13]

2–5 years

Children of this age tend to rationalise experiences through fantasy, daydreaming and magical thinking. They lack a concept of permanence and believe that death is reversible. For example, they might dig up a dead animal's body to see if it has come back to life.

Children may think that they wished a person dead or caused their death in some way, so there is a need to dispel magical thinking with an honest and rational explanation (this also applies to 5- to 8-year-olds). In addition, they may become confused by explanations of death – for example, 'like going to sleep' or 'not waking up again.' They need to be told repeatedly about the loss, and in play they may act out reunion with the deceased person.

This child clearly demonstrates the illogical reasoning that is common at this age and gives

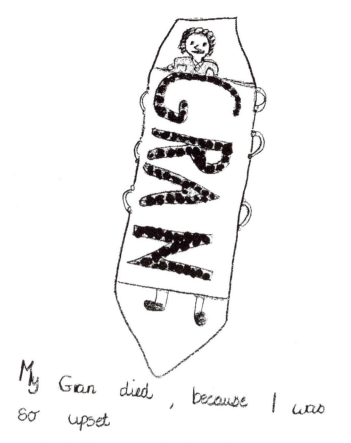

My Gran died, because I was so upset

Figure 2.3. Reproduced with permission from Brown.[13]

'I was so upset' as the reason for gran's death, not the consequence of her death. If during the emotional turmoil that adults are experiencing at the time of a death this goes unnoticed, the child's perception will be that he or she has caused the death by wrongdoing.

5–9 years

This is an age of fears and fantasies. Children may personalise death as skeletons, monsters or ghosts. They also develop a curiosity about the rituals surrounding death (*see* figure at the top of page 20).

Children at this stage of development are mastering or have already mastered some bodily functions, so they wonder about dead bodies and the need for food, clothing and to be looked after. Children are very perceptive with regard to adult reactions, and will deny their own grief in order to protect adults. There is often a fear that they were responsible for the death, and illogical reasoning is common.

9–12 years

At this age children have greater cognitive ability. They can grasp the finality of death and that this fate is common to all living things. Towards 10–12 years of age, children become aware that death is final, universal and inevitable.

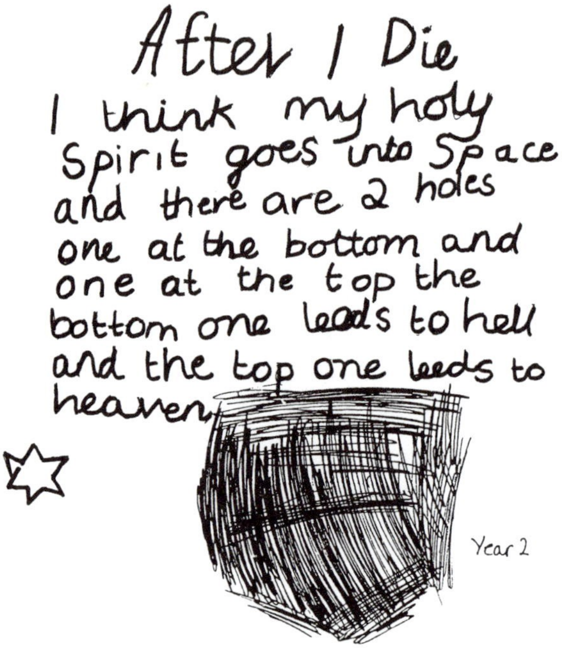

After I Die

I think my holy
Spirit goes into Space
and there are 2 holes
one at the bottom and
one at the top the
bottom one leads to hell
and the top one leeds to
heaven

Year 2

Figure 2.4. Reproduced with permission from Brown.[13]

Children grieve as adults do, but might be in denial and 'get on with life.' They perceive death as an injustice – as 'not fair.' They also recognise the possibility of their own death, and this can be a frightening concept. Children may respond to a death by developing a psychosomatic illness.

Adolescence

Adolescents grieve as adults do and experience sadness, depression, crying and other emotions. They may have suicidal thoughts or mood swings.

Youngsters in this age group are going through a period of loss and asking the question 'Who am I?', so a death at this time is particularly challenging. They may take on adult roles. Peer expectations play an important part.

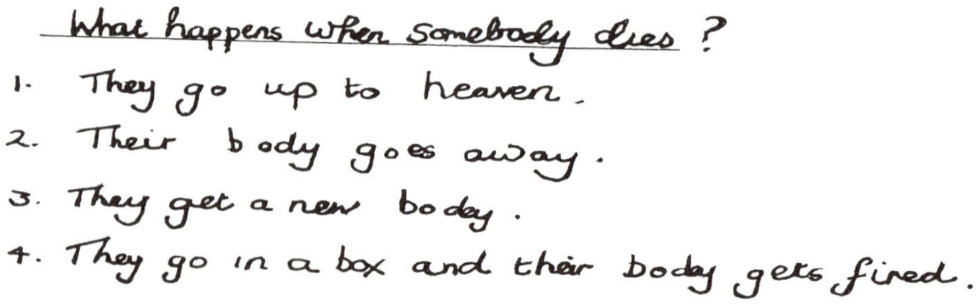

What happens when somebody dies?

1. *They go up to heaven.*
2. *Their body goes away.*
3. *They get a new body.*
4. *They go in a box and their body gets fired.*

Figure 2.5. Reproduced with permission of Oxford University Press from Brown E (2006) *Ritual and Religion.* In: A Goldman *et al.* (eds) (2006) *Oxford Textbook of Palliative Care for Children*, OUP, Oxford, p.209.

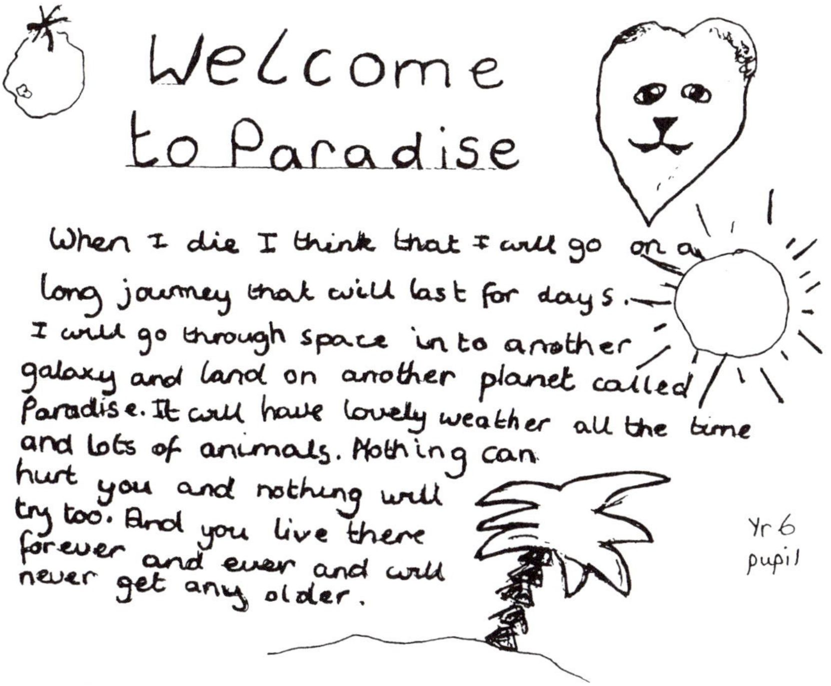

Welcome
to Paradise

When I die I think that I will go on a long journey that will last for days. I will go through space into another galaxy and land on another planet called Paradise. It will have lovely weather all the time and lots of animals. Nothing can hurt you and nothing will try too. And you live there forever and ever and will never get any older.

Yr 6
pupil

Figure 2.6. Reproduced with permission from Brown.[13]

Religious, cultural and spiritual context

Weaver *et al.*[14] reviewed adolescent research journals with regard to religion and found one article by Zeidner[15] that addressed psychological trauma and religious coping. Jewish teenagers in Israel who were threatened by missile attacks during the 1992 Persian Gulf War used religion and prayer to cope positively with traumatic stress. In the same review, an article by McIntosh *et al.*[16] found that greater religious participation was related to increased perception of social support, increased meaning to be found in loss, enhanced well-being, lower levels of distress, and faster and more effective cognitive restructuring.

Walker[17] explains that culture defines accepted ways of behaving for members of a particular society, and that such definitions vary from one society to another, leading to misunderstanding and a failure to engage therapeutically in a helping relationship. According to Walker culture is not static, but rather it is an organic living entity with an external and internal presence – and people, especially children and young people, are developing rapidly at many levels of physicality and consciousness. They do so in an equally fast-changing and bewildering societal context which, according to Walker, sets the scene for their understanding of culture, which is the medium within which human individuals grow and become competent.

Doka[18] clearly distinguishes religion from spirituality, offering a definition that includes religion, ethics, supernatural beliefs, love and non-materialistic philosophies as dimensions of spirituality. In this context Doka[18] defines a child in religious terms as Roman Catholic, Muslim or Baptist, with beliefs shaped by religious training harbouring a variety of interpretations that render sole reference to religious affiliation inadequate. Doka links spirituality to culture and asserts that each child's spirituality has to be understood within its own cultural context.

Garbarino and Bedard[19] use the term 'spirituality' to refer to the inner life of children and adolescents as the cradle for construction of meaning. They describe the core of spirituality as a recognition of oneself as having a physical as well as a spiritual identity or existence.

Bradford[20] considers the spirituality of the child to be a dynamic, tripartite and interrelated concept with three interlinked dimensions (see table below).

Spiritual dimensions of the child (adapted from Bradford[20])

The human spirituality of the child	The devotional spirituality of the child	The practical spirituality of the child
Receiving love	Sharing membership	Forming relationships
Having security	Sharing creed and moral code	Having resilience

These dimensions represent 'human spirituality', which is developed through love and affection, security and new experiences. These can be external, such as play and exploration, or internal, such as opportunities for stillness, reflection, awe and wonder, praise and recognition, and participation and responsibility. According to Bradford, the 'devotional spirituality' of the child is about belonging and refers to the formation of a corporate and personal religious life, offering the religious identity and warmth of membership, the security of established creed and moral code, possibilities for growth and discovery, the support of pastoral encouragement, and multiple opportunities for taking part within the local faith community. The third dimension, namely the 'practical spirituality' of the child, describes signs of the integration of human and devotional spirituality into everyday life. Bradford refers here to the frame of mind and activating emotions of a person who is engaging and participating in life.

Like Walker in a cultural context, Garbarino and Bedard[19] suggest that spirituality in childhood is developmental, as children's cognitive skills are less well developed and have a shorter time span than those of adults in which to build a solid framework of 'meaning.' Yet Doka[18] is critical of the use of Piagetian models because children do not have the abstract thinking necessary to embrace religion. Piagetian models highlight what children are unable to do without stressing what they are trying to do – that is, make sense of their world, incorporating many of the beliefs that they are exposed to even when they are very young. Doka[18] proposes that the question is not at what age or developmental level children can understand spiritual concepts, but how the child, at his or her particular age and developmental level, understands and expresses spirituality. According to Garbarino and Bedard,[19] children have a significant openness to spirituality, due to their being less constricted by social conventions with regard to reality, which leaves them more vulnerable to believing in spirits than most adults, who can distinguish between the acceptable spirit world of religion and the 'unacceptable' world of fantasy. Garbarino and Bedard propose that this leaves children not only more vulnerable to harm, but also more open to developmentally enhancing experiences, because children imagine God as a protective, ideal parent figure, which is magnified by the child's absolute need for care, protection and love, and their need to believe that a parent is almighty.

When exploring what a child is expressing in a picture, the emphasis is on the 'emotional safety' that a child expresses rather than on the 'political correctness' of the picture. In the picture below a child expresses factually what she believes will happen to her. From a faith perspective, Muslim children are not permitted to draw images of themselves, and a picture like this could be interpreted as offensive to the family's religion. In this example the parents were more interested in the emotional well-being of their daughter. The therapist who was exploring what the child had expressed in the picture was also confident enough not to worry unduly about a potential cultural rift between the family and the therapist.

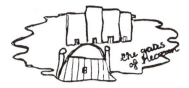

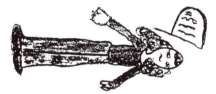

When I die my soul will go to Allah.
My body will stay in the ground.

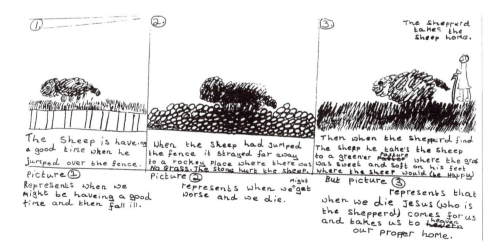

Figure 2.7. Reproduced with permission of Oxford University Press from Brown E (2006) Ritual and Religion. In: A Goldman *et al.* (eds) (2006) *Oxford Textbook of Palliative Care for Children*, OUP, Oxford, p.210.

The child in the picture below (Figure 2.8) uses metaphor as described in 'Therapeutic work with children' (below) to express her perception of feeling emotionally safe. This picture was handed out of context to the child's maths teacher. The child had 'chosen' the moment she needed to discuss what was on her mind, and we need to be alert to the cues that a child offers. If the teacher had chosen to reprimand her for not doing the work intended, this opportunity would have been missed.

Figure 2.8. Reproduced with permission of the young artist.

Pictures that are available for academic use which portray children's expression of their feelings and religious beliefs are few and far between. This does not mean that the authors of such articles have discriminated against one or another faith – far from it, it might simply mean that only a particular picture representing a particular faith community was available.

Brown (personal communication, 2005) described the potential minefield of providing community support for families of life-limited children in Northern Ireland during politically very troubled times. She wondered whether nurses of the same faith were allocated to care for families, and if so, how this was managed. She found that the common situation of all involved and the recognition of the overriding need of the children and their families outweighed the religious or political issues.

Therapeutic work with children

Storytelling

In 'The Wonderful World of Roald Dahl', broadcast on Channel 5,[21] the attraction of using stories for children was discussed:

> Being frightened is a very exciting place to be. When you are a child your deepest, darkest fears are something horrible happening to you or anybody you love, and you can face these fears very very safely, knowing it's all just in a story, it's not actually happening to you....They <children> are not going to be hurt really and they are not damaged psychologically, because they know it's a story. You know you can put the book away and it stays within the book and hopefully you won't have nightmares.

There are a number of books which help children to deal with separation from or the death of a loved one. Not all of the books that deal with difficult issues have been written as 'therapeutic texts', as the Magee poem at the beginning of this chapter illustrates.

A selection of books that can be used in a therapeutic context is discussed below. A number of the books have animals as the main characters, which firmly places the story in the realm of fantasy while exploring a very painful issue. The child remains in this 'safe place' and the book (and any disturbing thoughts associated with it) can just go away. Sunderland[22] points out that by and large children use metaphor and story as their natural language for feeling, and that they do so because this indirect expression offers them protection. Sunderland emphasises that all the healing work can take place entirely through empathising within the metaphor of the story. Therefore talking about real life is certainly not necessary for resolution and change.

The practical disadvantage of this approach is that it does not provide factual information, if we perceive that the child's distress is caused by not understanding the nature of the problem. In the context of how a child feels, Sunderland[22] advises that if we do venture into real life, we should do so tentatively and in a way that does not require an answer if the child does not wish to give one, and that we should respect a 'keep out' response or a resounding silence.

But what type of practical information might a child need to know? As an example, a story has been constructed that explains to a child aged 4 years or over what is happening to her little baby brother, who was born prematurely and does not survive. I do not suggest that this is a particularly good story, but it has a beginning, a journey and an end, and it follows some simple principles offered by Sunderland[22] for constructing a therapeutic story. However, the assumption here is that we are helping an otherwise well-adjusted child to make sense of a difficult situation, and we are not providing psychotherapy.

According to Sunderland,[22] construction of a therapeutic story should involve the following steps.

• Identify the emotional problem or issue with which the child is grappling.

- Think of characters, a place and a situation that can provide a metaphorical context for this.
- Present the main character as grappling with the same emotional problem or issue as the child.
- Show the main character using coping strategies.
- For a therapeutic story to have an impact on the child, it must speak to them about the emotional issues that they are busy grappling with, moving on to coping mechanisms and a way of being that feels better for the child.

However, it must be emphasised that I am not proposing that all of us can do any type of therapeutic work with children. This remains a highly skilled area, and children must be referred appropriately, as there is the potential for doing more harm than good. I am merely proposing that we need to be alert to the issues that children struggle with, and that simple means and explanations can often resolve a problem or empower parents to reopen communication channels with a child who might have unintentionally been pushed into the background.

My little baby brother

On Monday I went with dad to see my new baby brother.
I looked at him in the incubator.
Tubes went into him.
There were lots of beeping and buzzing machines.
He was really really small
Really really tiny.

I stood on a chair and reached
Through a peephole into his incubator.
I held his hand and his fingers and toes.
They were really small
Really really tiny.

Mum and dad said: 'he is very sick.
And because he is so very small
He might be with us only for a little while.'
You see:
He is really really small
Really really tiny.

I went to see him every day – he was really very tiny.
Tubes went into him to help him breathe and eat.
And even the tubes were tiny.
Machines were buzzing and beeping
For my little baby brother

Who was really really small
Really really tiny.

I drew a picture of him in his incubator.
Of his fingers and toes that were

Really really small
Really really tiny.

I gave him a teddy and stroked his face.
Dad put his picture up on the wall
And mum said how lucky my brother was
To have a big sister like me.

I went to see my brother every day, but he just stayed

Really really small
Really really tiny.

Mum and dad told me: 'he is not strong enough
To stay and live right here with us.
You see, his little body is really just too tiny.'

Then one last time my dad and I
Went and said 'good-bye' to my little baby brother.
His little body had not been strong enough.

You see, he was really really small
Really really tiny.

We all had a cuddle and I gave a big kiss
To my little baby brother.
On Friday we went to the graveyard
And had a funeral for my little baby brother.
He was in a small coffin.
And he had with him my picture and teddy.
We cried and hugged each other
And were really sad as we said 'good-bye'
to my little baby brother.

But the vicar told mum and dad and me
That we mustn't be sad,
And he doesn't need anymore
This really really tiny body.
For a tiny little while I had a little baby brother.
He'll always be with mum and dad and me
And live in our hearts.

I now have a picture on my wall
From my little baby brother.
He gave me a print of his hands and his toes
My clever little brother.

Who just was really really small
Really really tiny.

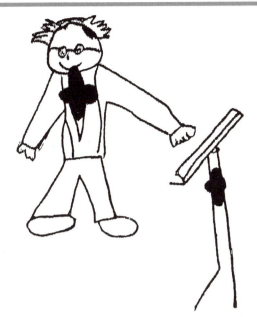

Figure 2.9. The vicar talking about my baby brother. Reproduced with permission from Brown.[13]

This poem explores bite-size issues at a pace that a child can understand. It guides the parent or professional to the type of information that a young child can take in. This includes the following:

- the concept of the physical setting where the brother is (i.e. an incubator)
- the fact that he is very small
- the fact that there are tubes and beeping machines
- once the child is used to the idea of tubes and beeping machines, a simple explanation of what they do
- the brother is there for some time
- the child is involved and encouraged
- a gradual dawning that the brother is not going to get better and that he is not coming home
- the child is actively involved by making a picture and giving her brother a teddy
- the child says goodbye to her brother
- the family is sad
- a simple explanation of where the brother is going to be
- the making of memories
- the funeral
- having memories.

This list is not exhaustive, and the poem can be approached in many different ways. Keeping the story simple allows the exploration of issues that the child may be particularly troubled by or interested in.

The following extract from a story intended for older children and teenagers attempts to deal with the type of questions an older child who is sick or his siblings or friends might be grappling with. An attempt has been made here to explain (from the perspective of the family dog) what happens when somebody is dying or has died.

Later that evening Mum, Dad, Daniel, me and Sue all went back to the hospice. Days passed, and Daniel got weaker and weaker. Daniel had enjoyed his day at home, but decided with his parents that he was happy at the hospice and wanted to stay there with them and me. I lost count how often we watched the video of Daniel's birthday. I just stayed right there with him. So did Mum and Dad. We did a lot of talking just by holding hands. One for Mum, one for Dad, and I was lying as close as I could. I wasn't going to leave him! I had promised!

And then Daniel died. He just stopped. I don't know what I had expected. It wasn't scary. He didn't hurt. He was so peaceful. I guess he didn't need his old tired body anymore, but I needed my Daniel. And I was so sad. We all were so sad.

The hospice had a special room, and we put Daniel's bed in there so Mum and Dad could see him as often as they liked. And I could stay on the bed there with him whilst Mum and Dad were in there, too. They kept telling me what a good dog I was, how I had helped, and that it was OK now not to be in his room all the time....

....So the next day they all came: Katja, her dad, Craig, Darren and Ben. The boys wanted to see the place again where Daniel had been for so long, but they didn't want to see Daniel. They wanted to remember him as they knew him and that was OK. But Katja wanted to say goodbye to Daniel. Katja's dad was not so sure about this: 'Is this really a good idea? You'll make yourself all upset.' Katja nodded: 'I just have to do this!' 'Do you want me to come with you?' asked her dad. 'No, no, I think I have to do this by myself!'

Sue was there and offered to take Katja. And of course I came, too! Sue explained that Daniel would be in his bed, and his eyes were closed. She explained that he wasn't breathing and that he'd look a bit paler than when she'd seen him before, because his heart was not beating. Katja was glad Sue was there and she could feel a reassuring hand on her shoulder.

Sue said: 'Daniel, Katja is here!' At first Katja thought that was odd, because she knew that Daniel couldn't hear her, but it felt right, so she started to chat, because it seemed the right thing to do.

'Please can I hold his hand?' asked Katja. 'Yes, that's OK, just remember, he can't respond. His hand will feel cold. This is only Daniel's shell.' 'Yes, I know', said Katja, her voice a bit wobbly. 'Daniel as we know him is no longer here. He is in our hearts and our minds now.'

Katja stayed a bit longer and Sue stayed in the room with her and couldn't help thinking what a lot of growing up these kids had done.

One consideration that is absolutely crucial when making up stories or explaining various issues to children and young people is the attitude of the person who is dealing with the youngster. It is worth exploring whether we are comfortable discussing with a young person what happens in these situations. Can we be frank and factual? Are children likely to pick up on the fact if we are not? Is there a more appropriate person to hold this conversation? Is a story a suitable medium or is a question-and-answer session more appropriate for an older child? A story can provide the starting point for a child to ask questions. The child might not be able to think of any questions to ask, but equally importantly it gives the child a chance to decide whether they are comfortable having this conversation with a particular person.

Books for children

These can be utilised in many different ways. Parents can be encouraged to read a book with the child. This fosters closeness between the parent and the child, and reading a book together can also provide a starting point for conversation.

Current thinking on child development suggests that a sick child or their sibling might have an understanding of the issues affecting the child that is beyond the expected stage of chronological cognitive development for their age.

Details of suitable books can be easily accessed via the section on recommended reading for children on the 'Winston's Wish' website.[23] This website lists 12 pages of books that are suitable for children and young people, grouped by age group, with a brief synopsis for each title. These include the following:

- Althea (2001) *When Uncle Bob Died*. Happy Cat Books, Bradfield.
- Connolly M (1999) *It Isn't Easy*. Oxford University Press, Oxford.
- Harrison S and Weiss L (1996) *My Book About Me*. Greenfield Publishing, Newport, Isle of Wight.
- Ironside V (1996) *The Huge Bag of Worries*. Hodder Wayland, Hong Kong.
- Isherwood S and Isherwood K (1996) *Remembering Grandad*. Oxford University Press, Oxford.
- Levete S (1997) *How Do I Feel About: when people die*. Franklin Watts, London.
- Magee W (2000) *The Boneyard Rap and Other Poems*. Hodder Wayland, Hong Kong.
- Stickney D (1983) *Waterbugs and Dragonflies*. Continuum International Publishing Group, London.
- Varley S (1992) *Badgers' Parting Gifts*. Picture Lions, London.
- White E (1993) *Charlotte's Web*. Puffin Books, Harmondsworth.
- Wild M and Vivas J (1989) *The Very Best of Friends*. Harcourt Children's Books, London.
- Wilhelm H (1985) *I'll Always Love You*. Hodder and Stoughton, London.

Books for adolescents

- O'Tool D (1995) *Facing Change: falling apart and coming together in the teen years*. Rainbow Publications, Burnsville, NC.
- Saint-Exupery A (1945) *The Little Prince*. Pan Books, London.
- Wilson J (2001) *Vicky Angel*. Corgi Children's Books, London.

A book with a cautionary note

- Kubler-Ross E (1982) *Remember the Secret*. Tricycle Press, Berkeley, CA.

My personal reservation about this book comes from the observation that not all people who die have been kind or have treated a bereaved child well. If a child concludes that such a person who has died is able to make contact with them, that child is no longer in an emotionally safe environment.

Children who need specialised professional support

Kinchin and Brown[24] state that there are occasions when the circumstances of death will almost inevitably cause a child to experience complicated grief. They explain that the way in which the child responds to the bereavement is generally much less significant than for how long they do so. These authors suggest that a child may be experiencing trauma if after several months they:

- appear sad or depressed all the time
- are unable to relax or to return to activities which interested them before the bereavement
- lack self-esteem or express feelings of self-recrimination or worthlessness
- become persistently aggressive
- appear withdrawn
- are suffering from bouts of physical illness
- are perpetually tired

- are experiencing flashbacks or night terrors
- become involved with drug or alcohol misuse, stealing, etc.
- pretend that nothing has happened.

Post-traumatic stress disorder (PTSD)

According to the National Institute for Clinical Excellence (NICE),[25] PTSD is characterised by the following:

- re-experiencing
- avoidance
- hyperarousal
- emotional numbing
- depression
- drug or alcohol misuse
- anger
- unexplained physical symptoms.

NICE (2005) also recommends screening for PTSD after major disasters, as well as screening refugees and asylum seekers.

Herbert[26] suggests that a child's family may need help to enable them to:

- accept and understand the child's difficulties
- express their feelings/emotions
- accept their child's feelings as normal
- deal with the 'tasks' that families have to get on with in life
- clarify distortions and misconceptions
- cope with family changes.

Suicide-bereaved children

Suicide and young people

According to statistics published by the Samaritans:

- 19% of deaths among young people are by suicide – second only to road accidents (the corresponding figure for suicide in the general population is 1%)
- there are 19,000 suicide attempts by adolescents (aged 10–19 years) every year in the UK – one every 30 minutes
- 11% of these young people will successfully kill themselves over the next few years
- there are two actual suicides by young people every day in the UK
- the suicide rate among young men has more than doubled since 1985
- suicide attempts among young people are 70% more likely to be fatal than road accidents.[27]

Cerel et al.[28] followed up 26 suicide-bereaved (SB) children aged 5 to 17 years and compared their progress with 332 children bereaved due to paternal death not caused by suicide (NSB) with regard to emotional reaction to the death, psychiatric symptomatology and psychosocial functioning. The results are briefly summarised below.

- Many children experienced feelings of sadness, anxiety and anger, as well as acceptance. The similarities between the two groups with regard to the grief reaction might reflect a societal trend towards decreased stigma associated with mental illness as well as with suicide, helping to normalise the grief process somewhat for SB families, and making their experience more similar to the kind of grief that is experienced whenever a parent dies.

- None of the SB children had witnessed the suicide. Contrary to expectations, Cerel *et al.*[28] stated that SB children were no more likely than NSB children to experience symptoms of PTSD as a result of the death. Having expected that the SB children would experience the kind of post-traumatic stress that is experienced by survivors of violent natural disasters or interpersonal violence, the authors concluded that suicide per se is not necessarily associated with trauma but, like any other traumatic event, requires direct exposure for trauma to occur.
- Overall, SB children showed more symptoms of psychopathology than NSB children at every point of follow-up, and appeared to show more global behavioural dysfunction than NSB children, which the authors attributed in part to the disruption experienced at home before the death.
- SB children made fewer visits to the doctor and missed fewer days of school than NSB children. Cerel *et al.*[28] attributed this to the nature of the deaths experienced by the NSB children. For example, a child who had observed a parent's long fight with cancer might be more likely to somatise and to complain of pains in the area of the parent's tumour.
- In a follow-up comparison of SB children and the surviving parent, Cerel *et al.*[29] found that before the death SB families were less stable than NSB families, and relationships with the deceased were compromised. No difference in the relationship with the surviving parent was found between the SB and NSB groups. Also, few differences were found with regard to social support or changes in religious beliefs between the SB and NSB groups.

Refugee children and victims of public disaster and terrorism

Heptinstall *et al.*[30] have provided a general overview of asylum seekers from a healthcare professional's perspective. Their article is not written in relation to children, but it includes an excellent reference and resource list.

Jaycox *et al.*[31] surveyed 1004 recent immigrant schoolchildren in the USA aged 8–15 years about their previous exposure to violence and symptoms of PTSD and depression. According to the authors, immigrant children are particularly vulnerable for the following reasons.

- They may have been exposed to violence in their country of origin. This is clearest among refugee children whose families have fled their country of origin due to a well-founded fear of persecution for reasons of race, religion, nationality, membership of a particular social group or political opinion. Often these children have been witness to violence or war.
- Non-refugee immigrant children come from areas where poverty, crime and social unrest are common.
- Some immigrant children have experienced violence during the actual migration process. Although for some the migration is uneventful, others experience life-threatening events such as assault and robbery.
- Once they are settled, many recent immigrant children are impoverished. A third of immigrant children live in poverty, 45% have mothers who have not received a high-school education, and 62% live in overcrowded housing. Such stressful living situations are in turn associated with an increased risk of exposure to violence.
- The findings of the study were as follows:

  - immigrants, who are not necessarily refugees, also have high levels of PTSD symptoms; many children also reported higher levels of depressive symptoms than are found in the general population
  - older children reported witnessing more violence than younger children, but there was no significant difference between children of different ages in their levels of depressive or PTSD symptoms
  - PTSD symptoms were related to victimisation, witnessing of violence in the previous year and, to a lesser extent, lifetime exposure to violence before the previous year.

- The clinical implications identified by Jaycox *et al.*[31] are that both adult and child immigrants are less likely to receive mental health services than their non-immigrant peers, with large gaps in existing services as well as a shortage of bilingual/bicultural mental health professionals. Many parents are unaware of their child's exposure to violent or traumatic events and the emotional consequences of this.

A final point, cited by Heptinstall *et al.*[30] and originally made by Papadopoulos,[32] is that human suffering is not always synonymous with psychological trauma. We also need to take into account other phases of the asylum seeker and refugee experience, such as 'survival' and 'adjustment', which can be painful.

Walker[17] is sceptical about proposed changes in the law in relation to the UN Convention on the Rights of the Child, as they are not in the best interest of the child and will very probably harm their development and mental health. He states that it is doubtful whether the quality of education offered in accommodation centres would properly meet even basic standards of teaching practice. Walker[17] asserts that children who have suffered extreme trauma, anxiety and hardship need to feel safe, included and part of their community with their peers if they are to thrive and rebuild their fragile mental health.

Whoever we are, wherever we live,

These rights belong to all children
under the sun and the moon and the stars,
whether we live in cities or towns or villages
or in mountains or valleys or deserts or forests or jungles.
Anywhere and everywhere in the big, wide world,
these are the rights of every child.

....

In times of war do not make us part of any battle
But shelter us and protect us from all harm,

....

Do your best to let everyone know that
Whoever we are, wherever we live,
These are the rights of every child.

Castle, *For Every Child*[33]

Swick *et al.*[34] have explored the likely reactions and the consequences of children's pain and suffering following the loss of one or both parents as a result of an act of terrorism, in the wake of the 9/11 attack in New York in 2001. Their article is essential reading on this subject, exploring depression, the role of the surviving parent and the nature of the parent's death. It includes an extensive discussion of developmental considerations as well as risk and protective factors. The authors' conclusions with regard to what can be done for these children are briefly summarised below.

- The effect of this event will resurface in different ways throughout the development of these children into adulthood. They will re-experience their loss on birthdays, the anniversary of September 11th, getting a good grade at school or kicking the winning goal in a soccer game. It is not a loss that can be put behind them – it will become a part of them.
- The struggle to make sense of any death is formidable, but especially so for children whose parents were lost in a senseless, hostile and violent act.
- Children are endowed with a capacity for resilience that enables them not only to survive, but also to develop competence in the face of adversity so that they can deal with life's transitions, difficulties and hardships (both expected and unexpected).

- The capacity for resilience is partly endowed by innate temperament, talents and intelligence, and is also influenced by a child's interactions with people and the environment, including their parents, other adults, peers, school and social support. Swick *et al.*[34] quote Silverman's statement[35] that resilience is 'not protective in the classic sense of insulating children from negative forces in their world', but provides children with the 'tools that promote their ability to cope and adapt positively to the vicissitudes of life.'
- Protective factors include the following.

  - A surviving parent who is physically and emotionally available to provide consistent and patient support for the child.
  - The surviving parent or primary caregiver will need financial, emotional and practical assistance. Support includes support groups, access to treatment if needed, and education about the particular needs of children of different ages.
  - Parents can be greatly supported by supplementary childcare, excellent schooling and supportive community resources, as having a stable home and community without economically driven relocations is helpful. Bringing in additional family support, such as a grandparent, is very beneficial, even if it means funding the move.
  - Children need as much consistency as possible, and to be in an environment where they can safely express distress and intense emotion. Being able to attend a stimulating, enriching, safe and stable school will be crucial for these children, so that they can develop competency, identity and self-esteem, and find new adult role models.[34]

Bromet *et al.*[36] investigated the well-being of children 11 years after the Chernobyl disaster (in which 120,000 people were abruptly and permanently evacuated following a nuclear accident at the Chernobyl nuclear power plant in 1986). A number of studies of Hiroshima and Nagasaki as well as Chernobyl have identified elevated levels of somatisation, anxiety, depression and PTSD symptoms during the first decade after the accident. The children who were studied by Bromet *et al.*[36] were infants at the time of the explosion, and perceived their own well-being as being similar to that of their classmates. This was found to be consistent with neuropsychological testing as well as physical examination, although the children's mothers reported significantly more somatic symptoms in their children.

The authors describe how the Chernobyl disaster had unleashed a cascade of stressors, such as harrowing experiences during evacuation, battles for residency permits, government benefits, social stigma, and irreversible loss of home, belongings and lifestyle. They cite the Armenian earthquake of 1988 in identifying the multiple stressors as a distinctive characteristic to which the children were exposed as a result of the traumatisation. These multiple stressors make it difficult to disentangle the web of stress and pinpoint specific experiences that increased the children's vulnerability.

Bromet *et al.*[36] identified as the key factor in the resilience of these children the fact that they had grown up with consistent and loving parents with whom they had a positive relationship. Although the trauma in this case was inflicted primarily on the parents and only secondarily on the children, the children are the focus of parental anxiety. According to Bromet *et al.*, the way in which trauma is handled in these families is by open discussion and grieving, rather than a conspiracy of silence.

Clinical governance: suggestions for work-based learning and networking

Explore with your colleagues how the NSF and the ACT Care Pathway might be implemented in your working environment in relation to the issues raised in this chapter. What are the challenges? How can they be overcome?

Departments for children and young people usually have members of staff with a des-

END OF LIFE AND BEREAVEMENT

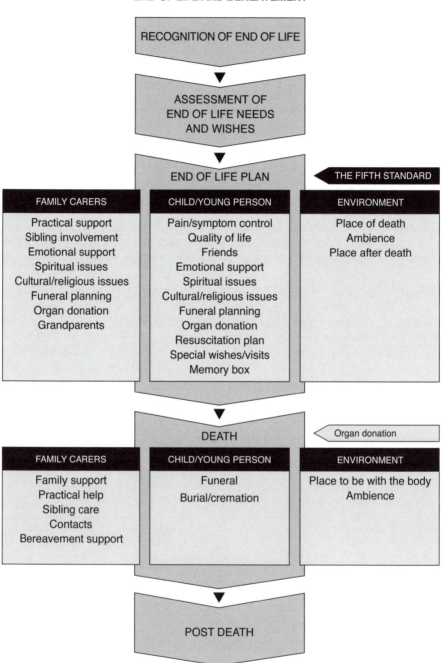

ignated role and/or special interest, such as play specialist, schoolteacher, funeral directors and bereavement centre (covers chaplaincy, patient services, mortuary, funerals, etc.).

Summary

This chapter has considered issues relating to children and young people who are experiencing either personal or public tragedy or disaster. We have explored the exposure to trauma of children and young people in everyday life through personal experience, formal learning at school and the media. 'Grief' has been linked to personal experience and cognitive development, and has been explored in a religious, cultural and spiritual context. Therapeutic work has been examined in the context of what we as individuals can do to help children to understand difficult situations, using examples of therapeutic storytelling. However, some children need specialised professional support if they have developed post-traumatic stress disorder. Particular consideration has been given to rare but harrowing situations that might be experienced by children and young people, such as suicide-related bereavement, becoming refugees and being caught up in acts of terrorism or natural disasters.

SWOT

It might be useful to revisit the SWOT analysis (*see* chart on next page) at this point in order to determine any further learning needs in relation to this chapter and the Knowledge and Skills Framework (KSF) requirements, namely:

1. communication
2. personal and people development
3. health, safety and security
4. service improvement
5. quality
6. equality and diversity.

Action plan for further learning

| |
| |
| |

References

1. Magee W (2000) *The Boneyard Rap and Other Poems.* Hodder Wayland, Hong Kong. Poems reproduced with the permission of the author.
2. For details of the NSF standard, *see* Appendix.
3. For details of the KSF, *see* Appendix.
4. For details of the ACT Care Pathway, *see* Appendix.
5. House of Commons (2003–04) *Health Committee Report on Palliative Care. Fourth report;* www.dh.gov.uk/assetRoot/04/08/91/61/04089161.pdf
6. http://news.bbc.co.uk/cbbcnews/
7. www.curesearch.org

Strengths	Weaknesses
Opportunities	Threats

8. Lindsay B and Elsegood J (1996) *Working with Children in Grief and Loss.* Bailliere Tindall, London.
9. Faulkner K (1997) Talking about death with a dying child. *Am J Nurs.* **97:** 64, 66, 68–9.
10. Harrislord J, McNeil T and Froggs S (1999) *Victims: helping children cope with death;* www.madd.org/VICTIMS/children-cope.shtml
11. Sources B (1996) The broken heart: anticipatory grief in the child facing death. *J Palliat Care.* **12:** 56–9.
12. Bee H and Boyd D (2005) *Lifespan Development.* Addison-Wesley, Menlo Park, CA.
13. Brown E (1999) *Loss, Change and Grief: an educational perspective.* David Fulton Publishers, London.
14. Weaver A, Samford J, Morgan V *et al.* (2000) Research on religious variables in five major adolescent research journals, 1992–1996. *J Nerv Ment Dis.* **188:** 36–44.
15. Zeidner M (1993) Coping with disaster. *J Youth Adolesc.* **22:** 89–108.
16. McIntosh D, Silver R and Wortman C (1993) Religious role in adjustment to a negative life event. *J Pers Soc Psychol.* **65:** 812–21.
17. Walker S (2005) *Culturally Competent Therapy.* Palgrave Macmillan, Basingstoke.
18. Doka K (1994) Suffer the little children: the child and spirituality. In: B Dane and C Levine (eds) *AIDS and the New Orphans.* Auburn House, Westport.
19. Garbarino J and Bedard C (1996) Spiritual challenges to children facing violent trauma. *Childhood.* **3:** 467–78.
20. Bradford J (1995) *Caring for the Whole Child: a holistic approach to spirituality.* The Children's Society, London.
21. *The Wonderful World of Roald Dahl.* Broadcast on Channel 5 on 24 July 2005; www.freeatlasttv.co.uk/credits_dahl.html
22. Sunderland M (2000) *Using Storytelling as a Therapeutic Tool with Children.* Speechmark, Bicester.
23. Winston's Wish recommended reading for children; www/winstonswish.org/ukbookshop.asp
24. Kinchin D and Brown E (2001) *Supporting Children with Post-Traumatic Stress Disorder.* David Fulton Publishers, London.
25. National Institute for Clinical Excellence (NICE) (2005) *Post-Traumatic Stress Disorder (PTSD): the management of PTSD in adults and children in primary and secondary care.* NICE, London.
26. Herbert M (1996) *Post-Traumatic Stress Disorder in Children.* British Psychological Society, Leicester.

27. The Samaritans; www.samaritans.org
28. Cerel J, Fristad M, Weller E *et al.* (1999) Suicide-bereaved children and adolescents: a controlled longitudinal examination. *J Child Adolesc Psychiatry.* **38:** 672–9.
29. Cerel J, Fristad M, Weller E *et al.* (2000) Suicide-bereaved children and adolescents. II. Parental and family functioning. *J Child Adolesc Psychiatry.* **39:** 437–44.
30. Heptinstall T, Kralj L and Lee G (2004) Asylum seekers: a health professional perspective. *Nurs Standard.* **18:** 44–54, 56.
31. Jaycox L, Stein B, Kataoka S *et al.* (2002) Violence exposure, post-traumatic stress disorder, and depressive symptoms among recent immigrant schoolchildren. *J Child Adolesc Psychiatry.* **41:** 1104–10.
32. Papadopoulos R (2002) Therapeutic care for refugees: no place like home. In: T Heptinstall, L Kralj and G Lee (2004) Asylum seekers: a health professional perspective. *Nurs Standard.* **18:** 44–54, 56.
33. Castle C (2000) *For Every Child.* Hutchinson Children's Books, London.
34. Swick S, Dechant E and Jellinek M (2002) Children of victims of September 11th: a perspective on the emotional and developmental challenges they face and how to meet them. *J Dev Behav Pediatr.* **23:** 377–84.
35. Silverman P (2000) *Never Too Young to Know: death in children's lives.* Oxford University Press, New York.
36. Bromet E, Goldaber D, Carlson G *et al.* (2000) Children's well-being 11 years after the Chernobyl catastrophe. *Arch Gen Psychiatry.* **57:** 563–71.

Part Two

Life-limited illness according to different palliative care categories

Chapter 3

A sudden, unexpected death in infancy

This chapter covers

Content	Related to disease
Scenario	• Contemporary issues in children's palliative care pertaining to neonates
• Infant suffering sudden infant death syndrome (SIDS)	• Clinical governance and suggestions for work-based learning
• Setting the scene	• Summary
• The National Service Framework	
• The Knowledge and Skills Framework	
• The ACT Care Pathway	
Contemporary issues	*Relevant topics in other chapters*
• Unexpected, unexplained deaths in early childhood	• Chapter 2: if there are siblings
• Emergency baptism	• Chapter 11: social care and schooling in relation to siblings
• EPICure study	• Chapter 11: complex disability
• Viability issues	
• The very young patient	
• Argument for the ACT Pathway	

Infant suffering sudden infant death syndrome (SIDS)

For more information, a definition and details of the risk factors, the reader is referred to a number of useful websites.[1–8]

Setting the scene

Emily had been born prematurely at 32 weeks' gestation. After a very difficult start and six weeks on the neonatal intensive-care unit, she was finally discharged. Emily was David and Debbie's first baby, but they gradually gained confidence in handling her. Both parents had been well prepared for her coming home, and they had also been trained in infant resuscitation prior to her discharge. The family gradually settled into a routine. Emily was beginning to thrive and displaying a very lovable nature, compensating some-what for the sleepless nights and fraught feeding times.

One night, Debbie woke at 3 a.m., realising that Emily had not been crying for her feed. When she looked into the cot Emily was blue and not breathing. Frantic attempts by the parents to resuscitate her were to no avail, and Emily was pronounced dead on arrival at hospital.

Jot down your initial reaction to this situation.

<table>
<tr><td></td></tr>
<tr><td></td></tr>
<tr><td></td></tr>
</table>

Does this bring back memories of a situation you have encountered?

Does this help or hinder?

SWOT

What are your learning needs when considering this scenario? They could look similar to those in the chart below. There might be issues that you wish to explore, in which case feel free to do so, but also think about the following.

Strengths	*Weaknesses*
• Good knowledge of CONI (Care of Next Infant) scheme. • We have a critical care pathway. • We have a good liaison team that follows up families in the community.	• I don't know what the NSF says in relation to sudden infant death.
Opportunities	*Threats*
• In clinical supervision we have agreed that I can spend some time with 'liaison' to evaluate how effective our pathway is.	• I am very aware of recent publicity about diagnosing sudden infant death syndrome, and am worried about how parents might respond to professionals.

What are the immediate needs of David and Debbie?

Have you considered any of these?

1. Privacy and support on a one-to-one basis. David and Debbie will most certainly need to spend time with Emily and to cuddle her. They need someone to be there with them to provide support, to answer any immediate questions that they have and to reassure them. Any explanations might need to be repeated more than once, as parents who are very distressed are unlikely to take in or remember much of what has been said.
2. Although parents often don't remember what has been said, they do remember the manner in which support has been offered. A silence shared can be more supportive than conducting a polite conversation just for the sake of it.
3. Basic comfort and safety. The parents might like a relative or friend to come in to give support. They might also like to speak to a chaplain of an appropriate faith.
4. If Emily has not been baptised they might wish her to be named. Any offer of spiritual support needs to be given in such a way that the parents do not think this is a hospital procedure with which they are expected to comply (for a discussion of emergency naming, blessing and baptism, see below).
5. When the parents are ready, they will need safe transport home.

What are the legal implications of cot death?

Have you considered any of these?

1. A more detailed explanation is given below. In summary, if there is a sudden, unexpected death there will have to be a post-mortem examination of the baby and an inquest. This means that information needed by professionals and parents is simply not available at this point. Explanations of the likely cause of death and what needs to happen next must be honest.

2. Very distressingly for the parents, a cot death will invariably involve the police. After speaking to a senior member of the medical staff, the police will need to speak to the parents and possibly check the environment in which the baby died before the area has been 'touched.' It is important to ensure that the parents understand that this is a routine procedure.

3. A one-to-one care approach for the parents therefore has the double role of providing support but also ensuring that the parents can be observed with their baby.

What support is available for parents who have lost a baby?

Have you considered any of these?

1. Most neonatal units provide support for bereaved parents. In addition, in many areas health visitors run parent support groups.

2. A particularly helpful organisation in this situation is CONI (Care of the Next Infant).[9]

How is cot death handled in the Emergency department both from a managerial point of view and in terms of staff support?

Have you considered any of these?

1. This is obviously an especially stressful situation for the staff. The particular emotional challenge stems from being unable to prepare for this situation. There are ambivalent emotions of needing to support the parents who are devastated by the unexpected death of their baby, while bearing in mind that the death might not be a true case of SIDS, and therefore the need to establish the true cause.

2. For this reason, usually two members of staff deal with a cot death. Staff can then support each other and ensure that support for the family and liaison with various agencies take place smoothly.

3. In the spirit of true multi-disciplinary teamwork, it is appropriate in the scenario

described above to contact the baby unit and involve Emily's named nurse or another member of staff whom the family know well. Emily's consultant will also be informed while the family is still in the department.

4. Emergency departments keep protocols for dealing with sudden paediatric deaths. One item on this list will be notification of the family's GP and health visitor. This will not only ensure good communication and therefore support for the family, but will also avoid mistakes such as sending out appointments for vaccinations, etc.

5. There is an obvious need for thorough debriefing of staff and effective clinical supervision.

What are the long-term needs of David and Debbie?

> Folk who have babies who die...are parents. They have lived with the idea, and the reality, of their baby for a long time. Perhaps they lived with the idea for many years before it was conceived....They have carried it in their bodies and minds and hearts and souls since conception and perhaps for a good time before that. Because of this they need to be treated as bereaved parents....Men whose babies are born dead or die after birth need to be treated as fathers who have lost a baby...
>
> Fairbairn[10]

Have you considered any of these?

1. Parents who have lost a child can feel very isolated. Friends and family often do not know how to respond, and tend to avoid a bereaved family. Another stereotypical response can be the suggestion that the family can have another baby. However, the grief that is experienced is for the baby who has died, and any consequent child will not and cannot replace him or her. Parents never forget a child. I have spoken to an elderly woman who had lost a baby 70 years previously. As she talked about her baby it became clear that she was still grieving for the child she had never seen grow up.

2. Many nurses shy away from offering support to bereaved parents, due to a fear of 'over-involvement.' This can be clarified through effective clinical supervision. Most units welcome the involvement of members of staff by maintaining telephone contact with a family in the period immediately after a death, and are happy for staff involved in the care of the baby to attend the funeral.

3. It is up to the unit's discretion how long-term contact is maintained. Families tend to appreciate receiving a card at critical times, such as the anniversary of the baby's birthday, the anniversary of the death and at Christmas.

4. Families require extra support at critical times with the next baby, as they are likely to be very worried about the recurrence of a cot death.

5. A particularly helpful organisation in this situation is CONI (Care of the Next Infant), which can be accessed via its website.[9] CONI offers practical help by systematically monitoring the progress of the family's next baby in order to boost the confidence of

parents who are worried that the new baby might also suffer a cot death. Support includes resuscitation training, provision of monitoring equipment, and extra support at the stage of development of the previous baby's cot death, as well as additional support when the time comes to wean the next child off any monitoring equipment.

6, Some health authorities practise a type of 'risk assessment' for babies who are considered to be at particularly high risk of cot death, and proactively target extra support for these families by using a similar approach to monitoring to CONI, through the health-visiting system.

The National Service Framework

- No section of the NSF could be identified that refers specifically to SIDS.
- There is reference to neonatal death in the NSF under Maternity Services,[11] where it is stipulated that:

> Women, their partners and sibling children who have suffered a bereavement arising from…neonatal or infant death or the death of the mother herself will need supportive information and choices which are:
>
> – responsive to the individual needs and those of the family
> – easily accessible and available for as long as required
> – consistent in content across all sectors of the health service
> – appropriate and based on relevant guidelines and
> – respectful of culture and diversity.

Frank et al.[12] discuss neonatal intensive-care units (NICU) in relation to the NSF (2003) Standards for Hospital Services in the context of assessing parental emotional and psychosocial needs. The NSF specifies that generic and specialised support should be made available to parents. It also sets standards for staff training and communication to enable parents to be active partners in their child's care. Frank et al.[12] apply this to the NICU environment in terms of providing greater opportunities for parents to hold their infant, give basic care and learn to read their infant's behavioural cues, and improving staff–parent communication and parent participation in decision making.

Skills and knowledge

- This addresses how to deal with sudden infant death.
- Particularly helpful here are the principles presented by the Royal College of Paediatrics and Child Health and the 'Common Core' – which also refers to local policies.
- In 2004, the Royal College of Pathologists and the Royal College of Paediatrics and Child Health issued clear guidelines, including a flow diagram for multi-professional working.[13]

The ACT Care Pathway

In the scenario described above, Emily enters the ACT Care Pathway on Diagram 3. Organisations which the NSF for Maternity Services suggests can be contacted in the event of infant death[11] provide resources for professionals and bereaved parents and are voluntary organisations only (Child Bereavement Trust, CRUSE, Compassionate Friends, Stillbirth and Neonatal Death Society).

Contemporary issues in children's palliative care pertaining to neonates

Unexpected and unexplained deaths in early childhood

On 16 July 2005 Professor Sir Roy Meadows was struck off the register as a practising paediatrician for giving misleading evidence that resulted in unsafe convictions for a number of mothers. On 17 February 2006 he was reinstated as a paediatrician.

The Royal College of Pathologists and the Royal College of Paediatrics and Child Health[13] have raised concerns about the potential standard of proof and quality of evidence, and about the procedures adopted for the investigation of sudden unexpected deaths of children. It is highly recommended that practitioners access the full report for the proposed protocol and flow chart. The salient points of the report are briefly summarised below.

- In the vast majority of cases where babies die suddenly, nothing unlawful has happened.
- Children are four times more likely to die in the first year of life, from either natural or unnatural causes, than at any other time.
- Parents who are suffering a terrible tragedy need sensitive support to help them to deal with their loss.
- It is every family's right to have their baby's death properly investigated. Families desperately want to know what happened, how the event could have occurred, what the cause of death was and whether it could have been prevented.
- This is important in terms of grieving, but it is also relevant to a family's high level of anxiety about future pregnancies, and may identify some hidden underlying cause, such as a genetic problem.
- If there happens to be another sudden infant death in the family, carefully conducted investigations of an earlier death also help to prevent miscarriages of justice.
- There are 43 police forces in England and Wales, each with its own procedures, and there are 28 strategic health authorities, as well as many social work departments. The geographical remits of these different agencies do not coincide with each other, and they have different operational methods.
- This sometimes results in insensitivity and failure, with parents being treated with inappropriate suspicion.
- About 600 babies die suddenly every year in the UK.
- The proposed protocol has the following elements.

  - A paediatrician working with a specially trained senior police officer visits the bereaved family at home within 24 hours of the death to take a complete history and offer initial support.
  - This provides an opportunity for the family to explain events in the setting in which they took place, and the sleeping arrangements can be seen *in situ*. In contrast to the situation in most adult deaths, parents usually lift the child and attempt all manner of resuscitation, clean away sputum and vomit from the airways, and blow into the mouth. These descriptions come back as parents relive the event and help to explain the absence or presence of different features. It is important that the doctor at the heart of this investigation of the scene is someone who understands the normal care of babies.
  - This home visit is at the centre of the protocol and is not a negotiable element.
  - The post-mortem examination is performed by a paediatric pathologist or by a forensic pathologist with some training in paediatric pathology. The pathologist also has evidence gathered at the home visit. The post-mortem examination includes a skeletal survey, tissue sampling and clear records kept for any future need.

- Similar protocols with regard to record keeping should be a requirement of Accident and Emergency departments.
- All of the professionals involved meet after full information about the family and the death is available, to agree what factors might have contributed to the death. They provide a multi-disciplinary report for the coroner, and plan further support for the family.
- For the full protocol, the reader is referred to pages 18–45 of the original document.[13]

Why is it so difficult to distinguish SIDS from child abuse fatalities? Hockenberry et al.[14] assert that post-mortem findings in SIDS and accidental suffocation or intentional suffocation, such as that observed in Münchausen's syndrome by proxy, are practically the same.

The Committee on Child Abuse and Neglect[15] describes how almost 50 years ago the medical community began a search to understand and prevent SIDS, and almost simultaneously was awakened to the realities of child abuse and infanticide, perpetrated by suffocation and masqueraded as apparent life-threatening events (ALTE). Their article, which reviews 70 references, is a very helpful introduction to the subject and can be summarised as follows.

- Our understanding of the aetiology of SIDS remains incomplete. However, some SIDS victims show abnormalities in the arcuate nucleus of the brainstem, which suggests that true SIDS deaths are linked to a delayed development of arousal, cardiorespiratory control or cardiovascular control. It is suspected that when the physiological stability of these infants becomes compromised during sleep, they may not become aroused sufficiently to avoid the noxious insult or condition.
- The diagnosis of SIDS is by exclusion, and requires a post-mortem examination and a review of records that fail to reveal another cause of death and remain 'undetermined.' 'Undetermined' includes suspected (but unproven) infant death attributable to infection, metabolic disease, accidental asphyxiation or child abuse.
- If the infant has previously been healthy and there is no external evidence of injury, a preliminary diagnosis of 'probably SIDS' is given. With this diagnosis it is possible to convey to the parents that they could not have prevented their infant's death.
- The parents should be informed that other causes of death will be excluded by a thorough investigation of the death scene, a post-mortem examination and a review of the case notes. However, it should be emphasised that this might help to show why their infant died and how other children in the family might be affected.
- The family should be given every opportunity to see and hold their infant once death has been pronounced. Most units will have protocols pertaining to issues such as the following:

  - baptism
  - grief counselling
  - funeral arrangements and religious support
  - cessation of breastfeeding
  - reaction of the surviving siblings
  - information about SIDS and the local SIDS support group.

The Committee on Child Abuse and Neglect[15] warns that failure to differentiate fatal child abuse from SIDS is costly, as it might overlook child maltreatment, genetic disease, threats to public health, inadequate medical care, product safety issues and progress in understanding the aetiology of SIDS and other causes of unexpected infant death.

Emergency baptism

Campbell and Campbell[16] discuss emergency baptism by healthcare professionals. This is an area rarely written about, and I would strongly recommend the reader to consult the article. It is briefly summarised below.

- The holistic duty of care to the child and their family involves body, mind and spirit.
- As 70% of the UK population consider themselves to be Christian according to the 2001 census,[17] the most commonly requested religious ceremony when a child is seriously ill is emergency baptism.
- Campbell and Campbell explain that in the past some Christians held the view that the soul of unbaptised children could not be admitted to heaven. However, this is not the official view of the major churches today. It is important to dispel this fear, especially if baptism has been requested but has not been administered.
- Although there can be a strong desire to have a child properly named, a name is not strictly necessary at baptism. Campbell and Campbell state that from a more explicit theological perspective, baptism puts the child into God's care in the fullest possible sense, and expresses a family's faith and trust even if the situation is desperate.
- In a situation where a child is deteriorating rapidly and a priest or spiritual leader is not available, a layperson may perform emergency baptism. The major Christian churches do generally recognise each other's baptism ceremonies, as baptism implies membership of a Christian denomination.
- Provided that a baptism is validly administered, it neither needs to be nor can be repeated.
- The principle of beneficence applies, as does the Code of Conduct.[18] Emergency baptism is performed by request of the parents, and cannot be initiated as a result of the personal beliefs held by staff and without consent by a parent.
- Campbell and Campbell[16] describe the emergency baptism procedure at Great Ormond Street Hospital:

  - Initially contact on-call chaplain.
  - If the chaplain agrees to the baptism taking place before he/she arrives, any member of staff may proceed as follows:
    Fill in baptism form (chaplain will use this to complete the registers).
    Place small amount of warm tap water in suitable bowl.
    Dip thumb in water, make the sign of a cross on the child's forehead (if possible) or on another suitable part of the body, and say:
    <Christian names> I baptise you in the name of the Father, and of the Son, and of the Holy Spirit. Amen.
    Invite all present to join in the Lord's Prayer.
    When the chaplain arrives, he/she will meet the family and give them the baptism certificate.

Hemstock (personal communication, 2005) explains that in reality emergency baptism by a layperson is a very rare event, as larger hospitals have a 24-hour on-call service. At Queen's Medical Centre in Nottingham the wards hold emergency baptism equipment on the wards and will prepare a trolley with a white cloth and a silver bowl ready for baptism. The emphasis is on having a simple service that will be a family occasion. Photographs are taken and a baptism certificate is given to the family to keep in the child's memory box. No promises are made and no godparents are required to see the child through to adulthood.

According to Hemstock, in the case of stillbirth or sudden infant death a brief blessing or naming ceremony is a pastorally sensitive rite of passage. It is something that a pastor can do for a child who has died and who therefore cannot be baptised. By a parent giving a child a name, it is acknowledged that the child has been a person in his or her own right. Again, a certificate is given to the parents for the child's memory box.

Although there are no rights of passage associated with death in the other major faiths, there are rituals related to death, such as the washing of the child and positioning of the child in Islam, where the head is turned to the right and then to face Mecca, and prayers are said in a special way.

Jewish boys are traditionally circumcised on the eighth day after birth. However, this can be postponed if there are concerns about the child's health, and it is not considered a rite of passage should the child not survive. Very practical guides to the rites and rituals surrounding death have been provided by Brown,[19,20] who also points out that there are differences in the geographical spread of people from different cultures, and we therefore need to be conversant with local need (Brown, personal communication, 2005).

The EPICure study

The EPICure study[21] was established in 1995 to determine the long-term outcomes for all infants born in the UK during a 10-month period at 20 to 25 weeks of gestational age. The advantage of a longitudinal study such as this one is that it allows planning for the long-term management of these children. The findings are summarised briefly below.

- A total of 4004 births were recorded.
- A total of 811 infants were cared for in 276 neonatal units.
- Of these, 497 infants (61%) died before discharge.
- Of these, intensive care was actively withdrawn in 269 cases (55%).
- A total of 314 infants (39%) survived to discharge.
- At 1 year of age, 95 of the children (31%) had significant problems in areas such as development, neurology and need for oxygen, and 40 children had more than two major disabilities.
- At 2½ years of age, six of the 314 children had died (2%, and no data were available for 1% of the children leaving).
- At 2½ years of age, 283 children were assessed. In total, 64 children (24%) had severe disabilities, 64 (24%) had non-severe disability, and 49% had no disability.
- The commonest medical problems related to the chest, with 45% of children needing treatment for wheeze and cough.
- In total, 40 of the children required readmission after discharge, mainly for chest problems. This was more common if the child had needed oxygen for a long time after birth. Wood *et al.*[22] found a direct link between chronic lung disease and growth failure in the children in the EPICure study.
- At 6 years of age, 241 children were assessed again. The distribution of disabilities had remained roughly the same, with about half of the children having no disabilities, a quarter having moderate disability and a quarter having severe disability.
- When these figures were compared with the ability of the children's classmates at school, the scores were somewhat more favourable. In total, 22% had severe disability, 24% had moderate disability, 32% had low–normal scores/mild impairment and 20% had no problems.
- These results help us to understand the problems of prematurity, and they provide a guideline from which to assess how long-term outcomes change with new types of care or treatment.
- They also provide a basis on which we can give information to parents so that they can make informed choices for their children.

Markestad *et al.*[23] also describe a longitudinal study of infants born between 22 and 27 weeks' gestation in 1999 and 2000 in Norway. Whilst first outcomes in this study incorporate recent developments, such as antenatal steroids for the mother, and demonstrate slightly better outcomes than the EPICure study, Markestad *et al.* also look back at an earlier lon-gitudinal study, conducted from 1986 to 1988 and assessing children at the ages of 5 and 11 years. They found that socio-economic status was a much stronger predictor of outcome than birth weight. This highlights the interrelationship between factors that affect outcomes for all children, and the need for inter-professional assessment and teamworking.

Lastly, but most importantly, these findings guide us as professionals to see the long-term needs of these children and their families that must be addressed and planned for with the parents well before the child is discharged into the community.

The viability issue

In June 2005, the British Medical Association[24] reviewed and rejected a proposal for low-ering the maximum time permitted for legal terminations of pregnancy. There are no plans by the Government to review the current laws,[25] and the upper limit remains at 24 weeks' gestation. This means that a fine line is drawn between this upper limit and the lower end of the spectrum at which premature babies can be kept alive.

Ramer-Chrastek and Thygeson[26] describe perinatal hospice care for an unborn child with a life-limiting condition. The philosophy and multi-disciplinary working in this situation offer psychological support, information and resources to families as they plan for both the birth and the probable death of their child. Families are supported in parenting their child *in utero* by talking to the baby, playing music to him or her, and even seeing the pregnancy as 'taking the baby' wherever the parents go. Care includes individual birth classes, so that parents whose baby is not expected to survive can address both issues related to the birth process and issues that they may encounter due to their child's con-dition. A birth plan can be formulated to meet their very individual needs – for example, being able to hold the baby after birth until (and after) death occurs.

The very young parent

In July 2005, Sue Axton, a mother who herself regrets an abortion she had 20 years ago, brought a legal challenge to terminations of pregnancy without parental knowledge in girls as young as 12 years.[27] She argues that this precludes any support which a young per-son might receive from her family. Hazen[28] speaks of the complexities of reproduction and mothering, such as pregnancy, fertility and infertility, miscarriage, abortion, etc., and the physical, sexual and emotional aspects of these topics that are taboo.

Although it is far beyond the scope of this book to discuss the issues of termination of pregnancy, it is worth considering the psychosocial and emotional impact on the young person. She and her partner potentially have to deal with an unforeseen bereavement (and in the case of termination the emotional aftermath might not have been discussed and therefore has to be faced unsupported).

Hazen[28] states that trauma can accompany perinatal loss. Symptoms that are encountered include hyperarousal, anxiety, and intrusive memories that are encoded in wordless images.

Young people might also potentially have to cope as parents with a very premature baby or the loss of a baby. Hazen[28] points to our knowledge about attachment, loss, trau-ma and healing. She states that the women in her research (the youngest of whom was 22 years of age) who experienced perinatal death were supported in connecting with their bodies and feelings, their children's bodies or spirits, and the family and community. Statistics for maternal age in relation to prematurely born infants are not easily accessi-ble. Within palliative care, statistics for parental age are not collected, as this can be viewed as being in conflict with the Data Protection Act.[29]

It is implied in the NSF for Maternity Services[11] that the young person should receive support. Provision of appropriate support for a teenage parent will be haphazard in prac-tical terms if their needs according to their cognitive age are not met.

A poignant description of meeting a 15-year-old mother of a SIDS victim surrounded by her family is given by Diamond,[30] who just 8 weeks previously had lost her son Sebastian to SIDS:

> On the floor, sitting dejectedly on one of the mattresses, was a young Maori girl. She looked all of 15. The skin on her face was blotched with pink and purple patches, and her eyes looked as though they had been crying forever...there were 12,000 miles, an entire culture and at least 20 years between this young mother and myself – but I had more in common with her at that moment than anyone else in the room.

Much research has been undertaken on the experience of bereavement, yet very little can be identified that is specific to very young parents. This is an area that requires further research, so we don't exclude this group of young parents from the following description by Hazen:[28]

> Just as no one brings a child into being alone and, in the words of African-American folk wisdom, 'it takes a village' to successfully rear a child to adulthood, no one heals alone from the death of a child. To heal from perinatal loss, a mother connects with her body and feelings, connects with her child physically or symbolically, and connects her child and herself with the social environment.

The argument for the ACT Care Pathway

It is pertinent here to scrutinise palliative care issues in neonatology more closely in relation to the following:

- outcomes of very premature babies
- the long-term reality – the argument for entering a 'premy' on Diagram 1.

Hockenberry et al.[14] cite an example of a critical care pathway for preterm infants which can be advanced to a 'Complex Discharge Path' if the infant is to be discharged home with high-tech needs. This approach successfully caters for the majority of infants who are discharged from neonatal units, who grow and develop into normal healthy children, but it also allows for those children who either do not survive into childhood or experience significant problems along the way.

Siden[31] describes several models of paediatric healthcare, namely the 'well child' model, the 'new morbidities' model, the 'disease' model and the 'chronic condition' model. He concedes that there are several moving targets in this scenario – one of them being the clinician, as he or she must work with patients who are potentially located in different models of enquiry. The second moving target is the patient, possibly as he or she moves from a curative to a non-curative state. The final moving target may be the underlying disease or condition, which may drift or relocate as we learn to intervene and change the natural course. According to Siden, the biggest challenge for palliative care is not that it is a 'particularly difficult arena', but rather it lies in defining the work in relation to models, where the patients, their families and sometimes the conditions themselves are shifting all the time, thus defining the work to be done for ourselves, for the programmes and commissioners, and for research.

Units working to a pathway similar to this, described by Hockenberry et al.,[14] will easily work with the ACT Pathway. Where no pathway is used, the ACT Pathway can be locally adapted to provide a seamless journey from neonatal intensive care/transitional care if required to support in the community, the pathway merely ensuring a minimum standard in tandem with Standard 8 of the NSF requirement. For example, children who are identified as having 'severe disabilities' in the EPICure study will now have moved on to Diagram 2, Standard 4 (multi-agency care plan with regular review of needs).

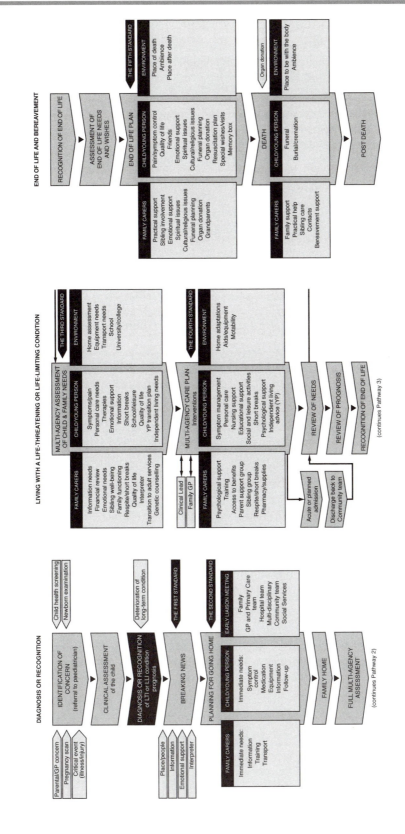

DIAGNOSIS OR RECOGNITION

Parental/GP concern
Pregnancy scan
Critical event (illness/injury)

Child health screening
Newborn examination

IDENTIFICATION OF CONCERN
(referral to paediatrician)

CLINICAL ASSESSMENT
of the child

DIAGNOSIS OR RECOGNITION
of LTI or LLI condition
prognosis

Deterioration of long-term condition

THE FIRST STANDARD

BREAKING NEWS

THE SECOND STANDARD

PLANNING FOR GOING HOME

Place/people
Information
Emotional support
Interpreter

CHILD/YOUNG PERSON
Immediate needs:
Symptom control
Medication
Equipment
Information
Follow-up

FAMILY CARERS
Immediate needs:
Information
Training
Transport

EARLY LIAISON MEETING
Family
GP and Primary Care team
Hospital team
Multi-disciplinary Community team
Social Services

FAMILY HOME

FULL MULTI-AGENCY ASSESSMENT

(continues Pathway 2)

LIVING WITH A LIFE-THREATENING OR LIFE-LIMITING CONDITION

THE THIRD STANDARD

MULTI-AGENCY ASSESSMENT
OF CHILD & FAMILY NEEDS

FAMILY CARERS
Information needs
Financial review
Emotional needs
Sibling well-being
Family functioning
Respite/short breaks
Quality of life
Interpreter
Transition to adult services
Genetic counselling

CHILD/YOUNG PERSON
Symptoms/pain
Personal care needs
Therapies
Emotional support
Information
Short breaks
School/leisure
Quality of life
YP transition plan
Independent living needs

ENVIRONMENT
Home assessment
Equipment needs
Transport needs
School
University/college

THE FOURTH STANDARD

MULTI-AGENCY CARE PLAN
Interventions

Clinical Lead
Family GP

FAMILY CARERS
Psychological support
Training
Access to benefits
Parent support group
Sibling group
Respite/short breaks
Pharmacy/supplies

CHILD/YOUNG PERSON
Symptom management
Personal care
Nursing care
Educational support
Social and leisure activities
Short breaks
Psychological support
Independent living advice (YP)

ENVIRONMENT
Home adaptations
Aids/equipment
Motability

Acute or planned admission

Discharge back to Community team

REVIEW OF NEEDS

REVIEW OF PROGNOSIS

RECOGNITION OF END OF LIFE

(continues Pathway 3)

END OF LIFE AND BEREAVEMENT

RECOGNITION OF END OF LIFE

ASSESSMENT OF
END OF LIFE NEEDS
AND WISHES

THE FIFTH STANDARD

END OF LIFE PLAN

FAMILY CARERS
Practical support
Sibling involvement
Emotional support
Spiritual issues
Cultural/religious issues
Funeral planning
Organ donation
Grandparents

CHILD/YOUNG PERSON
Pain/symptom control
Quality of life
Friends
Emotional support
Spiritual issues
Cultural/religious issues
Funeral planning
Organ donation
Resuscitation plan
Special wishes/visits
Memory box

ENVIRONMENT
Place of death
Ambience
Place after death

DEATH

FAMILY CARERS
Family support
Practical help
Sibling care
Contacts
Bereavement support

CHILD/YOUNG PERSON
Funeral
Burial/cremation

Organ donation

ENVIRONMENT
Place to be with the body
Ambience

POST DEATH

Clinical governance and suggestions for work-based learning

Explore with your colleagues how the NSF and the ACT Care Pathway can be implemented in your working environment in relation to Emily and her family. What are the difficulties? How can they be overcome?

- Speak to a member of staff in the Emergency department who has dealt with cot death.
- Find out what the regulations are regarding the release of the baby's body.
- Talk to a member of staff who has sat through an inquest.
- Contact bereavement/support groups.
- How is support organised locally for parents who have lost a baby? It might be suggested that you meet with parents who have lost a baby.
- How does the liaison health visitor facilitate multi-professional working?

You might decide to explore other issues surrounding infant death. Speak to a member of staff based at the Special Care Baby Unit, and find out from what age a non-viable fetus is classified as a stillbirth, and the implications of funeral arrangements for such babies.

What is the procedure within the delivery suite for dealing with fetuses that are considered to be non-viable? You might also wish to speak to a funeral director and chaplain in order to explore these issues further.

Draw up a workable care plan for Emily and her parents based on ACT Care Pathway 3.

Consider the feasibility of adapting the pathway for sudden infant deaths in your workplace so that it can be used jointly with other agencies, such as the police and emergency services.

Now consider how the ACT Care Pathway could be utilised both from a perinatal perspective for the very premature infant, and also considering the possibility that the baby might go on to have complex needs (like the child in Chapter 11).

Reflect on how the transfer from neonatal services to children's services can be planned for utilising Pathways 1 and 2.

Summary

This chapter has considered SIDS and also wider issues relating to life-threatening and life-limiting conditions in neonates. A rationale for using the ACT Care Pathway for 'high-risk' neonates has been suggested. Ongoing research (the EPICure study) into the long-term outcome of very premature babies has been identified. One area of further research identified pertains to effective support for very young parents in order to minimise adverse long-term effects.

SWOT

It might be useful to revisit the SWOT analysis (*see* chart on next page) at this point in order to determine any further learning needs in relation to this chapter and the Knowledge and Skills Framework (KSF) requirements, namely:

1. communication
2. personal and people development
3. health, safety and security
4. service improvement
5. quality
6. equality and diversity.

Strengths	Weaknesses
• We have a critical care pathway. • We have a good liaison team that follows up families in the community.	• I have never considered any of our babies as 'being palliative' or my work as in any way related to palliative care. • I don't know what the NSF says in relation to teenage parents.
Opportunities	Threats
• In clinical supervision we have agreed that I can: – spend some time with 'liaison' to evaluate how effective our pathway is – liaise with other units to find out what is good practice with very young parents.	• I find it difficult to strike a balance between the emphasis of being positive even with the sickest infants and realistically introducing strategies if all is not well.

Action plan for further learning

References

1. The Foundation for the Study of Infant Deaths; www.sids.org.uk
2. The SIDS Network; www.sids-network.org
3. Circle Solutions, Inc.; www.sidscenter.org/professionalrole.aspx
4. The Royal College of Pathologists; www.rcpath.org
5. The Royal College of Paediatrics and Child Health; www.rcpch.ac.uk
6. Health Online; www.sids-id-psc.org
7. Parenthood.com (parenting, parenthood and childcare resources); www.parenthood-web.com/parent_cfmfiles/pros.cfm/332
8. Healthfinder (a service of the National Health Information Center, US Department of Health and Human Services); www.healthfinder.gov/text/orgs/hr0985.htm

9. Care of the Next Infant (CONI), accessed via www.sids.org.uk
10. Fairbairn GW (1993) When a baby dies – a father's view. In: D Dickenson and M Johnson (eds) *Death, Dying and Bereavement.* Open University Press, Buckingham.
11. Department for Education and Skills and Department of Health (2004) *National Service Framework for Children, Young People and Maternity Services: maternity services.* Department of Health, London.
12. Franck L, Cox S, Allen A *et al.* (2005) Measuring neonatal intensive-care-unit-related parental stress. *J Adv Nurs.* **49:** 608–15.
13. Royal College of Pathologists and Royal College of Paediatrics and Child Health (2004) *Sudden Unexpected Death in Infancy: a multi-agency protocol for care and investigation.* Royal College of Paediatrics and Child Health, London; www.rcpath.org and http://rcpch.ac.uk
14. Hockenberry M, Wilson D, Winkelstein M *et al.* (2003) *Wong's Nursing Care of Infants and Children.* Mosby, St Louis, MO.
15. Kairys S, Randell A, Block R *et al.* for the Committee on Child Abuse and Neglect (2001) Distinguishing sudden infant death syndrome from child abuse fatalities. *Pediatrics.* **107:** 437–41.
16. Campbell A and Campbell D (2005) Emergency baptism by health professionals. *Paediatr Nurs.* **17:** 39–42.
17. National Statistics (2004) *Census 2001.* Office for National Statistics, London; www.statistics.gov.uk
18. Nursing and Midwifery Council (2002) *Code of Professional Conduct.* Nursing and Midwifery Council, London.
19. Brown E (2002) *The Death of a Child: care of the child, support for the family.* Acorns Children's Hospice Trust, Birmingham.
20. Brown E (2006) Ritual and religion. In: A Goldman, R Hain and S Liben (eds) *The Oxford Textbook of Paediatric Palliative Care.* Oxford University Press, Oxford.
21. School of Human Development, University of Nottingham; www.nottingham.ac.uk/human-development/EPICure/epicurehome/
22. Wood N, Costeloe K, Gibson A *et al.* (2003) The EPICure study: growth and associated problems in children born at 25 weeks of gestational age or less. *Arch Dis Child Fetal Neonatal Ed.* **88:** F492–500; http://fn.bmjjournals.com/cig/content/full/88/6/F492
23. Markestad T, Kaaresen P, Ronnestad A *et al.* (2005) Early death, morbidity and need of treatment among extremely premature infants. *Pediatrics.* **115:** 1289–98.
24. http://newsvote.bbc.uk/mpapps/pagetools/print/news.bbc.co.uk/2/hi/health/46399
25. http://news.bbc.uk/1/hi/uk_politics/4696315.stm
26. Ramer-Chrastek J and Thygeson M (2005) A perinatal hospice for an unborn child with a life-limiting condition. *Int J Palliat Nurs.* **11:** 274–6.
27. http://news.bbc.co.uk/1/hi/england/manchester/4095215.stm
28. Hazen M (2003) Societal and workplace responses to perinatal loss: disenfranchised grief or healing connection. *Hum Relations.* **56:** 147–66.
29. Data Protection Act 1998; www.opsi.gov.uk/acts/acts1998
30. Diamond A (1995) *A Gift from Sebastian: the story of a cot death.* Boxtree, London.
31. Siden (2003) Models of child health care and paediatric palliative care research. *Paed Pal Lit.* **12:** 5–9.

Chapter 4

A young child with sudden serious illness

This chapter covers

Content	Related to sudden serious illness
Scenario	• Contemporary issues relating to life-limited children and young people in an intensive-care environment
• Meningococcal septicaemia	• Clinical governance and suggestions for work-based learning and networking
• Setting the scene	• Summary
• The National Service Framework	
• The Knowledge and Skills Framework	*Relevant to other areas of palliative care for children and young people*
• The ACT Care Pathway	
	• Chapter 11: going home for terminal care
Contemporary issues	• Chapter 3: children seeing dead sibling and attending funerals
• End-of-life care in PICU	
• Symptom control in PICU	*Relevant topics in other chapters*
• How intensive care staff are affected by end-of-life care	
• Working within the multi-disciplinary team	• Chapter 3: the EPICure study
• Parental perspective on end-of-life decisions	• Chapters 5, 6 and 7: grandparents
• Family-sensitive care	• Chapter 11: social care and schooling
• Implementing NSF principles	• Chapter 12: witnessing resuscitation
• Perspective on organ donation	• Chapter 12: withholding and withdrawing treatment
	• Chapter 12: 'do not resuscitate' orders
	• Chapter 13: biology of the dying process

Meningococcal septicaemia

Further information on meningococcal disease, and a definition of meningococcal septi-caemia, can be found on the website of the Meningitis Research Foundation.[1] A very useful document that discusses a number of case studies by Ninis and Glennie[2] can be accessed via this website.

Definition

This is septicaemia caused by *Neisseria meningitidis* (meningococcus), which presents with severe, sudden and rapid onset and a petechial rash, and is characterised by overwhelming septic shock.

Setting the scene

Ben, aged 1 year, had shown signs of a slight cold and was consequently a little grumpy when attending a friend's first birthday party. His parents, Peter and Anne, were not particularly worried about this. They had five children, aged 1, 3, 5, 7 and 10 years, so there was rarely a time when someone didn't have a cold.

That evening Ben vomited several times, and by 10 p.m. he had started to develop a petechial rash. By the time he arrived in hospital he was unconscious and in severe septic shock. He was cared for in the paediatric intensive-care unit. He was ventilated and fully supported, and in fact there were so many tubes attached to him and items of equipment surrounding the cot that it was not easy to be with him and just hold his hand.

By the following evening it was apparent that Ben had multi-organ failure. He had developed several necrotic areas, and both parents were extremely distressed at the appearance of their child, who just over 24 hours ago was a happy healthy toddler. Extracorporeal membrane oxygenation (ECMO) had been considered, but Ben suffered a cardiac arrest before this could be arranged. Resuscitation was performed for 40 minutes, but proved unsuccessful, and Ben died at 2 a.m. Unfortunately, Peter and Anne had just gone for a break when this happened, and as the unit had no policy on parental presence during resuscitation, they were not allowed back until after Ben had died.

Special considerations

There should already have been follow-up of contacts for the type of meningococcal disease that Ben had. This would have meant confirmation of the vaccination status of the other siblings and tracing contacts from the birthday party. Ben might not have had type C meningococcal disease, so all of the contacts might need prophylactic antibiotics. The parents would definitely be given antibiotics. Meningococcal disease is a notifiable disease.

Jot down your initial reaction to this situation.

Does this bring back memories of a situation you have encountered?

Does this help or hinder?

SWOT

What are your learning needs when considering this scenario? They could look similar to those in the chart below.

Strengths	Weaknesses
• I work in a highly professional and supportive environment where all members of the multi-disciplinary team are seen to make a valuable contribution. • We have clear protocols that guide the care that we provide.	• Some families are transferred who are living a considerable distance away, which can make it difficult to give truly family-centred care. • We do not always know the long-term outcome for our children once they are transferred back to their local hospital.
Opportunities	Threats
• We shall review the ACT Care Pathway in the light of developing a section in the care plan that discusses parental wishes and needs with regard to being present during potential resuscitation.	• Sometimes the unit is very busy and we simply can't spare a member of staff to look after parents when their child is being resuscitated. • A number of staff feel uncomfortable having parents watch their child being resuscitated.

There might be issues that you wish to explore, in which case feel free to do so, but also think about the following.

What are the immediate needs of Peter and Anne?

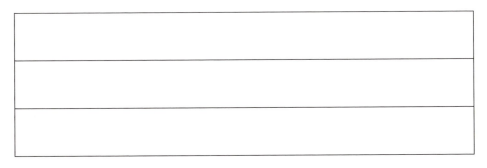

Have you considered any of these?

1. These parents are probably experiencing feelings of total devastation, exhaustion and guilt about not having acted on the symptoms that Ben had presented with earlier.
2. At this point they need support and empathetic responses to their questions. They should be allowed to stay with their child for as long as they need to do so.
3. Explain to the parents what practicalities have to be attended to next. They might want the other children to see their brother, and they might need support to make this decision, whether the siblings are brought in immediately or later the next day. There is no right or wrong answer here, and any decision needs to be guided by what feels right for this family. At the moment the parents are exhausted and might benefit from having a rest before facing the other children. The siblings might find it easier to come into hospital during the day, rather than being woken to be told the news.

Assuming that the other children are at present being cared for by their grandparents, what are their needs?

Have you considered any of these?

1. Point 3 under the previous question is obviously relevant. The grandparents will also feel devastated. Parents do not expect to outlive their children, and grandparents do not expect to outlive their grandchildren. Although grandparents usually make every effort to support their sons and daughters, they are doubly distressed by their own grief and the distress of the young family.
2. These children have to face major upheavals in their lives. Children are very dependent on how the adults in their lives cope. Therefore the way in which they are supported is very important. Their main need is to be provided with an emotionally safe environment.
3. In this respect it might be most helpful if the parents can tell the children the news themselves. If the parents are too distraught to do this, it might be more appropriate for the adults who are currently looking after them to tell them that Ben has died.
4. The children need to understand that although the parents are very upset, they love the children as much as they did before Ben died, and that they are still a family. Children also often feel that they are the cause of a family crisis, so they need to be reassured that they are not the cause of Ben's illness and death.

What is the likely understanding of the siblings about what has happened to Ben?

Have you considered any of these?

1. A child's concept of death is roughly linked to the developmental stage of the child (for an overview, see Chapter 2). A child's concept of illness is also linked to their stage of cognitive development. Children who are confronted with a very sick relative might show a rapid increase in their understanding. Whilst the younger children might still confuse cause and effect, the older children might well understand that Ben had caught germs which made him so ill that he died. We have to be careful not to take everything a child says at face value. Often children repeat what they have overheard adults saying, but it cannot be assumed that a child actually understands at the same level as an adult.

2. Children cannot distinguish between varying severities of illness, so may become very distressed if either they or another family member becomes ill, fearing that he or she will die as well.

How would you advise the parents with regard to the other children seeing their brother and participating at his funeral?

Have you considered any of these?

1. This decision has to be right for this family. We can guide, but we cannot prescribe. Children find it easier to come to terms with the death of a loved one if they have had the opportunity to say goodbye. The added difficulty in this case is that Ben's appearance is quite altered, and this could be distressing to the children. Invariably the children will be aware of the conversations that adults are having. This might mean that they imagine Ben to be totally mutilated, so seeing him might actually reassure them.

2. Children's coping abilities can be actively enhanced by giving them choices. Children can only make informed choices if explanations are given in a meaningful way. In this

scenario, they need to understand that Ben will be very still, that he won't be interacting with them, and that his body will be cold and pale and not soft as they are used to. Dressing Ben before the siblings see him will cover some of the marks, although warning them that Ben has 'black spots' and marks where various tubes have been can avoid unnecessary surprises and questions that adults find difficult to handle. Children can be very matter-of-fact about how they assimilate information.

3. The choice as to whether they wish to come to the hospital to see their brother or not should be balanced. For example, they should be offered the choice of coming to the hospital or staying with a significant other, rather than coming to the hospital or having a nice trip out as a treat. A child might opt for the treat and later regret it because at the time they had not realised the implications of the choice they were making.

4. With regard to attending funerals, Doka[3] holds the view that a child who is appropriately prepared and supported can gain psychological comfort from therapeutic rituals. Preparation should include giving the child information about what a funeral is, what is likely to occur, the purpose of the funeral, the physical setting, and the range of reactions that the child is likely to observe – people may cry because they miss the person, or they may laugh, remembering funny or happy stories about the person who has died.

5. Children should be allowed to participate in preparations for the funeral, by making drawings, writing stories or placing a favourite toy in the coffin. Doka[3] emphasises that rituals do not have to be overtly religious.

What methods could you use to help the children to express their feelings and needs? Reflect on the spirituality of children.

| |
| |
| |

Have you considered any of these?

1. According to Garbarino and Bedard,[4] traumatised children try to understand not only what has happened, but also why it did so. A concept of death can be roughly linked to the developmental stages of a child with regard to abstract thinking. We know that young children tend to interpret illness and death as punishment for wrongdoing, yet according to Pehler[5] we do not know whether a need for forgiveness in spiritual terms is found in children (this issue is explored further in Chapter 11).

2. Attig[6] suggests that the child should be helped by creating a safe and secure space that is permeated with trust, in which expression of their existential anguish is allowed and even welcomed, and the need for comfort is recognised. Attig[6] suggests that children's fears of separation can be addressed through a carer's presence. Support through the unknown that lies ahead can be given by providing reassurance that the child who has died will always be in our hearts and will not be forgotten. Questions can be answered honestly, acknowledging the limit of the carer's knowledge, exploring what the child believes and

not dissuading where belief comforts and consoles, but reality testing and providing assurance about forgiveness if a child is troubled by feelings of guilt and punishment.

3. Play – both active and passive – can be used to help children to express and act out their feelings. Bereavement work is hard work, and children who are challenged by this often have a reduced attention span and may respond to comfort measures (e.g. participating in activities that they might have enjoyed in earlier, happier times). This may involve a temporary regression in their development. Appetites might be small and comfort food welcome, while comfort eating at the other extreme might also need to be addressed. White[7] offers parents some practical ideas on how to cope with bereaved children so as to foster security. These include very basic comfort measures, such as providing warm, soft bedding and clothing to deal with the coldness of shock and provide the sensation of being lovingly wrapped against harm. Providing a nightlight or leaving a light on at night, and possibly allowing a tape player or television to play softly, may help to address fear of the dark. Children benefit from the opportunity to play, and this needs to be provided even if schoolwork suffers temporarily. Falling behind with schoolwork can usually be attributed to inability to concentrate, and the opportunity to unwind through play is likely to improve concentration.

The National Service Framework

No specific reference to paediatric intensive care has been found in the NSF. However, the recommendations of the National Coordinating Group on Paediatric Intensive Care[8] for audit and organisation of the service were put forward to the NHS Executive, detailing service requirements and interfaces with other services that meet the needs of children. It can be anticipated that many current developments are on their way with regard to implementing the NSF. Of relevance to paediatric intensive care is the pathway for the ventilator-dependent child[9] (this is explored further in Chapters 6 and 10). It is also worth noting that the National Coordinating Group on Paediatric Intensive Care[8] acknowledges the varying needs of young people by extending the definition of 'child' up to the age of 19 years. This may be particularly relevant in the context of life-limiting illness, where late adolescence might be the critical time in the young person's disease process.

Skills and knowledge

The National Coordinating Group on Paediatric Intensive Care[8] is specific about the organisation of high-dependency and intensive care and the required commitment at each level. This not only puts the onus on individuals and organisations to keep the required skills up to date, but also requires advocacy at all levels so that provision is made appropriate for each setting, from district general hospitals to tertiary units.

The ACT Care Pathway

In the above scenario, Ben enters on Diagram 1. Staff on the unit will be realistic with the family about the seriousness of Ben's condition, and while not abandoning hope will be preparing the parents for the decreasing likelihood that Ben can survive this overwhelming infection. Diagram 3 can be followed for the final stage of Ben's care. Using a pathway here might have allowed for dialogue with the family about their wishes with regard to being present at Ben's resuscitation. Many parents anticipate that a crisis might occur, and both parents and staff can feel more comfortable if issues are out in the open.

Contemporary issues relating to life-limited children and young people in an intensive-care environment

End-of-life care in the paediatric intensive-care unit (PICU)

According to Meyer et al.,[10] the transition from aggressive curative care to palliative care can be especially abrupt and difficult to achieve for dying children. At present, according to the authors, most end-of-life care for children occurs in the acute hospital setting, often the PICU. Burns et al.[11] explain that during the last 15 years there has been a dramatic increase in the number of decisions to withhold or withdraw life-sustaining treatment in critically ill patients. In their study, the factors most commonly considered when making these decisions pertained to quality of life (e.g. quality of life viewed by the patient or the family, the likelihood of survival, or the potential for neurologically intact survival), whereas the financial cost to society and the availability of beds in the PICU were the least frequently cited factors.

Garros et al.[12] conducted an 8-month study that provided a detailed breakdown of circumstances surrounding death in their PICU. Using their findings as a starting point, four research studies of grief responses, attitudes, treatment decisions and parental perspectives will be summarised below.

Garros et al.[12] found that around 60% of deaths in their PICU followed limitation or withdrawal of life-sustaining treatment (W/LT). Of the total of 99 deaths that were observed, 27 followed cardiopulmonary resuscitation, 39 followed W/LT, 20 were 'do not resuscitate' (DNR) cases and 13 were brain deaths. Life-sustaining treatment (LST) was later withdrawn from 11 of the 20 DNR children. The family was present for 76% of children when LST was stopped, and the dying child was held by the family in 78% of these cases. The findings of the survey included the following.

- Decision making at the end of life is a dynamic process, with limitation of treatment considered in the earlier stages.
- Approximately 50% of the active withdrawal of LST evolved from earlier DNR decisions.
- It seems to be easier for the family to agree initially to limitation rather than active withdrawal of LST.
- As time passes the clinical situation may in some cases become increasingly difficult for both the family and the staff – waiting and watching is no longer a good option.
- This extra time may allow the family to come to terms with their child's inevitable death – a period that is needed for acceptance.

Symptom control issues in the PICU

With regard to symptom control, Garros et al.[12] state that almost all of the children in the W/LT group received analgesia with morphine, with an increasing dose in less than 20% of children, and 13% receiving anticipatory dosing with sedatives at the time of death. The reason for this approach to prescribing in the study by Garros et al.[12] was not explored with the prescribing physicians. Burns et al.[11] give similar figures for escalating symptom control (89% of children), explaining that patients who were comatose were less likely to receive these medications. The reasons cited for administering these drugs to non-comatose children were treatment of pain, anxiety and air hunger. Yet in another study by Burns et al.,[13] only 20% of the same cohort of parents agreed that their child was comfortable in their final days in the PICU. This is in contrast with 87% of nurses and doctors agreeing with the decision about the medication that the children should be given.[11]

Burns et al.[11] found that 91% of doctors and nurses viewed hastening death as an 'acceptable, unintended side-effect' of terminal care. In this study the mean dose of sedatives and analgesia nearly doubled as LST was withdrawn. The degree of escalation in dose did not correlate with the doctor's views on hastening death. Burns *et al.*[11] concluded that care of the dying patient after withdrawal of life-sustaining treatment remains under-analysed and needs more rigorous examination by the critical care community.

This series of articles by Burns *et al.*[11,13] and Meyer *et al.*[10] (who belonged to the same team) makes very useful reading. One of the areas explored highlights the difficulties surrounding symptom control in the critical care environment. Unlike other areas of palliative care for children and young people, withdrawal of life-sustaining treatment poses further challenges to maintaining the comfort of the child who is undergoing terminal weaning off ventilator support, in terms of the timing of administration of neuromuscular blocking (NMB) agents. These agents are frequently used to prevent patient–ventilator dyssynchrony leading to severe patient discomfort and deleterious increases in alveolar pressure.[11] However, they also prevent spontaneous respiration on removal of ventilator support, and they render the child unable to express any discomfort, due to the fact that they are paralysed.

In anticipation of the discomfort of pain, anxiety and air hunger, and the difficulty of assessing these, an aggressive approach to the management of these symptoms is needed. According to Burns *et al.*,[11] the sedation and analgesia that are adequate for a patient who is receiving mechanical ventilation are usually inadequate for treating the air hunger experienced by imminently dying patients without neurological injury as controlled ventilation is removed.

The use and timing of NMB agents during terminal weaning have been discussed by the Royal College of Paediatrics and Child Health,[14] as has the use of analgesia and sedation (see also Chapter 12).

Burns *et al.*[11] found that in no case in their study were analgesia or sedation withheld due to fear of hastening death, a reasoning that is frequently attributed to the principle of double effect. Burns *et al.* stated that critics of the principle argue that it is neither morally relevant nor logically valid. It relies on an overly simplistic notion of intent that is impossible to verify externally, and may have the paradoxical effect of constraining some clinicians from providing adequate medication for relief of suffering, due to their fear of violating the principles of absolute prohibition against intentionally causing death. Burns *et al.* found that clinicians believed that they were allowing an inexorably moribund patient to die. They did not attribute the cause of death to the absence of life-support modalities or the provision of sedation and analgesia, but rather to the underlying disease itself.

Burns *et al.*[11] highlighted the following specific areas for improvement of end-of-life care.

- An open discussion with the family and all members of the care team on how palliative care measures will be provided should take place before the withdrawal of life-sustaining treatment.
- This should be followed by clear documentation of these decisions and the subsequent care provided in the patient's record.
- There should be regularly scheduled case reviews in which the palliative care that is being provided is thoroughly examined.
- Consensus guidelines are needed on medically indicated dosing of sedatives and analgesics for signs and symptoms of patient suffering during the withholding or withdrawal of life-sustaining treatment.

How intensive-care staff are affected by end-of life care

Rider[15] has provided the following reflection:

> I have come to accept that death is a part of life and to know that we have not failed as doctors when a patient dies. We only fail if we avoid our dying patients and their families or allow our patients to die alone without our compassion

and emotional presence. We cannot always control the outcome, but we can provide empathy and comfort.

We have choices about how we work with dying patients and their families, the time we spend with them, and how we help them with decisions about the life that is left. We can learn to empower parents and children to live well despite terminal illness, create a safe place for patients and their families to grieve and help them say goodbye.

Although the underlying philosophy of admission to intensive care is preservation of life, intensive-care nurses frequently find themselves in the situation of supporting dying children and their families. Rashotte *et al.*[16] have observed that this makes nurses vulnerable to emotional, physical and intellectual repercussions which may not be recognised or acknowledged. The grief responses of nurses who are working in a critical care area are influenced by a number of factors. Some aspects of the research study by Rashotte *et al.*[16] on the context of intensive-care work are highlighted below.

- Some participants had not wanted to work with chronically ill patients.
- They perceived that children in a critical care environment recovered more quickly from the acute phase of their illness, and were quickly transferred to another unit.
- Nurses expected to function at a high level of professional competence.
- The child's illness, level of cognitive development and therapeutic interventions placed the nurses at the front line for anticipation and swift detection of any life-threatening problems.
- It was important for the nurses to integrate comfort and supportive components of care with the cure or therapeutic goals of the intensive-care unit. The primary concern of their care was the physical and emotional comfort of the child and their family, and a strong desire to eliminate the suffering of the child and the family, as well as to help the family to cope with the crisis of their child's illness.
- Having a relationship with the family made caring for the child less technical, more personal and more humane.
- Nurses often faced ethical dilemmas. For example, if the technology is available, does it have to be used? If not, who should make the decision to withhold treatment, when enough is enough?

These results might have direct implications for nurses working with an increasing number of technology-dependent children with chronic problems who remain in an intensive-care environment for prolonged periods of time (this issue is explored further in Chapters 9 and 10).

Additional findings of the research by Rashotte *et al.*[16] include the following.

- Nurses who are working in a paediatric intensive-care environment face multiple, accumulated losses as part of their working life, and may be exposed to several deaths at one time or within a short period of time.
- Five themes emerged from the study data:
  - self-expression
  - self-nurturance
  - termination of relationship activities
  - engaging in control-taking activities
  - self-reflection (summarised in more detail below).

- Self-reflection helped the nurses to:
  - come to terms with the child's death
  - create meaning
  - accept their own feelings of emotional pain when a child died.

- All of these aspects are necessary to enable the nurses to cope with their exposure to multiple deaths.
- Through the process of self-reflection nurses had learned:
  - to understand how they reacted to the death of a child
  - to identify what factors related to the death affected their grief response
  - to understand which coping strategies helped them to manage their grief
  - that reflecting on past experiences of deaths, and reliving them in the light of new feelings and new knowledge, led to new understanding and changed perspectives.

Juggling care and family support involves complex issues, and one of the issues highlighted in the study by Rashotte et al.[16] is the need for nurses who are new to the PICU to have role modelling at every stage from the child's admission through to supporting the family through the child's death and finding their own coping strategy. 'Role modelling' and reflection in action appear to be recurring themes for a nurse to become an 'expert' practitioner – both in delivering what Tomlinson et al.[17] refer to as 'family-sensitive care' and in developing the coping strategies that will enable them to deliver this care.

Working within the multi-disciplinary team

One aspect of coping with end-of life care concerns how family care is practised within the multi-disciplinary team. Burns et al.[13] found serious perceptual differences between physicians and nurses in their assessment of end-of-life care as it is actually practised in their PICU.

- Nurses were significantly less likely to report that ethical issues are well discussed within the care team, and between the care team and the family, and that families are well informed about the advantages and limitations of further therapy.
- Nurses feel excluded from the decision-making process and the support for families facing end-of-life decisions for their children, despite the fact that it is nurses who bear the major responsibility for implementing end-of-life decisions, providing terminal care and helping families to cope with the death of a child.
- Nurses in the survey by Burns et al. were significantly more likely to advocate an increase in narcotics as life support was withdrawn.
- Some nurses reported that physicians were not always or frequently at the bedside as life support was withdrawn. This removed a significant source of reassurance both for the family and for the nurses, and might lead to suboptimal control of pain and other symptoms.
- Burns et al. conclude that the training of clinicians in end-of-life decision making has not kept up with the advances in critical care medicine, and they point to inadequacies in the ethics curriculum of medical and nursing education.
- They advocate unit-based education for less experienced clinicians, the identification and support of role models already on the staff, and greater interdisciplinary collaboration.

Parental perspectives on end-of life decisions

According to Meyers et al.,[10] the child's quality of life, their chances of getting better, and the amount of pain and discomfort were the most important factors when facing end-of life decisions. Their findings can be summarised as follows.

- Parents emphasised that they wanted to know the 'big picture' and the 'bottom line.'
- In line with other studies, Meyers et al. found that parental perception of the relief of the child's pain and suffering was critically important when facing end-of-life decisions. Parents may be more likely to withdraw support if they perceive their child to be in pain.

- From a psychological perspective, parents may gain reassurance from knowing that their child was kept comfortable and presumably did not suffer. This has implications for the bereavement process and long-term adaptive coping.
- Parents struggle with a loss of control as the main protector, and nearly a quarter of parents reported that, if they were able to do so, they would make decisions differently with regard to their child's care.
- Parents who harbour such feelings of loss of control and regret about their child's hospitalisation and circumstances before death may be at increased risk of unresolved grief and complicated bereavement.

Family-sensitive care

Tomlinson et al.[17] explored family care and found that it is widely accepted that complex care models which incorporate the whole family are seldom used in the PICU, except by expert family nurses who are not involved in primary care. Meyer et al.[10] conducted a study of parental perspectives on end-of life care in the PICU. Their main findings were as follows.

- Clinicians, usually initially unknown to the family, can be quickly drawn into the family's inner circle of support. This might be due to the clinician's expertise, availability and familiarity with the hospital culture in the context of a family's emotional needs and vulnerability.
- Nurses were considered to be more involved during the dying process than other family members or friends. They were described as 'wise, skilful and compassionate strangers' in recognition of the fact that they bear witness to and support families during medical crises.
- Whether they are prepared or not, staff members may be suddenly confronted with the intimate lives of families who are in considerable distress.
- In keeping with the principles of family-centred care and trends towards incorporation of patient perspectives into care delivery models, there are obligations to learn directly from families about what is important, and to deliver accordingly.
- In this context, Frager[18] suggests that tertiary centres should foster a selective reliance on their services and staff, which in most cases not only fade after the child's death, but also limit a family's access and use of potentially beneficial existing palliative care services. Meyer et al. therefore suggest that critical care practitioners need to keep their hospital-based roles and the attendant limitations in perspective and promote the development of a support network that can remain available throughout the bereavement process.
- After the child's death, the primary social support available to parents shifted abruptly from being dominated by staff to being provided mainly by family members, friends and religious sources. Just 40% of parents accessed support groups, and about half of these reported them to be helpful.

Implementing NSF principles: deciding on 'place of care' and recognising end of life

Taking up the points made by Meyer et al.,[10] cited above, Miller (personal communication, 2005) explained that in a small number of situations children were transferred from a PICU to their local children's hospice, either before or at some stage during withdrawal of life-sustaining treatment. The treatment was then withdrawn using the same techniques that were practised in the PICU, supported by the transferring anaesthetist. Miller describes how the calm environment of a children's hospice might help the child to 'let go.' Other factors cited by Meyer et al.,[10] pertaining to parental control and perception of their child's comfort as well as a clear protocol for bereavement support, can easily be achieved when relevant services work together. This is a clear example of imaginative implementation of the NSF and the Knowledge and Skills Framework.

This can also be achieved when treatment decisions have to be made involving intensive care. Miller (personal communication, 2005) suggests that it is necessary to keep 'one step ahead' when it becomes obvious that a child is approaching ACT Care Pathway 3. Planning ahead here can include a visit by parents to an intensive-care unit to make an informed decision as to whether they wish their child to be cared for in this environment – should the situation occur – in an attempt to prolong life, although it is unlikely that the child will survive.

Perspective on organ donation

Rashotte *et al.*[16] cites an interesting reflection on organ donation, in which a nurse recounted the story of her first and only experience of a child undergoing an organ donation procedure having died from a sudden and unexpected illness. The nurse had cared for the child during the diagnostic determination of brain death and the subsequent preparation of the body for organ donation. She experienced feelings of helplessness, unfairness and guilt, and found telling the story acutely painful. However, while she was caring for an organ recipient several months later, the same nurse found that she was extensively reviewing and possibly reinterpreting the death of the first child in the light of her new experience.

Clinical governance and suggestions for work-based learning and networking

Explore with your colleagues how the NSF and the ACT Care Pathway can be implemented in your working environment in relation to Ben and his family. What are the challenges? How can they be overcome?

Departments usually have members of staff who have a designated role and/or special interest (e.g. family bereavement, play specialist (some units organise siblings' weekends), schoolteacher, therapist, chaplaincy, patient services, mortuary, funerals, etc.).

Draw up a workable care plan for Ben and his parents based on ACT Care Pathways 1 and 3.

Assuming that the siblings and grandparents did not have an opportunity to see Ben again while he was alive, how would you accommodate their needs and their feelings when working with the pathways in this situation?

Reflect on your care plan. In what way did your actions pave the way for supporting the family through the death of their child and afterwards?

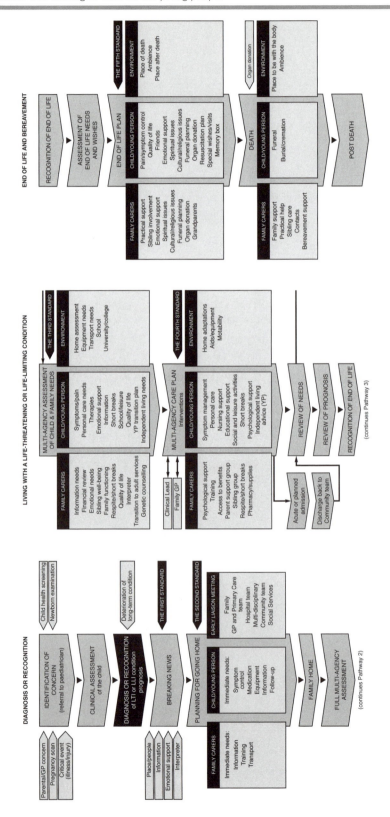

Summary

This chapter has considered life-limiting illness in an intensive-care context. As an example of this, issues of care for a young child dying from meningococcal disease have been explored in terms of family support extending to siblings and grandparents. Issues relating to children viewing the body and attending funerals have been highlighted. Contemporary issues in end-of life care pertaining to staff attitudes towards and ability to cope with end-of life decisions and symptom management, as well as parental attitudes to the care of their child, have also been explored.

SWOT

It might be useful to revisit the SWOT analysis at this point in order to determine any further learning needs in relation to this chapter and the Knowledge and Skills Framework (KSF) requirements, namely:

1. communication
2. personal and people development
3. health, safety and security
4. service improvement
5. quality
6. equality and diversity.

Strengths	Weaknesses
Opportunities	Threats

Action plan for further learning

References

1. Meningitis Research Foundation; www.meningitis.org
2. Ninis N and Glennie L (2004) *Lessons from Research for Doctors in Training;* www.meningitis.org
3. Doka K (1994) Suffer the little children: the child and spirituality. In: B Dane and C Levine (eds) *AIDS and the New Orphans.* Auburn House, Westport.
4. Garbarino J and Bedard C (1996) Spiritual challenges to children facing violent trauma. *Childhood.* **3:** 467–78.
5. Pehler S (1997) Children's spiritual response: validation of the nursing diagnosis spiritual distress. *Nurs Diagnosis.* **8:** 55–67.
6. Attig T (1996) Beyond pain: the existential suffering of children. *J Palliat Care.* **12:** 20–3.
7. White C (1995) Life crisis for children and their families. In: B Carter and A Dearmun (eds) *Child Health Care Nursing.* Blackwell, Oxford.
8. National Coordinating Group on Paediatric Intensive Care (1997) *Paediatric Intensive Care: a framework for the future.* NHS Executive, Wetherby.
9. Department of Health and Department for Education and Skills (2005) Care Pathway for the Discharge and Support of Children Requiring Long-Term Ventilation in the Community: National Service Framework for children, young people and maternity services. Department of Health, London.
10. Meyer E, Burns J, Griffith J *et al.* (2002) Parental perspectives on end-of-life care in the pediatric intensive-care unit. *Crit Care Med.* **30:** 226–31.
11. Burns J, Mitchell C, Outwater K *et al.* (2000) End-of-life care in the pediatric intensive-care unit after the forgoing of life-sustaining treatment. *Crit Care Med.* **28:** 3060–6.
12. Garros D, Rosychuk R and Cox P (2003) Circumstances surrounding end of life in a pediatric intensive care unit. *Pediatrics.* **112:** 371–80.
13. Burns J, Mitchell C, Griffith J *et al.* (2001) End-of-life care in the pediatric intensive-care unit: attitudes and practices of pediatric critical care physicians and nurses. *Crit Care Med.* **29:** 658–64.
14. Royal College of Paediatrics and Child Health (2004) *Withholding and Withdrawing Life-Saving Treatment in Children: a framework of practice.* Royal College of Paediatrics and Child Health, London.
15. Rider E (2003) Danny's mother – a lesson in humility. *Arch Pediatr Adolesc Med.* **157:** 228.
16. Rashotte J, Fothergill-Bourbonnais F and Chamberlain M (1997) Pediatric intensive-care nurses and their grief experience: a phenomenological study. *Heart Lung.* **26:** 372–86.
17. Tomlinson P, Tomlinson E, Peden-McAlpine C *et al.* (2002) Clinical innovation for promoting family care in paediatric intensive care: demonstration, role modelling and reflective practice. *J Adv Nurs.* **38:** 161–70.
18. Frager G (1996) Pediatric palliative care: building the model, bridging the gap. *J Palliat Care.* **12:** 9–12.

Chapter 5

An adolescent with cancer

This chapter covers

Content	Relevant to other areas of palliative care for children and young people
Scenario	
• Rhabdomyosarcoma	• Chapter 9: cognate children
• Setting the scene: Part 1	• Chapter 9: schooling
• The National Service Framework	• Chapter 6: transitions
• The ACT Care Pathway	
• The Knowledge and Skills Framework	
• Setting the scene: Part 2	
	Relevant topics in other chapters
Contemporary issues	• Chapter 4: organ transplantation
• Some alarming statistics	• Chapter 6: transition
• Palliative?	• Chapter 6: support for peers
• Improving outcomes for children and young people with cancer	• Chapter 9: the young person as a healthcare consumer
• The parents' perspective	• Chapter 11: social care and schooling
• The young person's perspective	
• Core elements of palliative care	
• Provisions for young people	
• The 'subculture' of adolescence	
• Resources	
• Symptoms, body image and teenage sexuality	
• Long-term follow-up	
• Bereavement: Winston's wish	
Related to oncological problems	
• Contemporary issues in palliative care for children and young people in relation to oncology	
• Resources	
• Clinical governance and suggestions for work-based learning and networking	
• Summary	

Rhabdomyosarcoma

Rhabdomyosarcoma[1] is a highly malignant soft tissue tumour that requires aggressive multimodal therapy. It has often metastasised by the time of diagnosis.

Setting the scene: Part I

Adam is 15 years old and has suffered from an orbital rhabdomyosarcoma for the past 2 years. He now has spinal secondaries and has been in severe and poorly controlled pain. He is receiving palliative care at home. A subcutaneous syringe driver with morphine sulphate and cyclizine was commenced 1 week ago, as well as an oral antidepressant, a muscle relaxant and an anticonvulsant. Adam is now much more comfortable. He has short bouts of energy, when he is able to be up in his electric wheelchair, which alternate with prolonged periods of exhaustion and very low mood. He feels that he has a lot of unfinished business to attend to, and he gets frustrated at the short time he has left. He is very keen on planning his own funeral and wants his friends from school to be involved. He has requested that his corneas be donated, but this request has been rejected emphatically by his adoptive parents.

Relationships among the family members have not always been happy. Adam's adoptive parents were initially overprotective of their son when he became ill, and Adam resented the imposed secrecy surrounding his illness. It has taken a long time for him to regain any trust in both his adoptive parents and the healthcare professionals. At times Adam has been physically and verbally aggressive towards his adoptive parents, Paula and James, and his 12-year-old sister, Helen.

Jot down your initial reaction to this situation.

| |
| |
| |
| |

Does this bring back memories of a situation you have encountered?

Does this help or hinder?

SWOT

What are your learning needs when considering this scenario? They could look similar to those in the chart opposite.

The National Service Framework

Standards 4, 6, 8 and 9 apply, as well as *Improving Outcomes in Children and Young People with Cancer*.[2] The latter document provides a care pathway for children and young people and their families, setting out effective interventions required to meet their needs, and indicating expected outcomes not only for survival, but also with regard to normal development into adulthood, in so far as that is possible. This document is discussed further below.

Strengths	Weaknesses
• We work in a supportive multi-disciplinary team. • We have regular multi-disciplinary meetings, including child psychology.	• Oncology services for children and young people have only recently been separated from the adult services locally. • Many parents and young people have not benefited from the same culture of involvement in decision making and information sharing that is promoted now.
Opportunities	Threats
• The NSF gives us the driving force to shape our new service in a way that best meets the needs of our families. • We can follow the ACT Care Pathway as a template to assess, plan, implement and evaluate care at critical points, making smooth transitions from hospital to home care, integrating health, education and social service support.	• We deal with a lot of residual mistrust from some of the older children. • This is hard to break through, particularly when time is running out for them. • This can be very stressful and disheartening, especially for less experienced staff.

The ACT Care Pathway

This can easily be applied alongside the principles set out in the above document.

The Knowledge and Skills Framework

1. *Communication.* This is the key aspect of multi-disciplinary working, especially as many families will access cancer services from a tertiary unit, given the fact that there are only eight designated units in the UK.[2] Links need to be established by a key worker and maintained within the child's local inpatient and community provisions. This might require development in the following areas.
2. *Personal and people development.* For both inpatient and community units there is the challenge of maintaining skills that might only be called upon infrequently, as well as learning new skills that are needed for newly referred children. It is vital that networking is optimised (e.g. staff may visit a tertiary unit and be 'trained up' in a particular skill so that care can be given safely either at home or in the child's local hospital). Issues around this link with the following areas.
3. *Health, safety and security.*
4. *Service improvement.*
5. *Quality.*
6. *Equality and diversity.*

There might be issues that you wish to explore, in which case feel free to do so, but also think about the following.

What are the issues that Adam and his family are likely to have to face?

Have you considered any of these?

1. Adam is at the formal operational stage of his development (for details of the different stages of cognitive development, refer to a child development text such as Bee and Boyd[3]), and he also faces the challenges of adolescence. Although he is desperately striving for independence, this is physically impossible. Although he can think and rationalise on an adult level, he lacks the life experience necessary to grasp his situation on an adult level. Ambivalent feelings are provoked by his becoming increasingly dependent on his family again for emotional support. He resents this.

2. There is much interpersonal stress within this family unit, and critical illness can make this worse. It is not unusual for communication between family members to almost completely break down in such a situation. There might be a sense of 'helplessness', as none of the family members can make anything feel any better at the moment. This situation might require a neutral person to 'interpret' and to help individuals to start talking again. Attig[4] suggests the creation of a safe and secure space that is permeated with trust, where expression of existential anguish is clearly allowed and welcomed, and the need for comfort is recognised. There can be a temptation to ignore unacceptable behaviour displayed by the young person, as an acknowledgement that they are acting out their frustration. However, this does not remove the frustration, because the reasons for it remain unresolved. Attig[4] identifies these as missing many potentially meaningful experiences, leaving much undone and unexpressed, and missing relationships that can never be and that will never flourish in adulthood. Adam's ability to cope with his situation is influenced by what Perrone[5] summarises as past childhood experiences, motivation level, present problem-solving abilities, family dynamics, cognitive function, and type of illness and treatment.

3. Depression can also be a feature of chronic, poorly controlled pain, to the point of consequent suicidal behaviour. Perrone[5] offers a useful discussion on the suicide risk of adolescents with cancer, highlighting the drive for life and the consequent will to live, looking at positive attitudes and outcomes. However, there is a need for individual assessment and also reassessment as the course of the disease progresses, so that the point at which the positive outlook changes into despair is not missed.

4. Sources[6] describes how through the terminal disease phase the young person is often aware of the diminishing or non-existent options that he faces, and thus experiences a profound sense of loss of control.

5. Depending on his own belief system and that of his family, Adam is likely to explore issues such as 'What is the meaning of life?' Physical pain, depression, anxiety and spiritual pain can potentiate each other, leaving the young person unsupported, in pain and in emotional isolation.

6. Hayout and Krulik[7] highlight the fragile, complex and apparently impossible existential limbo in which the parents of terminally ill children find themselves. This centres around the basic definition and purpose of parenthood, as well as a distortion of the

'time world.' Normal parenthood involves concentrating on and investing in the present as a way of preparing for the future. In the parenthood of a terminally ill child, the concentration on the present is to a certain extent opposed to preparing for the future. Another major factor identified by Hayout and Krulik[7] is the perceived helplessness of parents who are supposed to protect and defend the child and see him grow up, whereas they are being forced to watch many distressing situations during the child's decline. They must adapt to many unfamiliar norms of behaviour and to rapid changes related to the child's condition.

7. Helen is likely to feel very isolated, as her parents are so preoccupied with Adam and themselves. She might express this either by being very sensible, easygoing and grown up, or by rebelling against a very tense home situation. Her schoolwork may be suffering as a result of domestic problems. She might be subjected to bullying as a result of being very quiet, or she could be disruptive at school, acting out her frustrations outside the home as a way of asking for help. If her normal routine is very disrupted, this might interfere with maintaining contact with her friends or the social activities outside the home in which she might be participating. Helen might be torn between wanting to meet with her friends and feeling that she needs to be at home because Adam is so very ill and might die while she is not there. Feelings of loyalty might conflict with resentment of Adam's hurtful behaviour towards her, causing feelings of guilt. Nolbris and HellStrom[8] examined siblings' needs and issues when a brother or sister dies of cancer, and found that healthy siblings often felt included but not sufficiently prepared for what was happening. Siblings expressed feelings of anxiety, loneliness and jealousy of the parents, the sick child and the other siblings. In this study, healthy siblings reported that school and leisure activities sometimes provided a refuge to which they could retreat. Sidhu *et al.*[9] found that the experience of childhood cancer in a family is not completely destructive. There can be gains in empathy, maturity and self-esteem from increased trust and responsibility, particularly in older siblings.

How would you advise Paula and James, who are horrified by Adam's wish to plan his own funeral and donate his corneas?

| |
| |
| |
| |

Have you considered any of these?

1. It would be helpful to explore with Paula and James why they are horrified about both of these aspects.
2. Adam might wish to donate his corneas in order to have a part of him live on, and also to actively help someone else at a time when he is so dependent on others helping him.
3. The parents might benefit from discussing with a transplant coordinator whether Adam's corneas would in fact be suitable for transplanting. The Paediatric Intensive Care Society has published a useful document on this topic.[10] The parents might also benefit from being reassured that Adam would not be disfigured as a result of cornea

retrieval, and that retrieval would not take place until after his death. This type of donation is not dependent on a beating heart and normal circulation.

4. The National Organ Donor Register does not stipulate any age limits, and according to Dimond[11] any person who is capable within the law of consenting to treatment is capable of consenting to organ transplantation. Bijesterveld[12] asserts the instrumental value of autonomy – for a person who is able to determine his own choices and pursue his own values, it is more likely that life will be satisfying for him. In contrast to Adam's feelings are those of Paula and James. The issue here might not be so much a legal one as a matter of exploring the motivation of both sides and being able to reach a solution that is acceptable to all family members.

5. Although it might appear morbid to wish to plan his own funeral, this also gives Adam some control at a time when he is feeling that he is losing control over his life. It might be his way of wanting to say his 'goodbyes' and create some of the memories with which his family and friends will be left.

What are the issues that Adam's peers are likely to try to come to terms with?

Have you considered any of these?

1. Adolescents have an adult comprehension of death. However, it is commonly viewed as something that happens to others. To have a friend affected by an illness that is leading to his death can deeply shock and affect his peers.
2. Reactions are likely to range from avoiding him because the situation is so hard to bear, or because they feel embarrassed by his appearance, to rallying to support him and becoming very close to him.
3. Adam's care therefore needs to include close friends as part of the care that we offer to 'significant others.'

What are the issues with regard to schooling for the life-limited child or young person?

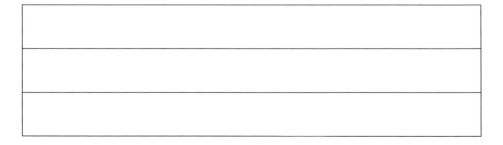

Have you considered any of these?

1. Many children and adolescents experience great anxiety on returning to school after the initial treatment. Although the element of 'normality' is comforting, children can be very self-conscious about their altered body image. They might be subjected to bullying or attract unwanted attention due to their altered appearance. These situations need careful handling, and good practice includes a visit by the liaison nurse before the child returns to school, to prepare the teacher and the child's peers, answer their questions and reassure them (the website of Teens Living With Cancer[13] contains useful information about this issue).
2. Bouffet[14] discusses schooling for the child with an oncological problem. There is a need for some young people to have 'normality' by succeeding and achieving set goals as well as being able to escape from their home and hospital routine.
3. Practical problems centre on the stress that teachers might experience as a result of trying to integrate the sick child's needs (e.g. short attention span, need for frequent rest periods) with those of the rest of the class. Vance and Eiser[15] found that schooling can be problematic for some children, who may be more sensitive and isolated than their peers, according to both peer and teacher report. Hindmarch[16] has written a very useful chapter on good practice and support for schools dealing with children with life-limiting illnesses. Lowton and Higginson[17] have reported the results of a study on how bereavement is handled in the classroom. Various activities are described, such as contact with other adults, 'time-out' cards and contact books. The management of bereavement was influenced by British culture, cultural issues and local communities. Servaty-Seib *et al.*[18] offer practical recommendations for schools on how to notify individual students of a death. The Winston's Wish charity also provides an example of good practice (see below).

Which palliative care category according to ACT and the Royal College of Paediatrics and Child Health[19] is applicable to Adam?

Group 1.

Setting the Scene: Part 2

The revised treatment is taking effect quickly, and Adam is able to go on short outings. A longer outing to a favourite beauty spot is planned, but that night Adam suffers a prolonged seizure and never regains consciousness before his death two days later.

What practical help is the family likely to need during the end stage of Adam's illness?

| |
| |
| |
| |

Have you considered any of these?

1. Given the tense situation within the family unit, this is a particularly stressful and emotionally loaded time. The respite period, during which Adam's symptoms were under control and the family could relax a little, was only short. There might be deep regret about what was not expressed, as well as feelings of resentment and anticipatory grief. There might also be anxiety about how Adam is likely to die.
2. As well as physical care for an unconscious child, the main focus of care needs to be psychological support for the family. Family members need to be made aware that hearing is the last sense to go, and that Adam is likely to be able to hear them. This means they should not have conversations that might distress him, but also that they should continue talking to him, and perhaps saying what previously remained unsaid.
3. At this stage the family needs 24-hour access to nursing care and medical intervention to act quickly as symptom control requires adjustment.
4. Provision must be in place through the paediatric community services, Diana nurses or the children's hospice service for the family to be supported at all times during this phase.
5. There might be grandparents, friends or other relatives available to offer support. Ideally, there should be one person available to support Helen if the parents are too distraught to do this.
6. If a child dies at home, the parents need to be aware of certain practicalities following the child's death, such as the need for confirmation of death by the general practitioner. Does the family want Adam to remain at home or to be taken to a chapel of rest until the funeral? Cooling units can be accessed to prevent deterioration of the body in hot weather. Can a relative or friend take on the role of informing others that Adam has died? Useful information for parents is offered in booklets such as *Precious Times*[20] and *Choices*.[21]

Contemporary issues in palliative care for children and young people in relation to oncology

Some alarming statistics

The Teenage Cancer Trust[22] provides statistics to put some of the issues faced by teenage cancer sufferers into context.

- Six teenagers are diagnosed with cancer each day in the UK. This means that there are over 2,200 new cases every year.
- Cancer is the commonest cause of non-accidental death in teenagers and young adults in the UK.

- One in 330 boys and 1 in 420 girls will contract cancer before their twentieth birthday.
- By the age of 15 years there is a 1 in 600 chance of developing cancer. By the age of 24 years this has increased to a 1 in 285 chance of developing cancer.
- In the last 30 years the incidence of cancer in the teenage and young adult age groups has increased by 50%, and for the first time ever the number of teenagers with cancer now exceeds the number of children with cancer.
- Teenagers contract some of the most aggressive cancers, which are made worse by their growth spurts.

Decker *et al.*[23] state that adolescents with cancer have poorer treatment outcomes as well as higher incidences and mortality rates compared with younger children. Figures for the USA show a 30% increase in cancers in the adolescent age group compared with younger children. In addition, according to Decker *et al.*[23] adolescents show lower rates of decreasing mortality and lower 5-year survival rates than younger children.

The National Institute for Clinical Excellence (NICE)[2] states that carcinomas and epithelial neoplasms and lymphomas are the most common types of cancer in the 15–24 years age group. The report points out that differences in coding and data collection between the 0–14 years and 15–24 years age groups hampers the calculation of comparable data. Consequently it might be difficult to plan for service provision, as some young people will be cared for by the children's services and some by adult services. This makes an overview of how they fare very difficult to assess, bearing in mind that the type of cancers that this age group contracts might lead to even greater problems to be addressed by the young person and their family, due to the developmental stage of the young person.

Palliative?

Having struggled with the term 'palliative' throughout this book, it appears that within children's oncology there is a very workable application of this term. Joy[24] states that with 70% survival rates, not all services that are offered to young cancer sufferers relate to life-limited children, although arguably nearly 100% of cancer cases are life-threatened.

As was mentioned earlier in this chapter, the document *Improving Outcomes in Children and Young People with Cancer*[2] provides a care pathway for children and young people and their families, setting out effective interventions required to meet their needs, and indicating expected outcomes, not only for survival, but also for normal development into adulthood, in so far as that is possible. The reader is urged to study this document in order to gain a full appreciation of the issues that affect children, young people and their families, as well as service providers, during the course of illness. The salient points of the palliative care aspects of this document are listed below.

- Most children with malignancy receive palliative care in the community, usually within the home.
- There are no routinely collected data that measure the use of palliative care services.
- Access to specialist paediatric palliative care expertise is provided from the oncology team, often from the paediatric oncology outreach nurse specialist (POONS) for end-of-life care.
- Healthcare professionals who provide palliative care for children with cancer are expected to be part of a wider paediatric palliative care network. Community children's nursing services provide much of the care of those dying at home.
- There is variable provision across the UK.
- There are very few dedicated services for teenagers and young people.
- In many centres POONS undertake or coordinate the palliative care of young people into their twenties.
- Some children's community nursing services do not accept referrals of patients over the age of 16 years.

- Adult Macmillan nursing services do not generally have experience in caring for this age group. At present there is very limited hospice provision for young people. Of the children's hospices, Douglas House (*see* Chapters 6, 7 and 9) and Martin House will consider new referrals of young people with malignancies up to the age of 23 years. This might expand, as a number of children's hospices are reviewing their admission ages. According to Joy,[24] the Ellenor Foundation is a hospice-at-home service which has been piloting a pathway for adolescents and young adults since 1994. This is based on persuading professionals in adult services to develop relationships with the young people who will come into their care, from the age of 16 years, two years before their transfer at the age of 18 years.

The parents' perspective

Clarke *et al.*[25] highlight the fact that treatment can continue for many years and this may include very aggressive chemotherapy, radiation, surgery, and/or bone-marrow transplant. Treatments take place both in hospital and at home, and as soon as a child is in remission, care is organised in the home. Clarke *et al.* examined the implications of mothers' healthcare work, and the salient points are summarised below.

- Mothers found that being with their children was not only a moral imperative, but also an assumption of the hospital system.
- Caring for their children was a full-time job that consumed their lives and left no time for outside employment or other activities.
- Extra work resulted from the effects of the cancer and associated treatment, such as pain, suffering and behaviour changes. Immune suppression resulted in having to stay away from school, thus requiring the parent to become a play provider and educator.
- About 40% of the mothers' time was spent in hospital or outpatient clinics and 60% at home.
- Mothers needed to be constantly alert for fever and other potentially dangerous and even fatal side-effects of treatment.
- The authors quote a study by Lozowkski *et al.*[26] which described the parental perspective and found that parents played an active and assertive role during hospital treatment. In total, 56% of the parents in this study reported intervening at some point in the treatment process to prevent or correct a medical mistake.
- There were specific healthcare tasks, such as the taking of numerous pills every day, often with comprehensive instructions for taking the medication. These medications frequently had physical and psychological side-effects.
- Getting children to take their medication was time consuming and required innovative means to facilitate the process.
- Part of the home healthcare work involved record keeping.

Svavarsdottir[27] examined parents' most difficult caregiving tasks over an 18-month period and found that although caregiving responsibility was shared between the parents, most mothers either worked part-time or did not work outside the home. Mothers reported that it was both difficult and time consuming to manage behavioural problems, to coordinate, arrange, organise and manage services for family members, to provide personal care for the child with cancer and to structure and plan activities for the family. Fathers found working outside the home, organising care for the child at the same time, and providing emotional support for their spouse both difficult and time-consuming caregiving tasks. Bjork *et al.*[28] described how families found their normal routine turned upside down, becoming dependent on other people as chaos entered their lives. However, by experiencing hope, focusing on positive aspects and learning about cancer and its treatment, family members acquired new knowledge, gained control and maintained some kind of normality in their family life. Bjork *et al.*[28] point out that although the entire family is negatively affected by the child's disease, the experience can at the same time bring the family members closer together as they start to examine their values and priorities. Ward-Smith et al.[29] report that time spent simply being with the child was valued. Hannan and Gibson[30] found that parents value the time that their child has to live when they know that their disease is incurable. Consequently, any decision with regard to place of care is purely about that, not about place of death. Parents described their decision to be at home as a reaction, rather than as the result of consideration of a number of different alternatives. However, the authors found that families valued the same types of support from staff regardless of the setting in which care was provided. They needed to feel safe and secure, and one parent spoke of needing someone else to be in control. Parents found the same deficiencies difficult regardless of where the child was being cared for at the time of death. The findings of this study have implications with regard to the ACT Care Pathway.[31] According to Hannan and Gibson,[30] the importance of the place of death is a major concern for healthcare professionals when planning ahead to ensure adequate service provision, whereas it is the quality of care in the time leading up to death that is important to families.

The young person's perspective

According to Freyer et al.,[32] the developmental issues relate to the ways in which life-threatening illness alters the normal physical and psychological changes associated with adolescence, including attainment of independence, social skills, peer acceptance and a healthy self-image. Their article examines the different stages of adolescence and ethical and legal issues from a very practical perspective. Young et al.[33] studied the way in which disclosure of a potentially life-threatening condition was managed. The views of the young people ranged from wanting to be told at the same time as the parents to believing that it was more appropriate for their parents to know first. By choosing to disclose to the parents first, doctors could take into consideration the parents' special knowledge of their child's personality when planning how communication with the patient should be managed. This also gave the parents an opportunity to compose themselves and to manage their identity as strong and optimistic, as many of them expressed a fear of 'breaking down' in front of their child. Young et al.[33] recommend that healthcare professionals should be aware of how the social position of young people in relation to adults and the executive role of parents can contribute to the marginalisation of young people, and can hamper the development of successful relationships between healthcare professionals and young patients. Penson et al.[34] studied negotiation between the parent and the young person and describe how a 19-year-old, as she became more ill, gradually started to function more like a teenager and deferred treatment decisions to her mother. In this case a minor regression returned her to a dependent status. The authors explain that paediatric units routinely work with parents and older children, presenting medical information to both, but looking to the parents to be the final decision makers, with the child's consent or assent to the treatment plan. Penson et al.[34] concede that the normal fluctuation between autonomous decision maker and dependent child makes treatment of the older adolescent or young adult challenging, whether on a paediatric or adult unit. According to Penson et al., this can leave the staff of an adult unit feeling particularly uncomfortable. A parent may not be seen as having authority to make decisions on behalf of a 'child' aged 18 years or older, whereas in developmental terms a 19-year-old may present more like a younger teenager in the face of the demands of life-limiting illness.

Decker et al.[23] have explored the information needs of young people with cancer. Based on the findings of their study they propose the following strategy for information giving.

- The opening discussion should cover the implications of the diagnosis, treatment and the psychosocial implications of the cancer.

- Ongoing probing for concerns is required.
- What is discussed immediately at diagnosis may not be absorbed or seen as relevant by the young person, but may become more of a concern during the course of the cancer experience.
- Information technology resources, such as the Teens Living With Cancer website,[13] may enable teenagers to explore questions that are often difficult for them to ask.
- Although young women in the study had higher ratings for the need to receive information, the authors question whether young men need to receive information in a different way, because they are less inclined to seek it directly.
- One issue raised by young people was the lack of individually tailored information and the inadequacy of written materials (particularly with regard to readability and the use of medical terms).

Core elements of palliative care

NICE[2] cites a number of core elements of palliative care:

- timely and open communication and information
- choice/options in all aspects of care, including complementary therapies
- death in the place of choice
- coordination of services at home, where this is the chosen place of care, including provision of specialist equipment
- expert symptom management, including radiotherapy and chemotherapy
- access to 24-hour specialist advice and expertise
- emotional, spiritual and practical support for all family members
- respite care, with medical and nursing input, when required.

Provision for young people

In addition to the core elements listed above, NICE[2] states that teenagers and young adults with palliative care needs require individual packages of care that:

- recognise teenagers and young adults as a distinct group with special needs
- give them full involvement in all aspects of decision making
- are provided by multi-disciplinary, multi-agency services
- provide coordinated joint working or transitional care with adult services where appropriate
- address specific staff training needs with regard to both palliative care and the management of young people.

The 'subculture' of adolescence

Rosenbaum[35] explored beliefs about care, health and individuation in adolescents, and found that 'care' meant 'being there' for listening in confidence, helping, gift giving, humour and demonstrating love in time of need. 'Health' was interpreted as well-being, absence of illness, being fit, dealing with problems and taking responsibility. Rosenbaum[35] also established that adolescents valued family, friends, education, money, sports and honesty. Clothes, hair and music were metaphors for adolescents' emerging identities. Adolescents who are struggling with their complex environments create challenges for professionals who are providing care in hospital as well as community environments, and Rosenbaum urges healthcare professionals to understand the meanings and experiences of adolescents within their subculture, in order to provide culturally relevant care.

Sheldon[36] analysed the concept of humour in children's nursing and found that although it is delicate and may be inappropriate in certain settings, it appears to have a positive correlation with information giving (it leads to improved recall) and reduces anxiety levels when used appropriately. When used as an 'ice-breaker' it can help to establish rapport with patients and families, and it can also communicate a message of caring and humanity. Sheldon quotes a study by Hinds[37] which found that the more an adolescent experiences humour in their care, the more hopeful they will become. According to Sheldon's concept analysis, there are several other benefits of using humour that can be helpful when dealing with young people.

• It fosters harmonious integrity.
• It can initiate 'togetherness', warmth and friendliness.
• A notion of trust emerges.
• It creates a relaxed atmosphere.
• It allows the participants to set aside institutional rules or assumptions and it therefore encourages open conversation.

Resources

I have found many excellent resources while researching the oncology aspects of this book – and they just keep coming! It therefore seems appropriate to offer an annotated resource list rather than discuss individual aspects of palliative care relating to oncological problems in children and young people.

UK Children's Cancer Study Group (UKCCSG)[38]

This organisation's website provides information on areas such as the following:

• clinical trials
• a newsletter ('*Contact*') with articles aimed at young people, families and healthcare professionals (there are also special issues with an international focus)
• the grandparents' perspective
• the siblings' perspective – booklets can be downloaded both for siblings ('*My Brother has Cancer*') and also as a guide for parents ('*Brothers and Sisters*').

International Confederation of Childhood Cancer Parent Organisations[39]

• When adequately treated, approximately 70% of childhood cancers are curable.
• However, at present only 20% of the world's children benefit from advanced medical care.
• The UN Charter on the Rights of the Child states that children have a right to life, to treatment when ill, and to rehabilitation following illness. Worldwide, around 80% of children with cancer do not currently have access to adequate diagnosis or treatment. Rehabilitation needs to be improved everywhere.[40]

Symptoms, body image and teenage sexuality

The West Midlands Paediatric Macmillan Team has produced an excellent resource[41] for professionals caring for children and young people suffering from malignant disease. It includes a very useful chapter on teenage sexuality. Issues relating to symptoms experienced while undergoing treatment are also addressed, and this information will be helpful to professionals who do not have contact with this age group on a daily basis. Sheldon[36] suggests that humour can be used to negotiate difficult topics because it can break down barriers. This is particularly valuable when caring for young people, in whom high levels of anxiety, loss of confidence and loss of control are recurrent themes that are consistently identified.

Teens Living With Cancer[42] also has a useful website. For example:

Weird Body Issues

Are you losing hair, growing hair in strange places…feeling fat or looking scrawny? These and many other strange things may happen to your body while undergoing chemo and/or radiation. There aren't always easy ways to solve some of these problems, but let's talk about them and learn from other teens what helps.

This website includes a number of useful sections on symptoms and body image, such as the following:

- *Plumbing Problems. What's that gurgling noise inside of me?* This section helps the teenager to look at embarrassing problems of nausea/vomiting, diarrhoea/constipation, mouth problems, etc.
- *Mirror, Mirror on the Wall. How long will I look like this?* This section tackles central lines, hair loss ('having a shaving party'), skin problems and steroids.
- *Do I Look Cool or What? How to look 'hot' even if you don't feel it.* This section explores 'health esteem' (keeping healthy), 'about face' (self-care), 'head way' (wig tips, working with your stylist), 'social circles' (how to deal with relationships and going out), going back to school, dealing with others, and family and friends.

Long-term follow-up

The Children's Oncology Group has published *Long-Term Follow-Up Guidelines for Survivors of Childhood, Adolescent and Young Adult Cancers*.[43] The website states that the purpose of these guidelines is to provide recommendations for screening and management of late effects that may potentially arise as a result of therapeutic exposure during treatment for paediatric malignancies. These guidelines represent a consensus statement by a panel of experts on the late effects of paediatric cancer treatment. It is intended that implementation of the guidelines will increase awareness of potential late effects and standardise and improve follow-up care provided for survivors of paediatric malignancies throughout the lifespan. The guidelines are intended as a resource for clinicians who provide ongoing healthcare for survivors of paediatric malignancies. This website also contains many useful links, one of which covers emotional issues after childhood cancer.

The After Cure website[44] discusses a range of issues, from clinic attendance and schooling missed while ill to questions such as whether prospective employers should be informed that the person has had cancer, and whether future children are likely to have cancer. There are also many links to other websites of which practitioners should be aware.

CLIC Sargent Cancer Care[45]

Services provided by CLIC Sargent Cancer Care include social care in hospitals, family support in the community, youth programmes (responding to the need of young people to build confidence), financial support (ensuring that families are made aware of their entitlements) and respite holidays.

Bereavement[46]

'Winston's Wish',[47] a charity based in Gloucestershire, is a grief support programme that accepts children who have experienced the death of a parent, brother or sister. It provides a range of services, including individual work, group work and residential weekends. Children are helped to acknowledge and express their feelings, to understand more about illness and the cause of death, to learn that it is still OK to have fun and, most importantly, to meet other children who have had a similar experience. Gloucester schools have been invited to join a support programme to ensure that they are prepared for the death of a pupil, a pupil's friend, a relative or a teacher.

This excellent website is strongly recommended for young people. There is a Chat forum, 'See, talk, ask, say, play, try', as well as various activities, such as *'Skyscape of memories'* (this is just wonderful!), *'Jar of memories'* and *'Calendar of memories.'*

Clinical governance and suggestions for work-based learning and networking

Explore with your colleagues how the NSF and the ACT Care Pathway as well as the Knowledge and Skills Framework standards can be implemented in your working environment in relation to Adam, his parents and Helen. What are the challenges? How can they be overcome?

Departments usually have members of staff who have a designated role and/or special interest (e.g. oncology liaison nurse, transplant coordinator, local children's hospice, family bereavement service, play specialist (some units organise siblings' weekends), schoolteacher, therapist, chaplaincy, patient services, mortuary, funerals, etc.).

Draw up a workable care plan for Adam, his parents and Helen based on ACT Care Pathway 3.

Now reflect on Pathway 2.

- To what extent was the pathway followed in the case of Adam and his family?
- To what extent does this pave the way for Pathway 3?

Now turn your attention to Pathway 1.

Which considerations of this pathway would have been useful at the point of diagnosis to facilitate advance planning for Adam and his family?

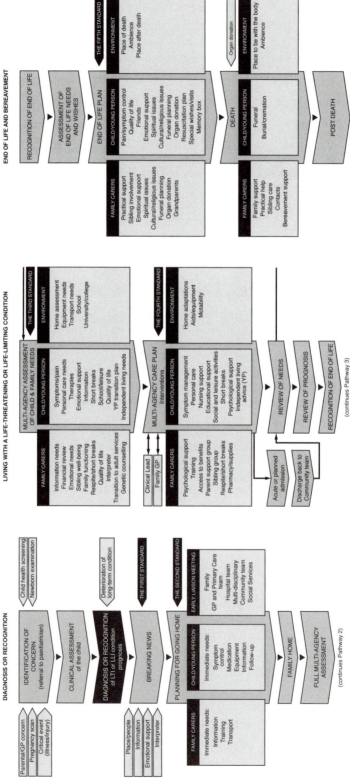

Summary

This chapter has considered the adolescent in the end stage of malignant disease, as well as wider issues relating to life-threatening and life-limiting issues in adolescents, such as the NICE guidelines, statistics on malignancies in young people, and the perspectives of both young people and their parents. Resources available for both healthcare professionals and families have been found to be well developed and easily accessible.

SWOT

It might be useful to revisit the SWOT analysis (*see* chart on page 75) at this point in order to determine any further learning needs in relation to this chapter and the Knowledge and Skills Framework (KSF) requirements, namely:

1. communication
2. personal and people development
3. health, safety and security
4. service improvement
5. quality
6. equality and diversity.

Strengths	Weaknesses
Opportunities	Threats

Action plan for further learning

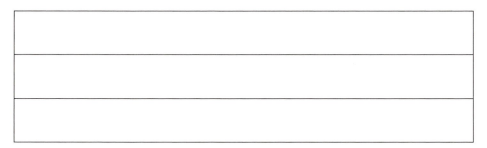

References

1. Hockenberry M, Wilson D, Winkelstein M *et al.* (2003) *Wong's Nursing Care of Infants and Children.* Mosby, St Louis, MO.
2. National Institute for Clinical Excellence (2005) *Improving Outcomes in Children and Young People with Cancer;* www.nice.org.uk
3. Bee H and Boyd D (2005) *Lifespan Development.* Addison-Wesley, Menlo Park, CA.
4. Attig T (1996) Beyond pain: the existential suffering of children. *J Palliat Care.* **12:** 20–3.
5. Perrone J (1993) Adolescents with cancer: are they at risk of suicide? *Pediatr Nurs.* **19:** 22–4.
6. Sources B (1996) The broken heart: anticipatory grief in the child facing death. *J Palliat Care.* **12:** 56–9.
7. Hayout I and Krulik T (1999) A test of parenthood: dilemmas of parents of terminally ill adolescents. *Cancer Nurs.* **22:** 71–9.
8. Nolbris M and HellStrom A (2005) Siblings' needs and issues when a brother or sister dies of cancer. *J Pediatr Oncol Nurs.* **22:** 227–33.
9. Sidhu R, Passmore A and Baker D (2005) An investigation into parent perceptions of the needs of siblings of children with cancer. *J Pediatr Oncol.* **22:** 276–87.
10. Paediatric Intensive Care Society (2002) *Standards for Bereavement Care.* Paediatric Intensive Care Society, London.
11. Dimond B (1996) *The Legal Aspects of Child Health Care.* Mosby, London.
12. Bijesterveld P (2000) Competent to refuse? *Paediatr Nurs.* **12:** 33–5.
13. Teens Living With Cancer; www.teenslivingwithcancer.org/dealing/weird/
14. Bouffet E, Zuchinelli V and Constanzo P (1997) Schooling as a part of palliative care in paediatric oncology. *Palliat Med.* **11:** 133–9.
15. Vance Y and Eiser C (2002) The school experience of the child with cancer. *Child Care Health Dev.* **28:** 5–19.
16. Hindmarch C (2000) *On the Death of a Child.* Radcliffe Medical Press, Oxford.
17. Lowton K and Higginson I (2003) Managing bereavement in the classroom. *Death Stud.* **27:** 717–41.
18. Servaty-Seib H, Perterson J and Spang D (2003) Notifying individual students of a death loss: practical recommendations for schools and school counsellors. *Death Stud.* **27:** 167–86.
19. Association for Children with Life-Threatening or Terminal Conditions and their Families (ACT) and the Royal College of Paediatrics and Child Health (2003) *A Guide to the Development of Children's Palliative Care Services.* ACT, Bristol.
20. *Precious Times;* www.cancer.ie
21. *Choices;* www.lrf.org.uk
22. Teenage Cancer Trust; www.teenagecancertrust.org/fysot/
23. Decker C, Phillips C and Haase J (2004) Information needs of adolescents with cancer. *J Pediatr Oncol Nurs.* **21:** 327–34.
24. Joy I (2005) *Valuing Short Lives: children with terminal conditions.* New Philanthropy Capital, London.
25. Clarke J, Fletcher P and Schneider M (2005) Mothers' home health care work when their children have cancer. *J Pediatr Oncol Nurs.* **22:** 365–73.
26. Lozowski S, Chesler MA and Chesney BK (1993) Parental intervention in the medical care of children with cancer. *J Psychosocial Oncol.* **11:** 63–88.
27. Svavarsdottir E (2005) Caring for a child with cancer: a longitudinal perspective. *J Adv Nurs.* **50:** 153–63.
28. Bjork M, Wiebe T and Hallstrom I (2005) Striving to survive: families' lived experiences when a child is diagnosed with cancer. *J Pediatr Oncol Nurs.* **22:** 265–75.

29. Ward-Smith P, Kirk S, Hetherington M *et al.* (2005) Having a child diagnosed with cancer: an assessment of values from the mother's viewpoint. *J Pediatr Oncol Nurs.* **22:** 320–7.
30. Hannan J and Gibson F (2005) Advanced cancer in children: how parents decide on final place of care for their dying child. *Int J Palliat Nurs.* **11:** 284–91.
31. Elston S (2004) *Integrated Multi-Agency Care Pathways for Children with Life-Threatening and Life-Limiting Conditions.* ACT, Bristol.
32. Freyer D (2004) Care of the dying adolescent: special considerations. *Pediatrics.* **113:** 381–8.
33. Young B, Dixon-Woods M and Heney D (2003) Managing communication with young people who have a potentially life-threatening chronic illness: qualitative study of patients and parents. *BMJ.* **326:** 305.
34. Penson R, Rauch P, McAfee S *et al.* (2002) Between parent and child: negotiating cancer treatment in adolescents. *Oncologist.* **7:** 154–62.
35. Rosenbaum J and Carty L (1996) The subculture of adolescence: beliefs about care, health and individuation within Leininger's theory. *J Adv Nurs.* **23:** 741–6.
36. Sheldon L (1996) An analysis of the concept of humour and its application to one aspect of children's nursing. *J Adv Nurs.* **24:** 1175–83.
37. Hinds P, Martin J and Vogel R (1984) Nursing strategies to influence adolescent hopefulness during oncologic illness. *J Paediatr Oncol Nurs.* **4:** 14–27.
38. UK Children's Cancer Study Group; www.ukccsg.org/
39. International Confederation of Childhood Cancer Parent Organisations; www.icc-cpo.org/
40. International Network for Cancer Treatment and Research (INCTR); www.inctr.org/publications/2003 v04 n01 s05.shtml
41. West Midlands Paediatric Macmillan Team (2005) *Palliative Care for Children with Malignant Disease.* Quay Books, London.
42. Teens Living With Cancer; www.teenslivingwithcancer.org/dealing/weird/
43. Children's Oncology Group; www.childrensoncologygroup.org/
44. After Cure; www.aftercure.org/intro
45. CLIC Sargent Cancer Care; www.clicsargent.org.uk/
46. Cure Search; www.curesearch.org
47. Winston's Wish; www.winstonswish.org.uk/foryoungpeople

Where to next? The transition to early adulthood: a young adult with Duchenne muscular dystrophy

This chapter covers

Content

Scenario

- Duchenne muscular dystrophy
- Setting the scene
- Carrying the 'guilt' of genetic disease
- The National Service Framework and the Knowledge and Skills Framework in context

Contemporary issues

- Quality of life: the sword of Damocles of a 'life-limited' label
- Treatment choices in late teenage
- Staying alive: relationships and families

Related to transition to early adulthood as well as Duchenne muscular dystrophy

- Respite care for young adults: the difference between children's hospice care and adult provision
- Too old and yet too young
- Transition to adult acute care
- Key issues when planning provision for young people
- Contemporary issues in young people's palliative care
- Clinical governance and suggestions for work-based learning and networking
- Summary

Relevant to other areas of palliative care for children and young people

- Chapter 8: neurological degenerative illness
- Chapter 9: contemporary issues
- Chapter 10: technology-dependent children
- Chapter 11: complex needs

Relevant topics in other chapters

- Chapter 9: parents' perspective
- Chapter 11: social care and schooling
- Chapter 12
- Chapter 13

Duchenne muscular dystrophy

Duchenne muscular dystrophy (DMD) affects 1 in 3500 male infants and is characterised by progressive loss of function due to muscle-fibre degeneration. Although the condition is variable, most boys lose the ability to walk at between 8 and 10 years of age. Progressive respiratory insufficiency begins early in the second decade of life. Scoliosis develops in 90% of boys who use a wheelchair full-time, and is likely to require surgery within two years.[1] Scoliosis, respiratory failure and cardiomyopathy that develop during the teenage years can all be managed, and Bushby[2] reports that survival into or beyond the late twenties is becoming more common.

The reader is also referred to the websites of the Department of Neurology at Washington University School of Medicine,[3] the Muscular Dystrophy Campaign[4] and UK Children on Long-Term Ventilation.[5]

Setting the scene

Stuart is coming up to his twenty-third birthday. He is the older of two brothers suffering from DMD. His younger brother Craig died at the age of 20 years at the local children's hospice last year. Both young men had been using the hospice for respite care since they were in their early teens. This had given a much-deserved break to their parents, who are now in their late fifties.

To the brothers the hospice has always been 'like a holiday camp', and a careful booking system ensured that they were in the company of other boys with DMD for the two weeks of their respite stay. The hospice usually allowed the boys to follow their own routines. If they wanted to stay up until 3 a.m., that was 'cool', and if the place was consequently like the Marie Celeste the following morning because they slept in late, that was also OK. It was a rare privilege being able to decide their own bedtime, because all of them had reached such a high level of dependence that practicalities at home dictated a much earlier bedtime.

Over the years Craig and Stuart have shared the triumphs (such as a wheelchair dancing championship and wheelchair painting) but also the sad times (such as losing good friends to DMD and having to face their own untimely mortality).

New treatments have become available over time, such as ventilation, and both Craig and Stuart chose non-invasive intermittent positive-pressure ventilation (IPPV)* when it became obvious that their respiratory effort was inadequate at night. Although Stuart adapted well to mask ventilation, Craig had struggled with this and also gradually developed serious heart failure. He requested that he receive no further intervention with his breathing, and died a few days later, surrounded by his family at the children's hospice.

Stuart has been missing his brother terribly, and has been diagnosed with depression, which is being treated with antidepressants. He is at a very low ebb at a point where he, too, is experiencing difficulty with his ventilation. He is aware that he is now the oldest young man accessing respite care at the children's hospice, and that the hospice is only licensed to take young people up to the age of 25 years. He has had poor experiences with the adult services at times of check-up, but has never had an acute inpatient admission. He is also worried that he might be considered a burden and is terrified of the future. He

---

* Patients commonly use a mouthpiece (for daytime use) or a mouthpiece with lip-seal retention or nasal IPPV (for night-time use) to maintain oxyhaemoglobin saturation above 94%. Mechanically assisted coughing (MAC) has been introduced following a study which found that 90% of episodes of pneumonia and respiratory failure occurred during otherwise benign upper respiratory tract infections due to inability to cough effectively.[6]

confides to you that he feels he should have died first, not Craig, and he is contemplating whether he, too, should refuse further respiratory support.

Jot down your initial reaction to this situation.

| |
| |
| |
| |

Does this bring back memories of a situation you have encountered?

Does this help or hinder?

SWOT

What are your learning needs when considering this scenario? They could look similar to those in the chart on the next page.

There might be issues that you wish to explore, in which case feel free to do so, but also think about the following:

What are the priorities in helping Stuart to deal with his current situation?

| |
| |
| |
| |

Have you considered any of these?

- Reviewing the treatment for depression.
- Exploring the causes of Stuart's depression:

  - the loss of his brother
  - uncertainty about his own future
  - his perception that he might be a burden
  - his lack of knowledge about the options for his own future care.

- Addressing Stuart's current problem with respiratory management.

Strengths	Weaknesses
• I enjoy working with older teenagers/young adults and believe that I can advocate effectively.	• I have no experience of using IPPV respiratory support. • I don't know where young adults go for respite care or what the upper age limit is for paediatric services.
Opportunities • I will be attending a 'moving and handling' update. • I'll have the opportunity to practise how to move someone safely who is of adult size and weight who has no muscle tone, with a hoist and sling.	**Threats** • I am not sure how I would react to a situation like this. I have a son at university and find the tragedy this family is going through overwhelming. • I am nervous that the young man might disclose something that will be disturbing, such as a wish for assisted suicide.

How can Stuart's parents best be supported through this very difficult time?

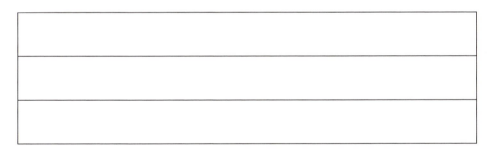

Have you considered any of these?

1 Provide information on a local branch of a DMD society that can provide support.
2. Explain how Stuart's respiratory failure is one cause of his depression.
3. Respect Stuart's decision-making capacity. Help him to reach his own decisions, but not based on pessimism.
4. What is the parents' own state of physical and mental health?
5. What is the level of 'togetherness' of the family?

This family faces the death of more than one family member because of the presence of X-linked recessive disease. They have already been through the death of their younger child, and realise that the time is now approaching for the older son. Hopefully the hospice can help to resolve grief from the first death and anticipate the grief process before

Stuart dies. Although the family at present feels a lack of control, the hospice can help to provide them with control over the physical environment where Stuart is going to die, how much care he will receive, and who will provide the care.

Carrying the 'guilt' of genetic disease

Price[7] provides an overview of inheritance and child health and explores the issue of probability in affected individuals. The emotional aspect of 'passing on a lethal gene', especially one that is sex-linked and therefore almost always passed on from the mother, must be taken into consideration when helping families to come to terms with genetic illness. Bushby[2] states that most cases of DMD are now born in families with no previous history of the disease. Blame can still be attributed within families as to 'who is responsible' for the misfortune of the life-limited child. Miller (personal communication, 2005) puts this in the context that we are all who we are, we all have good and bad genes, and a situation where a mother and father both randomly find themselves to have the same faulty genes is just extremely bad luck. This does not diminish the need for genetic counselling in families where a problem has been identified, but it can relieve the temptation to attribute or feel 'blame' (for a further discussion of inherited disease in relation to issues that may affect couples from different ethnic backgrounds, *see* Chapter 8).

The National Service Framework and the Knowledge and Skills Framework in context

The transition to adulthood is probably the greatest challenge facing palliative care for children and young people. The Association for Children with Life-Threatening or Terminal Conditions and their Families (ACT), the National Council for Hospice and Specialist Palliative Care Services (NCHSPCS) and the Scottish Partnership Agency for Palliative and Cancer Care (SPAPCC) examined palliative care for young people aged 13–24 years, and this document[8] is important background reading for this chapter.

The National Service Framework

Professionals in this context need not only to familiarise themselves with the section of the NSF that relates to their own area of work, but also to consider various NSFs in the context of where young people can be moving on to. For the purpose of this chapter, the children's NSF[9] as well as the children's NSF Standards 4, 6, 8 and 9,[10] the NSF for chronic conditions,[11] the older people's NSF[12] and Valuing People[13] were all found to be relevant.

The issues for transition to adult services are manifold, and it is doubtful whether we are even close to a workable model for young people who are experiencing long-term life-limiting illness. The Health Select Committee[14] refers to the children's NSF with regard to transition to adult services. An increasing number of exemplars are becoming available (e.g. UK Children on Long-Term Ventilation[5]) that aim to facilitate an agenda for local implementation.

The NSF[9] concedes that transition should be a guided, educational process rather than an administrative event, allowing for the fact that young people are experiencing life changes far beyond their clinical needs. Young people should not be transferred fully to adult services until they have the necessary skills to function in an adult service and have completed growth and puberty.[15]

Cancelliere and Widdas[16] suggest that community children's nurses (CCNs) have a pivotal role to play within the transition process. CCNs can influence the formation of local policy and act as key negotiators with the young person and their family. Effective and acceptable transition to adult services, according to Cancelliere and Widdas, is not only a key aspect of a young person's care but also, if timely, releases staff to provide services to new referrals of children and their families who require experienced child-focused care.

According to the Select Committee,[14] guidelines on transition should also consider social care, education and employment, rather than just hospital services.

The Association for Children with Life-Threatening or Terminal Conditions and their Families (ACT), the National Council for Hospice and Specialist Palliative Care Services (NCHSPCS) and the Scottish Partnership Agency for Palliative and Cancer Care (SPA-PCC)[8] have examined the successful model developed for cystic fibrosis in one locality, which involved the appointment of a chest physician and two respiratory nurse specialists, and a joint clinic involving the multi-disciplinary team. Young people attend the joint clinic for as long as they need to build up confidence in the new team, which can take anything from a few months to a year or more. ACT recommends the following principles for the transition process:

- an overall framework for guidance, so that the process is not open-ended
- a plan made with the young person and their family and set out so that the primary care team, consultants, therapists and everyone else involved have a clear direction
- an early start and a 'no-rush' policy.

The Department of Health states that there are specific issues relating to young people with serious long-term medical conditions when:[14]

- their condition has stabilised and they no longer have regular contact with a specialist, resulting in no planned handover
- appropriate services cannot be identified for them and they are transferred to inappropriate services.

The Department of Health recognises that current gaps in adult health services need to be addressed to make transition easier for young people who are at risk of or have genetic diseases.[10]

- Paediatric services for rare conditions are frequently more highly developed than adult services, making transition particularly problematic in these areas.
- New treatments mean that, for the first time, children and young people are surviving into adulthood, at which stage there are often no or only limited services.
- Young people will normally have experienced a more comprehensive approach to their problems through paediatric care services, whereas adult services are frequently organ or system specific. As many genetic diseases affect several organ systems, coordination can then become problematic.

The Royal College of Paediatrics and Child Health[15] states that where adult services do not exist for patients with less common conditions, it is not appropriate for paediatricians to follow up adults simply because they have a childhood illness. They suggest that where no adult specialty or service is active in providing long-term care for young people with specific health needs, new services should be developed to provide ongoing healthcare, which might require specialist commissioning of regional services.

Standard 8 of the children's NSF[10] concedes that assessment and planning for the transition from child to adult services are often unsatisfactory. A multi-agency transition group is in place which could be taken on by an existing group that has developed a multi-agency transition strategy and includes a 'transition champion' from the learning disability partnership board. However, training and development are restricted to 'specialist palliative care training for those working in paediatric palliative care.'

The *Government Response to the House of Commons Health Committee Report on Palliative Care*[17] includes the following salient points that are relevant in this context.

- There is a need for carers to have a break from caring. The Report cites the Carers and Disabled Children Act,[18] which strengthens the rights of carers to an assessment of their own needs as carers. (This point is elaborated on in the NSF for long-term conditions and the basis for assessment and planning for the welfare of the carer.[11])

- The range of services that can be commissioned by social services includes practical help inside and outside the home, such as cleaning and shopping, help with personal care, such as bathing and dressing, and ensuring a safe living environment.
- Provision of services should be based on a single assessment of need, be person centred and focus on the needs of most importance to the individual.
- Where there are multiple complex requirements as a result of one or more disabilities, there is no test for eligibility, and each individual case must be considered on the basis of the individual's own unique requirements.
- Palliative care for children poses different challenges to that for adults, and places greater emphasis on the involvement of the family as carers throughout the child's life, an issue that is addressed in the children's NSF (2004).
- 'The older people's NSF stresses the need for personal and professional behaviour to take account of dignity in end-of life care. The NSF also covers information and communication, pain control, supportive rehabilitation, spiritual care and bereavement support.'[17]

It appears that the NSF for long-term conditions[11] will take the lead for palliative care in non-cancer conditions, to take full account of recent NICE guidance in order to remove the distinction that is made between palliative care for cancer patients and that for patients dying from other diseases.[17] With regard to the transition to adult services, reference is made to the children's NSF, which in turn refers to this document.

Professionals who are involved in deciding at a grass-roots level which 'label' to give to a newly diagnosed child with a degenerative illness that will potentially continue into early adulthood need to be conversant not only with the children's NSF, but also with the older people's NSF and the NSF for long-term conditions.

However, there is a sense of urgency, as the *Government Response to the House of Commons Health Committee Report on Palliative Care*[17] states:

> We agree with the evidence received...that there are significant challenges in raising the skills and awareness of all healthcare staff in palliative care, whether they work in hospitals, care homes or the community. We recognise that steps towards this objective are already in progress in respect of the End-of-Life Care initiatives, but we recommend that these should be accelerated...that training in palliative care becomes part of continuing professional development, and consider making such modules a mandatory requirement for revalidation.

What is striking is that although close collaboration is desirable for sharing expertise, and is sought from cancer services in relation to palliative care, there is no reference to or tangible consultation with paediatric palliative care services, which after all have so far taken the lead in caring for young adults with DMD. After 25 years of paediatric palliative care the specialty still lacks the voice to assert that other services can benefit from a considerable body of knowledge in this specialty!

The NSF is a 10-year plan. It is well supported and supplemented through 'Every Child Matters',[19] and is given a legislative backbone via the Children Act 2004.[20] Although implementation takes time, time also passes fast. We are now 2 years into the 10-year plan for the first part of the children's NSF, and 1 year into the remainder of the document.

The Knowledge and Skills Framework[21]

1. There is a need for communication across the full spectrum of professional services both within the NHS and within the voluntary sector.
2. The competence is needed to give both skilled technical and psychological care to the young person and their family. These young people are 'displaced.' They do not fit with either the acute children's services or the acute adult services, and they face the

prospect of possibly outliving the rigid upper age limit of the children's hospice services, depending on geographical location.

Respite care for young adults: the difference between children's hospice care and adult provision

The Royal College of Paediatrics and Child Health[15] states that although excellent hospice and respite facilities exist for children and adults, there is little provision available for young people in respite and palliative care.

There are currently a number of children's and young people's hospices in the UK. For example, Martin House in Yorkshire currently takes young adults up to the age of 31 years, and there is an increase both in age reached by current patients and in the number of young adults requiring the service. Another such hospice, Douglas House in Oxford, has only recently opened full-time, and it is envisaged that it will provide care for young people up to the age of 40 years from anywhere in the country. A number of other children's hospices are also reviewing their provision at the higher end of the age range. This is positive news indeed, but on a practical level referral to these units will be dependent on healthcare professionals having the information and funding necessary to refer patients.

The model for adult hospice care does not necessarily meet the respite care needs of a young person. Brown (personal communication, 2005) highlights the difference by pointing out that the average end-of-life stay in an adult hospice is 2 weeks, whereas the average respite provision in a children's hospice is 2 weeks a year over several years. A practical consequence would be that young people who are receiving respite care would be nursed alongside terminally ill older patients. Within the children's hospice model, the majority of children are receiving respite care. This means that every effort is made to ensure that the child has a good time, including outings, etc. The scenario described earlier in this chapter, even down to arranging bookings of young people with similar needs to coincide, is not unusual.

If the model of respite provision that is currently practised in the majority of children's hospices is followed, allowing families to be together, respite care for young adults would encompass partners and possibly children, unless it is desirable to allow the partner a break from caring for the young person. Consideration also needs to be given to support during the terminal stages of life and bereavement care.

There is also a fundamental difference in the funding for adult hospice care. The *Government Response to the House of Commons Health Committee Report on Palliative Care*[17] highlights the fact that there is an anomaly in payment for adult hospice providers, which are funded per episode, thus making it more attractive to have patients with short terminal episodes rather than patients whose intermittent care needs may potentially extend over many years.

Too old and yet too young

Not all children's hospices take adolescents or young adults. Northern Ireland has an upper age limit of 10 years, and there are no children's hospice facilities at all in Southern Ireland.

Not all young people will be accessing children's hospices, either because they have not been referred or because they are outside the age limit or geographical catchment area.

According to the House of Commons,[14] patients who are in transition from children's to adult hospice services are denied continuity of care as a consequence of anomalies in standards regulation. There is a two-tier system in place whereby 18-year-olds with a new diagnosis are not eligible for services that are available to other 18-year-olds with a long-standing diagnosis.

In other words, if a young person has DMD and is referred to a children's hospice while under the age of 16 years, he is accepted under category 2, and depending on the age limit up to which the hospice is licensed, he can access its services for the rest of his life. However, if a referral is not made until he is 18 years of age, the same young man cannot be accepted into children's hospice care. He would at present be eligible for Douglas House in Oxford, which has seven beds and expects to be able to take 165 referrals in total. Other children's hospices which are already licensed for young adults can also use their discretion to be more flexible with regard to admission age. The Ellenor Foundation is a hospice-at-home service which is piloting a pathway for adolescents and young adults[22] (*see* Chapter 5).

Transition to adult acute care

Metules[23] states that due to greater attention to respiratory care and various forms of assisted ventilation and secretion management, including tracheostomy, young people with DMD are now living longer, into their late twenties and beyond. This is why hospital nurses are more likely to see adult patients with DMD, particularly because of their increased risk of respiratory and cardiac complications. Metules provides an excellent overview of the various stages that children and young people pass through. Although this chapter is restricted to the adult phase of the disease process, according to Metules[23] changes occur from the age of 15 years, when scoliosis together with weakening respiratory muscles, inactivity (due to loss of muscle function) and obesity (due to inactivity, usually despite a normal diet) combine to compromise both lung expansion and function. Another factor identified by Biggar *et al.*[1] is that patients with DMD have significant non-progressive abnormalities of the central nervous system, with a mean intelligence quotient of 82, 18 points below the normal mean. This is not a secondary effect due to loss of mobility and a disadvantaged lifestyle. According to Biggar *et al.*, verbal intelligence is primarily affected, while the other cognitive functions remain relatively intact. Metules[23] and Roccella *et al.*[24] report that the effect is seen particularly in attention focusing, verbal learning and memory and intellectual interaction.

Miller (personal communication, 2005) has observed another factor that contributes to the lack of control in the transition to adult care. Many of these young people have not been seeking active involvement in their management and have allowed their parents and carers to be 'in charge' of hospital visits.

Metules[23] also reports that many young people will struggle with bouts of depression and frustration as they become increasingly aware of the progressive functional loss that they face.

Key issues when planning provision for young people

The Royal College of Nursing[25] highlights a number of key issues to be considered when planning provision for this age group:

- concerns:
    - for adolescents, the desire for autonomy and involvement in decision making
    - for parents/carers, empowering the young person
    - for healthcare professionals, involving families, preparing and empowering the young person for transition, involving other professionals and working across boundaries

- potential problems and obstacles:
    - lack of specialist knowledge in adult teams and lack of confidence in knowledge
    - lack of specific service provision for young people
    - lack of understanding and appreciation of young people's needs and issues in both paediatric and adult healthcare sectors
    - healthcare professionals' attitudes

- specific issues for adolescents with disabilities:

  - low expectations of parents, the young person and healthcare professionals
  - lack of self-advocacy skills and lack of opportunity to practise these skills
  - different views of independence and success

- factors thought to enhance transition between services:

  - leadership
  - successful collaboration and cross-boundary working
  - adequate resources
  - acquisition of skills and knowledge
  - robust documentation and appropriate administration.

Contemporary issues in young people's palliative care

Quality of life: a 'life-limited' label – the sword of Damocles

Gjengedal et al.[26] conducted a number of focus groups with adults suffering from cystic fibrosis (CF) and also parents with children suffering from CF. They found a tendency for healthcare providers to underrate a patient's 'quality of life.' Nevertheless, according to these authors, one of the main challenges to chronic care seems to be the fact that the chronically ill have to live with their illness because no efficient cure is available. The CF patient group differs in one respect – although the life expectancy of CF sufferers is increasing, they still have to face the possibility of an early death. The authors reviewed two studies. The first study, by Tracy,[27] of adults aged 23–42 years, identified the following:

- 'being different' (from other children)
- 'don't call me terminal!' (referring to the medical establishment's tendency to treat CF patients as statistics rather than as individuals)
- 'will-power and faith' (expressing the wish to focus on goals rather than suffering).

The second study, by Christian and D'Aurial,[28] of adolescents aged 12–18 years, emphasised the need to 'reduce the sense of difference' by adopting the following protective strategies:

- keeping secrets
- hiding visible differences
- discovering a new baseline (in the struggle to regard themselves as 'normal').

Three themes emerged from the research by Gjengedal et al.:[26]

- moving from uncertainty to certainty:

  - a struggle to get a diagnosis

- a demanding but normal life:

  - participants spoke of having 'quite a normal childhood' and regarding themselves as 'normal.' Parents identified a sense that the child has a disease but is not ill
  - the daily regime involves a complex and time-consuming range of treatments
  - growing up with CF had been an unexpected experience
  - most had heard from early childhood that it was highly probable that they would face an early death
  - experts focus too much on statistics about life expectancy, and it was realised that they had poor prospects according to current statistics. One participant commented that 'it is strange to read statistics and realise that you are too old to die'

–   they have never been asked about their plans with regard to education and jobs
–   it is important to lead a normal life, even if the price paid in terms of effort is high

• a wish for continuity, stability and respect:

–   a feeling of being at the mercy of helpers
–   CF is extremely variable with regard to both the organs involved and clinical sever-
    ity – there is therefore a need for physicians and other healthcare workers to know
    individual patients well
–   the importance of healthcare professionals knowing patients, so that there is no
    need to start every consultation by telling their story
–   healthcare professionals then don't only care for the child, but also notice the
    strain on the rest of the family.

Although all the research described here relates to cystic fibrosis, it reflects many of the
issues faced by young people with neuromuscular disease, and in fact many of the issues
explored in this book where the 'label' attributed to a child's problems determines
whether or not the term 'palliative' should be awarded. Miller (personal communication,
2005) highlighted the fact that the label 'palliative' disrupts the processes and practices
that support a normal childhood and life. However, the overriding desire for 'normalisation' might prevent healthcare professionals from fully understanding the issues that are
faced when supporting services are being accessed by children and their families, and
therefore they might fail to provide effective support.

Knebel and Hudgings[29] cite an American study of the families of children with
Tay–Sachs' disease and related disorders which is symptomatic of this thought process. A
reluctance to acknowledge that the child was dying contributed to the low rate of referral for palliative care services. The authors state that the transition to palliative care services is particularly difficult when the prognosis is uncertain, because it is not clear when
the 'terminal' phase begins, and they cite a 'transitional model of end-of-life care' developed by Tonelli.[30] In a Canadian study of patients with CF by Mitchell,[31] cited by Knebel
and Hudgings,[32] 25% of physicians never discussed palliative care and 40% waited until
the patient's last month of life before discussing palliation. This resulted in 82% of patients
dying in hospital, with some receiving various aggressive treatments, including mechanical ventilatory support.

Treatment choices in the late teenage years

Sritippayawan et al.[33] reviewed the initiation of home mechanical ventilation in 73 children.
They found that for most children this treatment was initiated non-electively after acute respiratory failure caused by pneumonia, with many missed or mismanaged opportunities to
discuss therapeutic options prior to respiratory failure.

This study highlights many issues that are replicated within children's and young people's palliative care.

• The study is retrospective, covering the period from 1983 to 2001. This means the findings reflect the fact that home mechanical ventilation was not introduced locally until
  1987, and has increased significantly since 1995. There have also been advances in the
  technique for home ventilation, and the authors state that prior to this candidates for
  home ventilation were generally those with frequent, prolonged or severe episodes of
  lower respiratory tract infection, or those with complications secondary to hypoxaemia
  or hyperventilation.
• Although the average age for home ventilation is given as 8.5 ± 6.7 years, the actual
  range is 2 months to 24 years, although the outcomes for the young people are not
  described. This makes it difficult to draw long-term conclusions.

Eagle *et al.*[34] compared the outcome for 80 patients between 1986 and 2002 with regard to the effect of spinal surgery and nocturnal ventilation on lung function and survival in patients with scoliosis secondary to DMD. Their findings for the mean survival of patients were as follows:

- 19.7 years for patients who received neither surgery nor ventilation
- 24.3 years for patients who were ventilated but did not have surgery
- 26.4 years for patients who received both surgery and ventilation
- 16.3 years for patients who had early-onset cardiomyopathy.

The authors concluded that nocturnal ventilation was the most important factor in the improvement of survival in patients with DMD.

As in the study by Sritippayawan *et al.*,[33] which identified missed opportunities to discuss treatment options before a crisis occurred, a tendency to overestimate the relative hardship of the patient's lifestyle due to ventilator support, and a tendency to underestimate the patient's quality of life, Knebel and Hudgings[32] also reported that healthcare providers and the patient's family tend to view quality of life differently from the patient. They consider it more in terms of the physical dimensions, whereas patients put more emphasis on social and cognitive aspects, demonstrating that quality of life is deeply personal and family members might not be fully aware of the patient's wishes or values.

Metules[23] cites a small study which revealed that 25% of physicians who treat patients with DMD do not discuss long-term ventilation, due to the doctor's perception of the patient's poor quality of life.

Knebel and Hudgings[32] state that technological progress emphasises the need for advance care planning and directives. Ideally this should be done when the patient is not acutely ill, rather than in an emergency situation. In addition to the points already made above, the authors identify a number of considerations when faced with the need for ethical decision making.

- Medical indications (this includes knowing the patient's prognosis without further interventions).
- They cite a shift in ethical thinking. In the past, physicians hesitated to begin therapy which had only a small chance of success, because they did not want to withdraw that therapy if it failed, whereas the current view is that there is no moral or legal difference between withholding and withdrawing treatment. Therefore it is worth trying an intervention, and then withdrawing it if it does not meet the patient's goals.

Staying alive: relationships and families

Miller (personal communication, 2005) suggests that in this age group a strong motivating factor for staying alive is the hope of meeting somebody with whom the young person may form a close relationship. This highlights the area of sexuality in profoundly disabled young people. This is a difficult area for many able-bodied people, and even more so for young people who are not able to have a normal life in relation to any activity of living. Many young people with DMD remain highly dependent on their parents, often having little inclination to make their own decisions.

Opportunities to meet and build relationships with other young people tend to be limited and almost certainly require a lot of support. Bushby[2] states that boys with DMD do not often have children. This implies that young men with DMD are physiologically capable of having children and can have sexual intercourse. Sexual experimentation has its own unique difficulties because of taboos and the potential for embarrassing situations for both patient and carers. Sexuality in the teenage years and adulthood has been discussed within the contexts of oncology,[35] learning disability[36] and spinal injury.[37]

Clinical governance and suggestions for work-based learning and networking

Explore with your colleagues how the NSF and the ACT Care Pathway can be implemented in your working environment in relation to Stuart and his parents. What are the difficulties? How can they be overcome?

Departments usually have members of staff who have a designated role and/or special interest (e.g. nurse on both children's and adult unit, play specialist, school-teacher, therapist).

Where on the ACT Care Pathway would you locate Stuart, his parents, the staff at the children's hospice and the hospital staff in their thinking?

Stuart:
Parents:
Staff at the children's hospice:
Hospital staff:

Draw up a workable care plan for Stuart and his parents based on ACT Care Pathway 2.

Now turn your attention to Pathway 3.

What considerations in this pathway will be useful for advance planning for Stuart and his parents?

Summary

This chapter has considered the transition to adulthood. This is a complex issue that requires close cooperation between adult and paediatric services in both the state and voluntary sectors. It is difficult for these young people to achieve a reasonable degree of independence, and indeed they reach the level of greatest dependence both physically and emotionally in early adulthood, when the 'life-limited' reality hits particularly hard. Facilitation of the transition to adult services has been explored in the context of both quality of life and treatment choices available to the young person and their family. The provision of effective palliative care for this age group has been identified as a major challenge faced by both children's and young people's palliative care services, as well as the adult services.

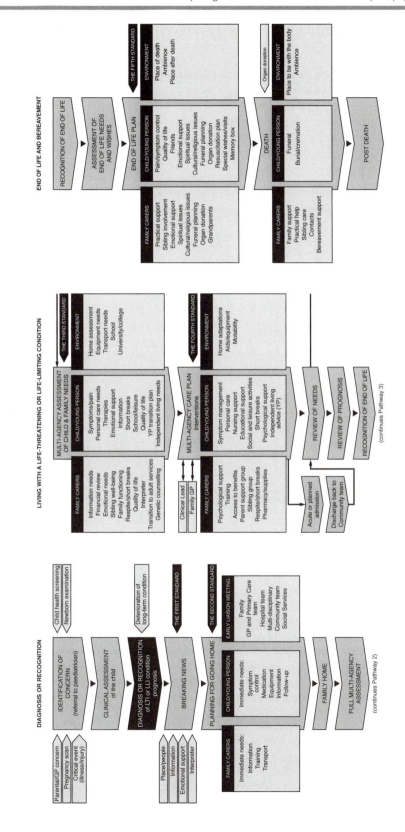

SWOT

It might be useful to revisit the SWOT analysis at this point in order to determine any further learning needs in relation to this chapter and the Knowledge and Skills Framework (KSF) requirements, namely:

1. communication
2. personal and people development
3. health, safety and security
4. service improvement
5. quality
6. equality and diversity.

Strengths	Weaknesses
Opportunities	Threats

Action plan for further learning

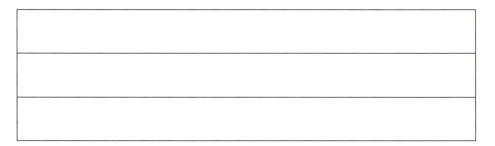

References

1. Biggar W, Klamut H, Demacio P *et al.* (2002) Duchenne muscular dystrophy: current knowledge, treatment, and future prospects. *Clin Orthop.* **401:** 88–106.
2. Bushby K (2003) Muscular dystrophy. In: D Warral, T Cox, J Firth *et al.* (eds) *Oxford Textbook of Medicine* (4e). Oxford University Press, Oxford.
3. Department of Neurology at Washington University School of Medicine; www.neuro.wustl.edu/neuromuscular
4. Muscular Dystrophy Campaign; www.muscular-dystrophy.org.uk/
5. UK Children on Long-Term Ventilation; www.longtermventilation.nhs.uk

6. Gomez-Merino E and Bach J (2002) Duchenne muscular dystrophy: prolongation of life by non-invasive ventilation and mechanically assisted coughing. *Am J Phys Med Rehabil.* **81:** 411–15.

7. Price S (2004) Inheritance and child health. In: S Neill and H Knowles (eds) *The Biology of Child Health.* Palgrave Macmillan, Basingstoke.

8. Association for Children with Life-Threatening or Terminal Conditions and their Families (ACT), National Council for Hospice and Specialist Palliative Care Services (NCHSPCS) and Scottish Partnership Agency for Palliative and Cancer Care (SPAPCC) (2001) *Palliative Care for Young People Aged 13–24 years.* ACT, Bristol.

9. All the documents for the National Service Framework for children can be accessed via the Department of Health website: www.dh.gov.uk/PolicyAndGuidance/ HealthAndSocialCareTopics/ChildrenServices/ChildrenServicesInformation/Children ServicesInformationArticle/fs/en?CONTENT_ID=4089111&chk=U8Ecln. See also Department of Education and Skills and Department of Health (2006) *National Service Framework for Children, Young People and Maternity Services Transition: getting it right for young people.* DES and DoH, London; www.dh.gov.uk/childrensnsf

10. Department of Health (2004) NSF National Service Framework for Children, Young People and Maternity Services: Core Standards Standard 4: Growing Up into Adulthood. DoH, London; www.dh.gov.uk/PolicyAndGuidance/HealthAndSocial CareTopics/ChildrenServices/ChildrenServicesInformation/ChildrenServicesInformati onArticle/fs/en?CONTENT_ID=4089111&chk=U8Ecln

11. Department of Health (2005) *National Service Framework for Long-Term Conditions.* DoH, London; www.dh.gov.uk/

12. Department of Health (2001) *National Service Framework for Older People.* DoH, London; www.dh.gov.uk/

13. Department of Health (2001) *Valuing People;* www.archive.official-documents.co.uk/ document/cm50/5086/5086.pdf

14. House of Commons Health Committee (2004) *Report on Palliative Care. Fourth report of session 2003–04.* The Stationery Office, London.

15. Royal College of Paediatrics and Child Health (2003) *The Intercollegiate Working Party on Adolescent Health: bridging the gaps. Health care for adolescents;* www.rcpch.ac.uk

16. Cancelliere L and Widdas D (2005) Transition from children's to adult services. In: A Sidey and D Widdas (eds) *Textbook of Community Children's Nursing* (2e). Elsevier, Edinburgh.

17. Department of Health (2004) Government Response to the House of Commons Health Committee Report on Palliative Care: fourth report of session 2003–04. The Stationery Office, London.

18. Carers and Disabled Children Act 2002; www.opsi.gov.uk/acts/acts2000/ 20000016.htm

19. 'Every Child Matters'; www.dfes.gov.uk/everychildmatters

20. Children Act 2004; www.opsi.gov.uk/acts/acts2004/20040031.htm

21. Department of Health (2004) *The NHS Knowledge and Skills Framework (NHS KSF) and the Development Review Process.* Department of Health, London.

22. Joy I (2005) *Valuing Short Lives: children with terminal conditions.* New Philanthropy Capital, London.

23. Metules T (2002) A new age for childhood diseases: Duchenne muscular dystrophy. *Registered Nurse.* **65:** 39–44, 47–8.

24. Roccella M, Pace R and De Gregorino M (2003) Psychopathological assessment in children affected by Duchenne Boulogne muscular dystrophy. *Minerva Pediatr.* **55:** 267–76.

25. Royal College of Nursing (2004) *Adolescent Transition Care: guidance for nursing staff.* Royal College of Nursing, London.

26. Gjengedal E, Rustoen T, Wahl A and Hanestad B (2003) Growing up and living with cystic fibrosis: everyday life and encounters with the health care and social services –

a qualitative study. *Adv Nurs Sci.* **26:** 149–59.

27. Tracy JP (1997) Growing up with chronic illness: the experience of growing up with cystic fibrosis. *Holist Nurs Pract.* **12:** 3–12.

28. Christian BJ and D'Auria JP (1997) The child's eye: memories of growing up with cystic fibrosis. *J Pediatric Nurs.* **12:** 3–12.

29. Knebel A and Hudgings C (2002) End-of-life issues in genetic disorders: literature and research directions. *Genet Med.* **4:** 366–72.

30. Tonelli M (1998) End-of-life care in cystic fibrosis. *Curr Opin Pulm Med.* **4:** 332–6.

31. Mitchell I, Nakielna T, Tullis E *et al.* (2000) Cystic fibrosis: end-stage care in Canada. *Chest.* **118:** 80–4.

32. Knebel A and Hudgings C (2002) End-of-life issues in genetic disorders: summary of workshop held at the National Institutes of Health on September 26, 2001. *Genet Med.* **4:** 373–8.

33. Sritippayawan S, Kun S, Keens T *et al.* (2003) Initiation of home mechanical ventilation in children with neuromuscular diseases. *J Pediatr.* **142:** 481–5.

34. Eagle M, Metha J, Bushby K *et al.* (2004) Improved survival in patients with scoliosis secondary to Duchenne muscular dystrophy: the role of spinal surgery and nocturnal ventilation. *J Bone Joint Surg.* **86-B (Suppl. II):** 117.

35. West Midlands Paediatric Macmillan Team (2005) *Palliative Care for Children with Malignant Disease.* Quay Books, London.

36. Outsiders (sex and disability helpline); www.outsiders.org.uk

37. Spinal Injuries Association; www.spinal.co.uk

Chapter 7

Trans-generational illness: a family affected by HIV/AIDS

This chapter covers

Content

Scenario

- Mothers and children affected by HIV and AIDS
- Setting the scene
- The National Service Framework
- The Knowledge and Skills Framework
- The ACT Care Pathway
- Clinical governance and suggestions for work-based learning and networking
- Helpful information on paediatric HIV infection
- The changing face of HIV and AIDS
- HIV and AIDS in the UK
- Entitlement to NHS services

Contemporary issues

- Trans-generational illness
- Normalisation strategies
- Stigma
- Disclosure
- Chronic disease
- Growing up with HIV/AIDS
- Compliance with treatment
- Safe passage to adulthood programme
- The global picture
- Giving care to adult children

Related to trans-generational illness as well as HIV/AIDS

- Contemporary issues in palliative care for children and young people in relation to HIV and AIDS
- The global picture
- Summary

Relevant to other areas of palliative care for children and young people

- This chapter: the stigma of having a child with a life-limiting illness in the family
- Chapter 6: transition to adulthood
- Chapter 11: child protection
- This chapter: giving care to adult children (Thailand)
- This chapter: trans-generational illness

Relevant topics in other chapters

- Chapter 2: post-traumatic stress disorder
- Chapter 3: reference to ritual and religion
- Chapter 6: transition to adulthood
- Chapter 9: compliance
- Chapter 11: social care and schooling

Mothers and children affected by HIV and AIDS

Background information

CHIVA[1] is the Children's HIV Association of the UK and Ireland and is a major resource that provides articles, protocols, further websites and other information. The following can be accessed via its website:

- the report by the London HIV Consortium Paediatric Subgroup, 'Developing clinical networks for paediatric HIV treatment and care in London'
- the Children's HIV National Network Review (CHINN) final draft report.

The Children With AIDS Charity (CWAC)[2] supports families that are affected by or infected with HIV or AIDS, and its website includes links to many other useful sites.

The Association for Children with Life-Threatening or Terminal Conditions and Their Families[3] has a website that offers a wide range of information on HIV and AIDS following an easy literature search in the 'for professionals' section.

The National Children's Bureau[4] provides information on various projects that it has commissioned relating to HIV and AIDS, including the following:

- HIV Forum for Children and Young People
- health projects – a huge range of topics, including the 'Childhood Bereavement Network', 'Young People from Minority Ethnic Background in Britain' and 'Building Resilience and Supporting Relationships in Families under Stress'
- Delivering Diversity – disabled children from black minority ethnic communities.

Setting the scene

Bibi is 8 months old and has lived with his mother Suhela, who is 18 years old, Suhela's sister Shamila, who is 25, and her son, his 6-year-old cousin Mohammed, in the UK for the last 6 months. They have escaped political persecution during which Suhela was raped repeatedly and several months later gave birth to Bibi. She loves Bibi, but is too ill to care for him unaided. Mohammed's father died while the family was being 'processed' for asylum.

Both Bibi and his mother are in poor health, and both are HIV positive. Suhela has rejected highly active antiretroviral therapy (HAART) due to fear of being deported and being shunned should the cause of her illness become known in the holding centre. She has had a prolonged hospital admission for *Pneumocystis carinii* pneumonia (PCP) and is not expected to survive. Shamila has been caring for Bibi, but is finding it very difficult. She does not speak any English, and is trying to fend for herself in an environment that is very different from her previous experience, where she was part of an extended family. She does not know what has happened to the older members of her family back home. Shamila is desperately grieving for her husband, is facing the prospect of losing her sister, and is expected to care for a terminally ill baby and her own child, who has just been assessed as having post-traumatic stress disorder.

Now Bibi has been admitted to his local children's ward, also suffering from severe PCP, profuse diarrhoea and neurological symptoms, in addition to his marked developmental delay and severe oral candidiasis.

Jot down your initial reaction to this situation.

| |
| |
| |
| |

Does this bring back memories of a situation you have encountered?

Does this help or hinder?

SWOT

What are your learning needs when considering this scenario? They could look similar to the following.

There might be issues that you wish to explore, in which case feel free to do so, but also think about the following:

Strengths	*Weaknesses*
• We have well-established policies and procedures with individual flow charts/standards for many situations. This helps us to respond to unusual situations.	• We feel out of our depth here. • We are not clear whether a child like Bibi can be referred to a children's hospice due to issues surrounding the family's immigration. • I was not aware of the 'Children's HIV National Network Review' (final draft report) and of the recommendations on how care for HIV-infected children should be commissioned.
Opportunities	*Threats*
• To review our standard for children with HIV in relation to family need. • Networking with various agencies.	• Time is running out and both the child and his mother are likely to die, in different wards.

What are the priorities when caring for Bibi and his family?

Have you considered any of these?

1. Bibi needs stabilisation and symptom control in relation to his physical condition (i.e. treatment of his pneumonia). He is likely to require fluid resuscitation and possibly ventilatory support. Dealing with the acute situation here is the priority while his general health status in relation to his HIV/AIDS disease is evaluated in order to determine further management. In a child like Bibi, treatment will probably lead to a significant improvement in quality and length of life. Therefore the emphasis must be on delivering that treatment, with other considerations (such as being with the mother) taking second place.

2. Depending on Bibi's response to the initial treatment, a decision about resuscitation status might have to be made. This is complicated by the fact that the mother, who holds parental responsibility, is critically ill herself. Legal advice might need to be obtained and issues of guardianship clarified. Although Shamila has assumed responsibility for Bibi should Suhela die, she will not automatically have parental responsibility. However, Shamila is the main carer for Bibi, with her own questions, fears, worries and views about the decision-making process. She therefore requires the same care and support that a parent would need. Effective communication is vital and an effective interpreter service is essential. White[5] states that the help of outside agencies, including interpreters, might be rejected because of fears that confidentiality might be compromised or Home Office knowledge of the diagnosis could lead to deportation.

3. Mohammed is also likely to be very distressed by the current situation, possibly wondering whether his mother and he himself will also become ill like Suhela and Bibi. Levenson and Sharma[6] have explored the health of refugee children and have written a useful section on reactions to trauma and loss (issues relating to post-traumatic stress disorder are explored further in Chapter 2). Support for both Suhela and Shamila needs to reflect their individual needs and must be acceptable to both.

This scenario is intended to stimulate discussion and further fact finding on the topic in the reader's own working environment.

- Once Bibi is no longer in a life-threatening situation, could the mother and child be cared for together locally on an infectious diseases ward, with support from both adult and children's unit staff?
  - Could they be transferred to a unit where this is possible?
  - Can you identify such a unit?
  - What practical support is available through the HIV clinical nurse specialist?
  - If at the moment no such provision can be identified, how can this situation be addressed?

The National Service Framework

At present there is no explicit reference to family services in relation to HIV and AIDS in the NSF for children. However, HIV and AIDS care has well-developed multi-disciplinary family services in the major centres that effectively facilitate the transition from child to adolescent and then to adult services. To this end, major centres are likely to be proactive in meeting NSF standards. In her document *Talking with Children, Young People and Families about Chronic Illness and Living with HIV*, Miah[7] discusses how children and young people are put at the centre of care by building services around their needs and promoting their voices.

Like the exemplars that are emerging for specific problems, such as ventilator-dependent children, published by the Department of Health (*see* Chapter 10), a pathway for HIV and AIDS would be extremely helpful to areas of the country where children are not primarily cared for in major centres.

The NSF evidence section[8] has identified a lack of evidence on interventions or services that are specifically designed for children, young people and women from disadvantaged groups such as minority ethnic groups, travellers, and women who abuse substances.

The Knowledge and Skills Framework[9]

1. *Communication.* Effective communication here is the key to successfully working within the multi-disciplinary team encompassing paediatric and adult services, possibly in the context of a family service.
2. *Personal and people development.*
3. *Health, safety and security.* This is likely to be new territory for all care and services providers in this scenario. Clear negotiation is vital to avoid healthcare professionals feeling out of their depth and to ensure that care is delivered safely both to Bibi and to his mother. It is likely that new skills will need to be developed. A supportive environment can be provided by allowing time for reflection and regular clinical supervision.
4. *Service improvement.*
5. *Quality.*
6. *Equality and diversity.*

Services need to be working together to deal with culturally sensitive and multilingual challenges as well as the fact that Bibi, Suhela, Shamila and Mohammed all find themselves in a very frightening situation of uncertainty, ranging from belonging to mere survival.

The ACT Care Pathway[10]

The ACT Care Pathway can be applied to Bibi as an individual, irrespective of where he is cared for. However, it would depend on a unit's interpretation of the pathway whether it is applied to the mother, and therefore in the context of the requirements of this family it is of limited value. The ACT Care Pathway is flexible enough to be applied across age ranges, but it implies that knowledge of the pathway is available on general children's wards as well as adult units. There are pathways for use with adults, such as the gold standard and the Liverpool pathway.[11]

Referral to a children's hospice has to be made by the time a young person is 18 years of age (*see* Chapter 9). Suhela therefore falls outside the reach of children's hospices other than Douglas House in Oxford. From a practical general perspective, children are referred to the nearest children's hospice. Educational provision will be local, and links will probably have to be made. This could cause problems if a child – and in the case of Bibi a refugee child – needs to cross district boundaries.

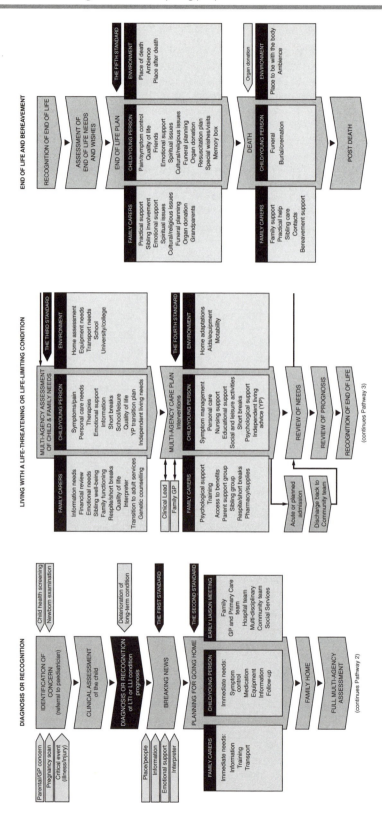

DIAGNOSIS OR RECOGNITION

Parental/GP concern
Pregnancy scan
Critical event (illness/injury)

Child health screening
Newborn examination

IDENTIFICATION OF CONCERN
(referral to paediatrician)

CLINICAL ASSESSMENT of the child

Deterioration of long-term condition

THE FIRST STANDARD

DIAGNOSIS OR RECOGNITION of LTI or LLI condition prognosis

BREAKING NEWS

Place/people
Information
Emotional support
Interpreter

PLANNING FOR GOING HOME

THE SECOND STANDARD

EARLY LIAISON MEETING
Family
GP and Primary Care team
Hospital team
Multi-disciplinary team
Community team
Social Services

CHILD/YOUNG PERSON
Immediate needs:
Symptom control
Medication
Equipment
Information
Follow-up

FAMILY CARERS
Immediate needs:
Information
Training
Transport

FAMILY HOME

FULL MULTI-AGENCY ASSESSMENT

(continues Pathway 2)

LIVING WITH A LIFE-THREATENING OR LIFE-LIMITING CONDITION

MULTI-AGENCY ASSESSMENT OF CHILD & FAMILY NEEDS

THE THIRD STANDARD

ENVIRONMENT
Home assessment
Equipment needs
Transport needs
School
University/college

CHILD/YOUNG PERSON
Symptoms/pain
Personal care needs
Therapies
Emotional support
Information
Short breaks
School/leisure
Quality of life
YP transition plan
Independent living needs

FAMILY CARERS
Information needs
Financial review
Emotional needs
Sibling well-being
Family functioning
Respite/short breaks
Quality of life
Interpreter
Transition to adult services
Genetic counselling

Clinical Lead
Family GP

MULTI-AGENCY CARE PLAN
Interventions

THE FOURTH STANDARD

ENVIRONMENT
Home adaptations
Aids/equipment
Motability

CHILD/YOUNG PERSON
Symptom management
Personal care
Nursing support
Educational support
Social and leisure activities
Short breaks
Psychological support
Independent living advice (YP)

FAMILY CARERS
Psychological support
Training
Access to benefits
Parent support group
Sibling group
Respite/short breaks
Pharmacy/supplies

Acute or planned admission

Discharge back to Community team

REVIEW OF NEEDS

REVIEW OF PROGNOSIS

RECOGNITION OF END OF LIFE

(continues Pathway 3)

END OF LIFE AND BEREAVEMENT

RECOGNITION OF END OF LIFE

ASSESSMENT OF END OF LIFE NEEDS AND WISHES

THE FIFTH STANDARD

ENVIRONMENT
Place of death
Ambience
Place after death

END OF LIFE PLAN

CHILD/YOUNG PERSON
Pain/symptom control
Quality of life
Friends
Emotional support
Spiritual issues
Cultural/religious issues
Funeral planning
Organ donation
Resuscitation plan
Special wishes/visits
Memory box

FAMILY CARERS
Practical support
Sibling involvement
Emotional support
Spiritual issues
Cultural/religious issues
Funeral planning
Organ donation
Grandparents

Organ donation

DEATH

ENVIRONMENT
Place to be with the body
Ambience

CHILD/YOUNG PERSON
Funeral
Burial/cremation

FAMILY CARERS
Family support
Practical help
Sibling care
Contacts
Bereavement support

POST DEATH

Clinical governance and suggestions for work-based learning and networking

Explore with your colleagues how the NSF and the ACT Care Pathway as well as the Knowledge and Skills Framework standards can be implemented in your working environment in relation to Bibi and his family.

Where on the ACT Care Pathway would you locate Bibi, Suhela, Shamila and Mohammed, the staff on the children's intensive-care unit and the social worker in their thinking?

Draw up a workable care plan for Bibi and his family based on ACT Care Pathway 1.

Bibi:
Suhela:
Shamila:
Mohammed:
Staff on the children's intensive care unit:
Social worker:

What are the challenges? How can they be overcome?

Now reflect on Pathway 2.

How can Pathway 2 be implemented, assuming that Bibi will survive this episode and be discharged into Shamila's care?

Now turn your attention to Pathway 3.

What considerations for Pathway 3 will be useful for advance planning for Bibi, Suhela, Shamila and Mohammed?

Include in your fact finding information on attitudes to western medicine, as well as rituals relating to loss and death. It might be helpful to include colleagues from other departments who have a designated role and/or special interest (e.g. nurse on the children's intensive-care unit, member of the care team at the local children's hospice, HIV clinical specialist, play specialist, community team, social services department, multi-faith centre/chaplaincy, interpreter service, dietitian, physiotherapist).

Helpful information on paediatric HIV infection

As mentioned earlier, the following can be accessed via CHIVA's website.[1]

- The report by the London HIV Consortium Paediatric Subgroup, 'Developing clinical networks for paediatric HIV treatment and care in London', gives an overview of the numbers, issues and commissioning in London.
- The Children's HIV National Network Review (CHINN) final draft report gives the national figures.

It is recommended that readers familiarise themselves with both reports. In the context of this chapter, the salient points can be summarised as follows.

- With regard to the distribution of children and their families with HIV infection, 70% live in and around London.
- The rising global epidemic, recent patterns of migration and the dispersal of asylum-seeking families have led to increasing numbers of children with HIV living in the UK outside London.
- There are currently no tertiary paediatric HIV centres outside London.
- Taking into account the informal networks that are already in place, the report proposes the development of a regional network structure for paediatric and perinatal HIV centres, with lead clinicians and nurses to be identified for each regional network linked to one of the London tertiary centres.
- Regional multi-disciplinary family HIV teams should be encouraged, including pharmacy, nursing, psychology, dietetics, allied health professionals and social work support.
- Commissioning arrangements for family HIV services need to be explicitly clarified for each region and for affiliated units. There will be limited but definite resource implications in developing both the regional centres and an audit programme, and these need to be identified at a commissioning level.

A very good overview of paediatric HIV infection in terms of epidemiology, routes of transmission, diagnosis, treatment and prognostic factors has been provided by Khoury and Kovacs.[12]

Many studies refer to the CD4 percentage count, which according to Hockenberry *et al.*[13] refers to lymphocyte counts and percentages. These authors describe common symptoms as shown in the table on the next page.

The multiple complications experienced by children are potentially very painful, and Hockenberry *et al.*[13] advocate aggressive pain management in order to ensure an acceptable quality of life. Pain may be due to infections (such as otitis media) or dental abscess, but may also be caused by encephalopathy (causing spasticity), adverse effects of medications (causing peripheral neuropathy) or an unknown source (e.g. deep musculoskeletal pain).

A very useful and still topical article, although now somewhat dated, is that by Rushton *et al.*[15] on ethical and legal issues pertaining to end-of-life care for infants with AIDS. Of relevance to the scenario described in this chapter, the authors explore dilemmas relating to the following:

- the emerging understanding of the trajectory of AIDS-related symptoms in children, and the resulting aggressive treatment versus potential lack of symptom control and possibly inappropriate prolonging of life at all costs
- in the absence of a person with parental responsibility to consent to treatment, a patient's status as a 'ward of state' might give rise to under- or over-treatment amidst concerns that this could be viewed as an effort on the part of the state either to save money, or at the other extreme lead to an avoidance to withdraw futile treatment.

This scenario has been explored further, both by Rushton[16] with regard to caregiver

Common clinical manifestations of HIV infection in children[13]	Common AIDS-defining conditions in children[13]	End-stage disease[14]
Lymphadenopathy	*Pneumocystis carinii* pneumonia	Severe clinical disease with substantial immune suppression
Hepatosplenomegaly	Lymphoid interstitial pneumonitis	
Oral candidiasis		HIV1 encephalopathy and wasting syndrome, which may be associated with cytomegalovirus infection
Chronic or recurrent diarrhoea	Recurrent bacterial infection	
Failure to thrive	Wasting syndrome	
Developmental delay	Candidal oesophagitis	
Parotitis	HIV encephalopathy	Cryptosporidiosis
	Cytomegalovirus disease	Atypical mycobacterial infection
	Mycobacterium avium-intracellulare complex infection	HIV1-specific malignant disease, such as leiomyosarcoma and central nervous system lymphoma
	Pulmonary candidiasis	
	Herpes simplex disease	Multi-organ failure
	Cryptosporidiosis	High HIV1 RNA load persists despite aggressive antiretroviral therapy with progressive loss of CD4 lymphocytes

suffering, and also by Carter *et al.*[14] in the same book. Carter *et al.* state that the aggressive and prophylactic treatment of children living with HIV has a significant impact on quality of life by improving survival, prolonging time free from opportunistic infection, and improving and maintaining immunological health. They also state that during end-stage disease, decisions relating to the continuation of antiretroviral therapy must balance the benefits against the side-effects of the medications and the ultimate futility of current treatment.

The changing face of HIV and AIDS

Young people affected by HIV in the 1980s and 1990s have grown up with a chronic illness that might still become life-threatening, but for the vast majority has not proved life-limiting. The shift from expecting to die to learning to live with HIV will be explored later in this chapter. Melvin (personal communication, 2005) cautions against dismissing the palliative care element that can continue over an uncertain period of time for these young people, due to the fact that we do not know the long-term outcome of the disease. There is a risk that both long-term effects of the actual treatment as well as a complex, persistent and increasingly resistant virus will alter the overall course of the disease.

Examining the situation for young people with HIV and AIDS in the UK results in two different pictures. In 2006, vertical transmission still represents the greatest risk of acquiring HIV in the UK. Prenatal screening, carefully screened blood products and the use of antiretroviral drugs have dramatically reduced infection rates. It is now possible to significantly reduce the risk for a baby born to an HIV-positive mother by giving antiretroviral drugs to the mother in labour and then to the baby for the first 6 weeks of life, starting within 8–12 hours of birth. The mean age of presentation is 6 months for children born in the UK, by which age it is possible to determine whether the antibodies found in the blood are those of the child, rather than those of the mother which still remain in the baby's bloodstream. To avert the risk of infecting the baby postnatally, HIV-positive mothers should not breastfeed. There can be difficult legal issues if the mother refuses treatment or insists on breastfeeding. However, the evidence that non-compliance puts the child at risk is now sufficiently strong for it to be likely that the child would be removed from the mother in such a situation.

In addition to HIV-infected children who are identified ante- and perinatally by screening, there are some children who are not identified via this route. The Children With AIDS Charity website[2] tells the story of a family in which the 12-year-old daughter died of AIDS, the mother died of AIDS, the father has AIDS and the 15-year-old son is not infected. The daughter was infected as a fetus by an intrauterine blood transfusion. Antenatal screening here would not detect the risk to the baby, the mother and the father. In addition, children might not be identified because the mothers did not have antenatal care for a variety of reasons, or because the children were not born in the UK. These infants are likely to come to medical attention when suffering their first, often overwhelming opportunistic infection, often requiring admission directly to a paediatric intensive-care unit (PICU), where the diagnosis is finally made.

While I was researching this chapter it became obvious that overall only relatively small numbers of children are affected, although no definite number could be identified. It is heartening to see the advances that have been made in the field of treatment of HIV and AIDS since the mid-1990s, and the fact that as a result only a comparatively small number of children are likely to require palliative care. Children and young people with HIV fall within category 2 of the ACT categories, which encompasses 'Conditions where there may be long periods of intensive treatment aimed at prolonging life and allowing participation in normal childhood activities, but premature death is still possible.' The needs of these children and their families are likely to be diverse. For a child and their family who are already being supported by an established HIV team, palliative care services are likely to play a mainly supportive and advisory role. Not all families have access to specialist centres, and for some their individual circumstances dictate a different approach to collaboration between HIV services and palliative care services.

HIV and AIDS in the UK

The Collaborative HIV Paediatric Study (CHIPS) collects long-term information on HAART, clinical HIV status, frequency of hospital admissions and virological and immunological status in children. Data are available from the CHIVA website.[1]

Gibb et al.[17] have provided the following figures:

- in total, there were 944 children with perinatally acquired HIV in the UK and Ireland in October 2002
- 628 of these cases were of black-African ethnic origin
- 205 cases were aged 10 years or older
- 39 cases were aged 15 years or older
- 193 affected children are known to have died
- the proportion of children presenting with HIV who were born abroad increased from 20% to 60% during the period 2000–2002
- the mortality rate before 1997 was 9.3 in 100
- this figure has fallen to 2 in 100 since 1997 due to antiretroviral therapy
- hospital admission rates declined by 80% since 1997; however, as the overall number of children diagnosed with HIV increased, the absolute number of admissions fell by only 26%

- the mean age at presentation is 6 months for children born in the UK and Ireland, and 5.2 years for children born abroad
- in total, 438 children developed AIDS indicator disease, and 13 of these children died before AIDS was diagnosed
- the proportion of children with opportunistic infections increased during the period 1997–2002
- since 1997 mortality has declined by 80% and progression to AIDS has declined by 50%, in parallel with the increased use of three- and four-drug combination anti-retroviral therapy
- the prognosis from the initial AIDS diagnosis varied; the mortality was higher in children with PCP or HIV encephalopathy than in children with other opportunistic infections, failure to thrive or severe recurrent bacterial infection.

More recent figures from the Health Protection Agency[18] indicate that by June 2004, a total of 4597 children were born to HIV-infected mothers according to the National Study of HIV in Pregnancy and Childhood (NSHPC). Of these, 89% (4091) were born in the UK. At that time, 25% (1136) were known to be HIV infected and 53% (2433) were uninfected. Of the remainder it is estimated that 98% are likely to be uninfected.

Cooper *et al.*[19] conducted a 10-year study of children admitted to intensive care with HIV. The authors state that 10 years ago the outcome for children admitted to intensive-care units was extremely poor, with a mortality rate of 84–100%, and the appropriateness of intensive-care treatment was questioned at that time. In their study, 42 children had 66 admission episodes during the 10-year study period. The main findings were as follows.

- There were no agreed admission criteria, but rather each child was considered on his or her own merits.
- No children were refused admission.
- Some children died outside the PICU. In these cases a decision had been made to give palliative care, and none of these children were referred to the PICU.
- The median length of PICU admission was 7 days and the median hospital stay was 25 days. One patient was discharged home on continuous positive airway pressure ventilation.
- In total, 16 children died in the PICU and 26 survived their last PICU admission (of these, five died at a later date).
- In total, 80% of the current survivors had good outcomes.
- The authors concluded that, despite a significant mortality rate among children admitted with HIV, admission to intensive-care units is appropriate as they have a good outcome with HAART and management by specialist multi-disciplinary teams.

White[5] describes the family HIV service at a London teaching hospital which provides multi-disciplinary, family-focused care that addresses the cultural, ethnic and social needs of service users, with the fundamental aim of helping families to live 'normal' lives in their homes and communities. White describes the service as having two components.

1. The inpatient service has two family 'suites' on the paediatric infectious diseases ward, and caters for parents and children who might require inpatient care at some time.
2. The outpatient service, known as the family clinic, caters for both parents and children, with multi-disciplinary input and on-site support from an adult physician.

Entitlement to NHS services

Levenson and Sharma[20] have summarised this as follows.

- The Home Office defines a 'child' as a person under the age of 18 years.
- All refugees, individuals with exceptional leave to remain (ELR) and asylum seekers

are entitled to all NHS services. Refugee children and adults should have access to the full range of primary, secondary and tertiary NHS services.

* All asylum seekers have the right to be registered with a NHS doctor. Doctors are not obliged or expected to check the immigration status of people who register to join their list.

* If a child tests positive for HIV, further specialist advice should be obtained from the Paediatric Infectious Diseases Unit at St George's Hospital, St Mary's Hospital or Great Ormond Street Hospital in London.

Contemporary issues in palliative care for children and young people in relation to HIV and AIDS

Trans-generational illness

Illness across different generations is not specific to HIV and AIDS, even though this example has been chosen for this chapter. Occasionally parents themselves have life-limiting illnesses and may die before their life-limited child. One example of this in the author's experience involved a child with a metabolic degenerative disease. The mother died of cancer when the girl was a young teenager, and the father had severe heart disease with a poor prognosis, not helped by the stress of having lost his wife and now being sole carer for a completely dependent teenage daughter.

According to Brown (personal communication, 2005), if both parents have died the responsibility can fall to the grandparents to become sole carers for the terminally ill grandchild, when they have already buried their own child and son- or daughter-in-law.

Practising family-centred care when both parent and child are in the terminal stages of their disease is logistically difficult, as the adult will be cared for within the adult services, and the child within paediatric services. Some detective work to ascertain where these families can be cared for at present revealed that only Douglas House in Oxford will potentially take patients across two generations, with the adult upper age limit being 40 years. When a scenario was suggested in which both child and parent require hospice care for HIV, it appears they would consider a referral from a family where both parent and child are affected by a life-limiting illness.

HIV is a comparatively new phenomenon, and it differs from other diseases in that both the illness and the treatment have undergone rapid changes within the paediatric field, but it also presents a very stubborn complicating factor, namely stigma.

It was not easy to choose a suitable scenario for this chapter. The original intention had been to explore how we care for a family unit in which both child and parent are affected by the same illness. It soon became apparent that in the case of HIV and AIDS the number of families that are experiencing acute life-threatening situations is declining. Because of treatments with antiretroviral drugs, HIV/AIDS is now considered to be a chronic illness, and some might question whether this is primarily an issue for palliative care. There are excellent examples of multi-disciplinary services and support for families affected by HIV and AIDS. A model that has been established here is that care is delivered by established multi-disciplinary teams which care for families for many years from the first contact. These teams prefer that palliative care services work very closely with them and act in a consultative rather than direct manner. Local adaptation of the ACT Care Pathway is an excellent example in this context. Where teams have clarified what the perceived issues are for families on each stage of the pathway, what each specialty can offer, and then decide what their involvement is likely to be, allowing for individual variations, the result should be working together without conflict or fear of one specialty 'taking over' or leaving gaps in provision.

Normalisation strategies for families affected by HIV/AIDS

Anderson[21] has provided an excellent overview entitled 'The needs of people living with HIV in the UK.' He summarises the needs of these people, and the problems that affect and create needs, as shown in the table below.

Key needs	Key problems and challenges	Key secondary needs
Physical health	Illness, pain and treatment side-effects	Knowledge of services
Mental health		Confidence, skills and resources to access services
Shelter and security	Uncertainty and anxiety	
Nourishment	Despair, depression and mental illness	Confidence and skills in dealing with professionals
Rest	Lack of energy	Knowledge and understanding of HIV treatment and care options
Mobility	Poor self-image	
Financial security and independence	Disclosure of HIV status	
Self-confidence	Bereavement and displacement	Skills, motivation and discipline to sustain a regular pattern of treatment taking
Relationships and friendships	Isolation and loneliness	
Sex and sexual well-being	Discrimination and inequality	
Children and family life	Poverty	
Education, skills and employment	Poor housing and living conditions	
Quality of life	Immigration and asylum problems	
	Infectivity and vulnerability	
	Sexual dysfunction	
	Services	
	Professionals	
	Treatment choices and treatment taking	

According to Rehm and Franck,[22] there is a growing population of parents and children who are long-term survivors of HIV/AIDS who use normalisation strategies, despite treatment complexity and the need for stigma management, to achieve the following goals:

- health maintenance
- facilitating children's participation in school activities
- enhancement of the emotional well-being of all family members.

Rehm and Franck[22] explain that families who are raising children with HIV/AIDS differ from families who are living with other chronic illnesses in the following ways.

- HIV is mainly acquired perinatally from the mother.
- Several family members may require extensive medical treatment. The parents need

to be organised and juggle multiple responsibilities in order to care for themselves, their children with HIV and other members of the family. Although Rehm and Franck[22] found that one parent neglected her own needs at times in order to prioritise those of her children, other parents with HIV stated that safeguarding their own health was absolutely essential if they were to keep their children healthy.

- The family may have experienced the death of one or more of its members.
- The problems are often compounded by stigma associated with drug use, poverty and minority ethnic status.
- Women, adolescents and young adults are currently among those with the highest new infection rates.
- Family care and support are gaining recognition as important topics of research for all populations affected by this disease.
- HIV/AIDS is a stigmatised condition that can isolate individuals and families from their usual sources of support.

Anderson[21] explains that the stresses which are placed on children and young people in these circumstances are considerable, and points out that a core issue for children and young people who are living with (or affected by) HIV is their own knowledge and understanding of the condition and its effects on the family.

Juhn et al.[23] surveyed 150 childcare centres about their willingness to accept children with HIV or hepatitis B. Of these, 58% would agree to accept a child with HIV and 23% would accept a child with hepatitis B.

Stigma

Joachim[24] discusses stigma in relation to chronic conditions. The salient points are summarised below.

- The term 'stigma' refers to signs that are perceived to indicate something out of the ordinary or bad about a person. These can be physical deformities, character blemishes (such as weak will, dishonesty, addiction or mental illness) or 'tribal stigma' (such as race or religion), and they can be passed down through family lines with all members of a group being equally stigmatised.
- According to Jones et al.,[25] there are six dimensions of stigma:
  - concealability (whether the condition is 'visible' or hidden)
  - the course of the condition (the extent to which the condition changes over time)
  - the strain that is placed on interpersonal relationships (by the visibility and aesthetically displeasing nature of the condition)
  - aesthetic qualities (the degree to which the condition affects appearance)
  - the cause of the stigma (e.g. whether the condition is congenitally acquired)
  - the dangers associated with stigmatised individuals (e.g. a Ugandan woman voiced her concern that maternity staff in rural Uganda might refuse to assist at the time of delivery because of her infected status).

Disclosure

One of the complicating factors with regard to disclosure is the fact that over 20 years into the AIDS epidemic most children with the virus have been vertically infected. Any disclosure of the child's condition is therefore potentially a revelation of both parental HIV status and lifestyle. For this reason, Rehm and Franck[22] identify HIV as a family disease, as the children's HIV infection cannot necessarily be separated from the effects of parental HIV disease. Not all children live with their birth parents, and Thorne et al.[26] reported children in their sample living with grandparents, foster parents and adoptive parents. Ledlie[27] found that the process of disclosure is ongoing and dynamic, with both parents searching for clues to their child's readiness to be told, sometimes leaving clues for the child and being ready to respond. When telling about their infection, parents struggled with aspects such as discussing the fatality and answering questions on perinatal transmission. Lester *et al.*[28] view disclosure as an ongoing process as the child develops cognitive and emotional awareness about the meaning of illness and death.

Rehm and Franck[22] found that in order to manage stigma, families perceived that silence about HIV preserved their ability to be treated normally and to blend in with others. Families disclosed the child's HIV status on a 'need-to-know' basis. For example, they would tell one or two responsible people at school, often the secretary or principal, and rely on them to guard the child's secret and to inform them if the child became sick while at school.

According to Ledlie,[27] the child in turn used 'selective telling' as a strategy for telling others, often in response to questions about the nature of their illness and the reasons for their treatments and medicines. Lee *et al.*[29] advocate that newly diagnosed seropositive parents should delay disclosing their own diagnosis to their children until the parent has dealt with their own feelings of anger, fear and/or depression.

Joachim[24] describes three different types of disclosure.

- Protective disclosure is used to enable individuals to control how, what, when and who to tell about their condition. This type of disclosure is planned and it protects the individual.
- Spontaneous disclosure is an emotional form of disclosure and is related to shock and disbelief.
- Preventive disclosure is used for an 'invisible' condition which is not under control (e.g. epilepsy), and might be based on the risk that another person will find out about the condition. Preventive disclosure might be used in the belief that social judgement of the person by others can be influenced by disclosure.

Sherman *et al.*[30] found that one of the most controversial topics of discussion among families of children who are infected with HIV/AIDS is whether or not to tell their child about the child's own diagnosis, and if they do, whether or not to allow the child to tell others. This can have both psychological and physiological consequences, which can be summarised as follows.

- Children who had disclosed their HIV status to friends had a significantly larger increase in CD4 percentage count than children who had not yet disclosed their HIV diagnosis to friends.
- This could be attributed to the fact that the repeated act of concealing personal secrets or traumatic information is thought to require inhibitory processes that are physically taxing and result in increased health costs. It also leads to rumination and increased worry – keeping difficult and painful information such as the HIV/AIDS diagnosis to themselves can be damaging to children's psychological well-being.
- Alternatively, disclosure may foster adaptation by promoting reinterpretation of the painful information, redefinition and accommodation into existing schemata.
- A child who is unable to discuss their diagnostic status with a friend loses an important means of testing how others may respond, or gaining a positive understanding of the illness in the face of the existing negative societal stigma.

In this context a worthwhile consideration is how a child's friends deal with the information that is disclosed to them.

Chronic disease

Although HIV/AIDS meets the criteria for a chronic illness since the advent of HAART, Siegel and Lekas[31] carefully spell out what this means in the context of a disease with an as yet indeterminable course. Common treatments can render a viral load undetectable, but cannot eradicate it from the body, and if left untreated, the viral load will rebound. These authors explain that although the natural history of the disease has been delineated, the course of HIV disease progression varies considerably among individuals. The salient points can be summarised as follows.

- As the disease is incurable, the goals of medical care are containment, slowing of disease progression and symptom management.
- The uncertain course of the disease is characterised by alternating periods of remission and recurrence or exacerbations.
- Adherence to a treatment regime is required, which varies across diseases with regard to complexity and efficacy.
- There is a need for considerable self-care and self-monitoring of symptoms.
- The disease carries a degree of stigma, which in turn depends on a variety of factors, such as:
  - whether the individual is perceived as being responsible for having acquired the illness
  - whether the disease is contagious
  - whether there is visible disfigurement.
- Siegel and Lekas[31] also describe changes in roles in relation to the following:
  - degree of dependency, certainly in the advanced stages of the illness
  - responsibility in families, which must be renegotiated in the light of the patient's limitations or disabilities
  - identity changes as the patient attempts to integrate illness into their own life and self-perception
  - psychological distress due to the uncertainty inherent in many chronic conditions.

Rehm and Franck[22] found that spiritual and religious beliefs were often cited as important coping strategies, with both children and adults talking about attending church, prayer or youth groups. Although they felt that church groups judged them or were afraid of individuals with HIV, it was the personal relationship with God or the act of prayer which they found reassuring or strengthening.

Growing up with HIV/AIDS

Siegel and Lekas[31] warn that the perception of HIV/AIDS as a manageable, chronic illness may significantly decrease the dread of acquiring the infection which historically motivated the adaptation of risk-reducing behaviour. They highlight the rapid spread of HIV and AIDS in rural areas among adolescents, heterosexual women and racial/ethnic minorities, and point out the need for future studies on prevention and intervention in these more recently affected populations.

Hockenberry et al.[13] suggest that children with HIV fall into one of three sub-populations:

- infants born to HIV-infected women (91%)
- children who received infected blood products before the initiation of HIV screening in 1985
- adolescents who became infected as a result of high-risk behaviour. Hockenberry et al.[13] warn that, given the fact that the progression from HIV infection to AIDS in adults takes around 10 years, most people in their twenties with AIDS were likely to have become infected with HIV/AIDS during their teenage years.

Lester et al.[28] suggest that 25–90% of schoolchildren with HIV have not been told about their illness. According to the authors, this might date back to a time when infants who were diagnosed with AIDS were expected to have a very short lifespan, and non-disclosure agreements were made. Medical providers still feel ethically bound by these, although there are now highly individualised disclosure attitudes and practices. Lester *et al.* suggest that delays in disclosure might result in negative consequences for the child, including impaired treatment and understanding, increased psychological and behavioural problems, decreased support services and a more complicated bereavement process.

As children reach adolescence and begin to engage in risk-taking behaviours, information about their own disease becomes an essential part not only of their own health maintenance, but also of HIV prevention within the larger population. This theme is echoed by several studies[26,32] that discuss the move towards a more independent life in adolescence, which for young people with HIV may be particularly difficult, with the associated stigma and discrimination, the impact of a strict treatment regimen, the burden of secrecy, the fear of rejection, regular visits to hospital and changes in physical appearance. Thorne *et al.*[26] found that older infected children who have been observed by the same paediatric clinic throughout their lives are benefiting from the continuity of close relationships between children, families and clinic staff. Many of the centres are taking a gradual approach to the transition from the paediatric clinic to adult HIV services. Gibb *et al.*[17] anticipate that the demand for specialist paediatric HIV services will continue to increase. Transitional links with adult services are required in order to deal with the medical, social and psychological needs of children entering adolescence and adult life.

Powderly *et al.*[33] have examined the ethical issues relating to perinatal HIV, which according to the authors represent some of the most pressing and unresolved issues in the bioethics literature, but also some new practical challenges for obstetric care providers, such as managing women with coexisting illness who might be faced with planning for the baby's future after the mother's death, or end-of-life decision making.

Compliance with treatment: child protection considerations

Cooper *et al.*[34] suggest that as most HIV-infected children are now surviving to adulthood with appropriate support, it may be that in recent years the onus on the family to take responsibility for their child's well-being and treatment has become such that non-compliance, such as insisting on breastfeeding or not giving medication to a young child with HIV, would be considered a child protection issue.

Safe passages to adulthood programme

This is coordinated jointly by the Centre for Sexual Health Research at the University of Southampton, the Thomas Coram Research Unit at the Institute for Education, University of London, and the Centre for Population Studies at the London School of Hygiene and Tropical Medicine, and details are available on the website of the Social Statistics Division, University of Southampton.[35]

The global picture

The global picture differs markedly from the experience of HIV/AIDS in the developed world. There are countries decimated by the disease, with the average life expectancy reduced to 39 years.[36] Some of this chapter was written in the same week that the Live8 concert organised by Bob Geldof took place around the world with the message 'make poverty history.' In the same week the G8 summit took place at Gleneagles, Scotland.

Fowler-Kerry[37] described the general perspective of child health in the context of the G8 summit, highlighting the fact that for many aspects of child health there are no accurate figures. However, some statistics do stand out. For example:

- only 0.08% of children who require it receive effective palliative care
- for carers and healthcare professionals in many countries, the only available treatment that they can give to patients infected with and dying of AIDS are their 'hearts, heads and hands', in the absence of affordable antiretroviral drugs.

Fowler-Kerry considers a child's needs to be a right, and as such this includes children's palliative care in the UN Convention on the Rights of the Child (ratified in 1991).

The United Nation's General Assembly in 2001[38] stated the following commitments:

- to attain the highest standard of treatment for HIV/AIDS
- to strengthen pharmaceutical policies and practices
- to improve by 2005 the effectiveness of the supply systems, financing plans and referral mechanisms required to provide access to affordable medicines, including antiretroviral drugs, diagnostics and related technologies, as well as quality medical, palliative and psychosocial care.

UNAIDS reports that earlier this year (2006), the Secretary-General presented the report to the General Assembly on progress made until the end of 2005. The main focus of the meeting was to review progress achieved in realising the commitments set out in the Declaration of Commitment and to:

- review progress in implementing the 2001 Declaration of Commitment on HIV/AIDS, focusing on both constraints and opportunities to full implementation
- consider recommendations on how the targets set in the Declaration may be reached, including through the 'towards universal access processes' and to renew political commitment; www.un.org.

Susman[39] has summarised the 16-page declaration, which aimed for a wide range of prevention programmes, taking into account local circumstances, ethics and cultural values, by 2005. These should be available in all countries, particularly those most severely affected, and include the following:

- education that encourages responsible sexual behaviour, including abstinence and fidelity
- expansion of access to essential commodities, including condoms and sterile injecting equipment
- access to education and services so that all young men and women aged 15–24 years can develop the life skills necessary to reduce their vulnerability to HIV infection
- a 20% reduction in the prevalence of HIV among infants
- the strengthening of healthcare systems and addressing of the affordability of HIV-related drugs, including antiretroviral drugs
- the elimination of all forms of discrimination against people living with HIV/AIDS and other vulnerable groups
- the creation of new national strategies to help those at greatest risk of new infection as indicated by local history of the epidemic, poverty, sexual practices, drug use, occupation, institutional location, disrupted social structures and population movement
- improvement of services for children orphaned and affected by HIV/AIDS
- increasing investment in research to develop an AIDS vaccine
- a concerted effort involving the full and active participation of the United Nations, the entire multilateral system, civil society, the business community and the private sector.

The urgency is obvious. Steinbrook[40] cites the following figures.

- By the end of 2003, between 34.6 million and 42.3 million people throughout the world were living with HIV.
- More than 20 million people had died of AIDS.
- The number of people living with HIV continues to rise steadily. Of the entire popula-

tion between 15 and 49 years of age, 1.1% are now infected with HIV.

- A total of 2.2 million people died of AIDS in sub-Saharan Africa in 2003 (representing 76% of the global total). By contrast, in Western Europe where effective treatment is widely available, 6000 people died of AIDS.
- In the same year a total of 12.1 million children in sub-Saharan Africa were orphaned by AIDS, representing an increase of 2.5 million from 2001.
- There are an estimated 2.1 million infected children under 15 years of age at the end of 2003, and 90% of these are living in Africa.
- In 2003, 490,000 children in this age group died of AIDS, including 440,000 in sub-Saharan Africa.
- There are 4 to 6 million people in developing countries who need treatment. Steinbrook estimates that the total number of people treated is around 400,000.

Gorbach *et al.*[41] have examined the impact of social, economic and political forces on emerging HIV epidemics, and cite the following figures.

Country	Declared cases	UN AIDS estimates	Specific factors
Russia	195,000	1.2 million	Mostly concentrated in socially vulnerable populations of intravenous drug users and commercial sex workers
China	850,000	1.5 million	A high percentage of these cases are in some of the provinces and attributed to intravenous drug use, as well as to illegal blood and plasma donor centres that often do not sterilise plasma-collecting apparatus between donors
Vietnam	48,762	140,000–165,000	High number of intravenous drug users

Giving care to adult children (Thailand)

Kespichayawattana and VanLangdingham[42] studied the effects of co-residence and caregiving of Thai parents of adult children, and found that it is widely recognised that young adults infected with HIV have children, but the fact that they also have parents is frequently ignored. Yet it is often the parents who care for their adult children and may be experiencing adverse effects on their own physical and mental health. Three findings by the above authors stand out in relation to trans-generational disease.

1. Their own poor physical or emotional health might be the reason why some parents did not engage in caregiving.
2. Grim as the experience of caregiving is for many parents, it gives them the opportu-

nity to fulfil their perceived duty as parents before their child dies. This is an opportunity denied to the AIDS-affected parents, who did not provide such care.

3. A 60-year-old mother was quoted as saying 'I was exhausted and in pretty bad shape. I didn't get enough sleep, either. I was worried about my son and my granddaughter.'

Summary

This chapter has considered trans-generational disease and the difficulties encountered in providing care for affected individuals within the framework of the paediatric services. HIV and AIDS have been examined in the contemporary context of 'living with HIV/AIDS' as a chronic and unpredictable illness. Complex issues pertaining to stigma and normalisation have been discussed, and a short overview of the global picture has been provided.

SWOT

It might be useful to revisit the SWOT analysis at this point in order to determine any further learning needs in relation to this chapter and the Knowledge and Skills Framework (KSF) requirements, namely:

1. communication
2. personal and people development
3. health, safety and security
4. service improvement
5. quality
6. equality and diversity.

Strengths	Weaknesses
Opportunities	Threats

Action plan for further learning

<table>
<tr><td></td></tr>
<tr><td></td></tr>
<tr><td></td></tr>
</table>

References

1. The Children's HIV Association of the UK and Ireland; www.bhiva.org/chiva/index.html
2. Children With AIDS Charity; www.cwac.org
3. Association for Children with Life-Threatening or Terminal Conditions and Their Families (ACT); www.act.org
4. National Children's Bureau; www.ncb.org.uk/projects
5. White J (2001) Sharing the care of children with HIV infection. *Nurs Standard.* **15**: 42–6.
6. Levenson R and Sharma A (1999) *The Health of Refugee Children: guidelines for paediatricians.* Royal College of Paediatrics and Child Health, London.
7. Miah J (ed.) (2004) *Talking with Children, Young People and Families about Chronic Illness and Living with HIV;* www.ncb.org.UK/HIV or www.bodyandsoulcharity.co.uk or www.bhiva.org./chiva
8. Department of Health and Department for Education and Skills (2005) *Evidence to Inform the National Service Framework for Children, Young People and Maternity Services.* Department of Health, London.
9. Department of Health (2004) *The NHS Knowledge and Skills Framework (NHS KSF) and the Development Review Process.* Department of Health, London.
10. Elston S (ed.) (2004) *Integrated Multi-Agency Care Pathways for Children with Life-Threatening and Life-Limiting Conditions.* ACT, Bristol.
11. Ellershaw J and Ward C (2003) *Care of the Dying: a pathway to excellence.* Oxford University Press, Oxford.
12. Khoury M and Kovacs A (2001) Paediatric HIV infection. *Clin Obstet Gynecol.* **44**: 243–75.
13. Hockenberry M, Wilson D, Winkelstein M *et al.* (2003) *Wong's Nursing Care of Infants and Children.* Mosby, St Louis, MO.
14. Carter B, Oleske J, Czarniecki L *et al.* (2004) The child with HIV infection. In: B Carter and M Leverton (eds) *Palliative Care for Infants, Children and Adolescents: a practical handbook.* The Johns Hopkins University Press, Baltimore, MD.
15. Rushton C, Hogue C, Billett K *et al.* (1993) End-of-life care for infants with AIDS: ethical and legal issues. *Pediatr Nurs.* **19**: 79–83, 94.
16. Rushton C (2004) The other side of caring: caregiver suffering. In: B Carter and M Leverton (eds) *Palliative Care for Infants, Children and Adolescents: a practical handbook.* The Johns Hopkins University Press, Baltimore, MD.
17. Gibb D, Duong T, Tookey P *et al.* (2003) Decline in mortality, AIDS and hospital admissions in perinatally HIV-1 infected children in the United Kingdom and Ireland. *BMJ.* **327**: 10; http://bmj.bmjjournals.com/cgi/content/full/327/7422/1019
18. Health Protection Agency; www.hpa.org.uk/infections/topicsaz/hiv_and_sti/publications/annual2004/ann

19. Cooper S, Lyall H, Walters S *et al.* (2004) Children with human immunodeficiency virus admitted to a paediatric intensive-care unit in the United Kingdom over a 10-year period. *Intensive Care Med.* **30:** 113–18.

20. Levenson R and Sharma A (1999) *The Health of Refugee Children: guidelines for paediatricians.* Royal College of Paediatrics and Child Health, London.

21. Anderson W (2004) *The Needs of People Living with HIV in the UK;* www.nat.org.uk

22. Rehm R and Franck L (2000) Long-term goals and normalisation strategies of children and families affected by HIV/AIDS. *Adv Nurs Sci.* **23:** 69–82.

23. Juhn Y, Shapiro E, McCarthy P *et al.* (2001) Willingness of directors of child care centers to care for children with chronic infections. *Pediatr Infect Dis J.* **20:** 77–9.

24. Joachim G and Acorn S (2000) Stigma of visible and invisible chronic conditions. *J Adv Nurs.* **32:** 243–8.

25. Jones E, Farina A, Hastorf A *et al.* (1984) *Social Stigma: the psychology of marked relationships.* Freeman, New York.

26. Thorne C, Newell M, Botet F *et al.* for the European Collaborative Study (2002) Older children and adolescents surviving with vertically acquired HIV infection. *J Acquir Immune Defic Syndr Hum Retrovirol.* **29:** 396–401.

27. Ledlie S (1999) Diagnosis disclosure by family caregivers to children who have perinatally acquired HIV disease: when the time comes. *Nurs Res.* **48:** 141–9.

28. Lester P, Chesney M, Cooke M *et al.* (2002) When the time comes to talk about HIV: factors associated with diagnostic disclosure and emotional distress in HIV-infected children. *J Acquir Immune Defic Syndr Hum Retrovirol.* **31:** 309–17.

29. Lee M and Rotheram-Borus M (2002) Parents' disclosure of HIV to their children. *AIDS.* **16:** 2201–7.

30. Sherman B, Bonanno G, Wiener L and Battles H (2000) When children tell their friends they have AIDS: possible consequences for psychological well-being and disease progression. *Psychosom Med.* **62:** 238–47.

31. Siegel K and Lekas H (2002) AIDS as a chronic illness: psychosocial implications. *AIDS.* **16:** S69–76.

32. Lyon M and D'Angelo L (2001) Parental disclosure of HIV status. *Pediatr Hematol Oncol.* **23:** 148–50.

33. Powderly K (2001) Ethical and legal issues in perinatal HIV. *Clin Obstet Gynecol.* **44:** 300–11.

34. Cooper S, Lyall H, Walters S *et al.* (2004) Children with human immunodeficiency virus admitted to a paediatric intensive-care unit in the United Kingdom over a 10-year period. *Intensive Care Med.* **30:** 113–18.

35. Social Statistics Division, School of Social Sciences, University of Southampton; www.socstats.soton.ac.uk/cshr/safepassages.htm

36. Action Aid report published in 2005; www.actionaid.org/wps/content/documents/UN%20World%20Summit%20Briefing_992005_11408.pdf

37. Fowler-Kerry S (2004) Conference presentation. *Evidence – Who Needs It?* International Conference in Paediatric Palliative Care, Cardiff, December 2004.

38. United Nation's General Assembly (2001) www.un.org/esa/coordination/ecosoc/wgga/home5.htm

39. Susman E (2001) Twenty years and counting: where will we be in 2021? *AIDS.* **15:** N17–18.

40. Steinbrook R (2004) Global health: the AIDS epidemic in 2004. *NEJM.* **351:** 115–17.

41. Gorbach P, Ryan C, Saphonn V *et al.* (2002) The impact of social, economic and political forces on emerging HIV epidemics. *AIDS.* **16:** S35–43.

42. Kespichayawattana J and VanLandingham M (2003) Effects of co-residence and caregiving on health of Thai parents of adult children with AIDS. *J Nurs Scholarship.* **35:** 217–24.

Chapter 8

Neurologically degenerative disease

This chapter covers

Content	Relevant to other areas of palliative care for children and young people
Scenario	
• Batten's disease	• This chapter: needs of parents and teenage brother
• Setting the scene	• This chapter: children as interpreters
• The National Service Framework	• This chapter: different settings for terminal care
• The ACT Care Pathway	• This chapter: childhood dementia
• The Knowledge and Skills Framework	• This chapter: restraining children
	• This chapter: children from different ethnic populations – competent cultural care in action
Contemporary issues	• This chapter: vCJD, PIND study
• Pain assessment in the child with severe neurological impairment	• Chapter 11: financial impact
• Bartiméus	
• Childhood dementia	*Relevant topics in other chapters*
• Restraining children	
• The PIND study	• Chapter 2: how grief and bereavements affect children
• Children from different ethnic populations: competent cultural care in action	• Chapter 3: religious, cultural and spiritual context
	• Chapter 3: therapeutic work with children
Related to neurologically degenerative disease	• Chapter 4: place of care
• Contemporary issues in palliative care for children in relation to neurologically degenerative illness	• Chapter 5: long-term emotional implications when planning for home care of a technology-dependent child
• Clinical governance and suggestions for work-based learning and networking	• Chapters 5 and 11: respite care
• Summary	• Chapter 11: social care and schooling
	• Chapter 11: families with disabled children and the Internet
	• Chapter 11: child protection

continues on p. 132

	Relevant topics in other chapters (cont.)
	• Chapter 11: maintaining a safe environment – children in their own home
	• Chapter 12: all aspects of this chapter, including limited knowledge base on which to draw – Creutzfeldt–Jakob disease
	• Chapter 13: all aspects of this chapter, including transporting children

Batten's disease

Batten's disease is a metabolic degenerative childhood encephalopathy. The progress of the disease is characterised by initial attainment of developmental milestones, followed by rapid regression, with death in middle childhood.

A full overview can be accessed through the website of SeeAbility.[1]

Setting the scene

Nadia, aged 7 years, is the youngest of three children. She was diagnosed as suffering from Batten's disease at the age of 18 months. By that time the middle child of the family, Saleem, then aged 4 years, was already affected by the same disease. Although the family had received genetic counselling and been informed that they had a 1 in 4 chance that the next child would also be affected by Batten's disease, the parents were delighted when Nadia came along, as they thought that they had had one sick child, and therefore Nadia would be fine. After all, their eldest child, Prakash, was unaffected by the disease. Both the parents and the extended family were distressed yet resigned to Nadia's prognosis, and the parents devoted their lives to caring for both sick children.

As Saleem and Nadia became increasingly dependent and heavy, their father had to stay at home more often to help to care for them. Within six months his employer noticed his increasing lateness and absence and how tired he was at work, and made him redundant. From that point onward the family lived exclusively on state benefit. Saleem died of a chest infection at the age of 8 years. Again, the parents were resigned to this and focused all their attention on Nadia.

Unfortunately, Nadia had been deteriorating rapidly over the past 6 weeks, after she had aspirated during a seizure. Although she had recovered from the resulting pneumonia, her swallow and cough reflex had been very poor since then, and she was admitted to her local children's ward for assessment. After careful discussion with the parents, a mutual decision was made to keep Nadia comfortable but not to treat the chest infection with which she presented.

Jot down your initial reaction to this situation.

```



```

Does this bring back memories of a situation you have encountered?

Does this help or hinder?

SWOT

What are your learning needs when considering this scenario? They could look similar to those in the chart on the next page.

There might be issues that you wish to explore, in which case feel free to do so, but also think about the following.

What are the immediate needs of the parents and of Prakash (now aged 15 years)?

```



```

Have you considered any of these?

1. This is the second time that this family has faced the death of a child after a long illness. Much of their perception of this situation will depend upon their previous experience. Witnessing a second child dying does not mean they are 'used' to this happening. These parents have the same need for our caring empathetic attention as any other parents. They might be absolutely terrified by the prospect of having to go through this situation a second time. They might also wish to change aspects of the way in which their child's terminal care is managed as a result of their previous experience with regard to professional involvement, setting, etc.
2. This situation could well be particularly difficult for Prakash. Developmentally, he is at a difficult stage at which to face mortality. He might try to hide away from this. On the other hand, older children often try to be brave and protect their parents, because they don't want the parents to be upset, and their own needs and grief can easily be overlooked as a result. Prakash might worry that he, too, has a terminal disease, and he

Strengths	Weaknesses
• We have a good rapport with families who have children with chronic problems requiring frequent admissions. • These families have direct access to the ward, and their medical notes are held on the ward in case a child is admitted 'out of hours.' • We work closely with our community team. • We suggest contact with the local children's hospice soon after the diagnosis of a life-limiting condition has been made, as we recognise the value of continuity of support throughout a child's illness.	• We have no statistics about the prevalence of autosomal-recessive diseases in our ethnic-minority population. • We have little experience of discussing difficult topics with children with a learning disability, and we leave this side of care to the expertise of the parents. • We do not normally discuss the financial implications of caring for a severely disabled child, and we assume that families are in touch with a social worker.
Opportunities	**Threats**
• This is a good opportunity to explore how the ACT Care Pathway would work in our unit. • There are elements of trans-cultural care that we have not considered and which we need to explore further.	• This is a very busy ward and caring for a child with severe learning difficulties is very time consuming. • We are aware that often we cannot give as much time and attention as is needed due to the constraints of the environment. • Often we have known families for many years, and the death of a child can be very upsetting for staff who have become very involved with the family.

needs to be reassured that he has not got Batten's disease. However, the need for genetic counselling for Prakash will have to be addressed at some point, as he might be a carrier of the disease.

What are the difficulties in relying on older children as interpreters in this type of situation?

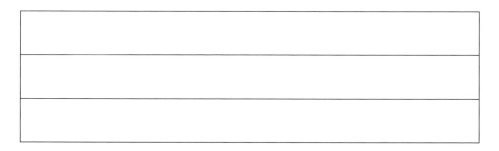

Have you considered any of these?

1. It is simply not acceptable to subject a child to the stress of having to give parents news and/or information in such a situation. The child might not be able to bring himself to pass on the prognosis to his parents, and he may instead state what he thinks they already know. Using a child as an interpreter renders the child the main means of support while he is denied this support for himself.
2. Older children often take on the role of 'grown-up supporter' to shield their family, who they observe to be struggling.

How can Nadia, who has childhood dementia, or any child with learning disabilities best be supported through the various stages of critical and terminal illness?

Have you considered any of these?

1. It is helpful if the level of cognitive development as opposed to the chronological level of a child with learning disabilities is known. Yoos[2] argues that this can be limiting if nurses assume that children are incapable of understanding medical information due to cognitive inability. Brown (personal communication, 2005) describes a current research project that aims to facilitate communication with children with severe learning disabilities. An example of how upsetting news can be communicated is demonstrated by Brown[3] – as is the effect on a person who is shielded from news altogether!
2. It cannot be assumed that because a child is unable to communicate, they are unaware of their situation or environment and therefore any conversation in the child's pres-

ence has to assume that they can understand. Like any other child, the learning-disabled child must be involved and given explanations on the basis of an assumed level of understanding. Hockenberry et al.[4] suggest several measures to avoid loneliness in the dying child who is unable to communicate. These include offering calm reassurance, talking to the child even though they might not appear to be awake, avoiding holding conversations about the child's condition in front of them, orientating the child to their surroundings when they are awake, and playing favourite music and reading stories to the child.

A particular problem that carers face when dealing with children with degenerative illnesses is that it is not known whether their cognitive ability deteriorates in line with their physical regression. This is particularly an issue in cases where more than one child in a family is affected by the same illness. A younger sibling might be aware that an older child is poorly or has even died, but might not be able to express his or her own anguish. This is one of many situations where we have to act on 'gut feeling' and use our observational capabilities and judgement. This is a key issue in the care of children with neurologically degenerative disease, and is further explored in the section on contemporary issues below.

3. Cues might be provided by uncharacteristic behaviour of the child, unexplained restlessness or separation anxiety. Carers need to be on their guard not to dismiss this as part of the disease process. If these cues are overlooked then the child will not be emotionally supported. Support and explanation of what lies ahead for the child then need to be given in the context of the relationship and normal interaction between the family and their child, as well as their specific cultural needs.

What are the resources (both material and manpower) required for effective palliative care for a highly dependent child both in hospital and in the community?

Have you considered any of these?

1. Any resources that a family needs can only be provided after thorough assessment of the family. An assessment framework has been described by Elston.[5]
2. Effective assessment will also take into consideration emotional resources and the support network that a family might have to care for a child with complex needs. Care provision can then be planned around these to avoid peaks and troughs. Good multidisciplinary teamwork is essential. Local provision of care and support is a factor that determines the physical setting in which the child receives care. For example, a fourth-floor flat in a house with no lift would not be a suitable setting.
3. Space to manoeuvre a wheelchair, a suitable bed and bathing facilities that can all be accessed with a hoist are necessary.

4. Twenty-four-hour professional support must be coordinated, ideally by a 'key person', so that the family's needs can be met effectively. If a family perceives that all these people come to 'check on them' then there is no support, but merely an extra burden on the family. Input is likely to be required from community paediatric nurses, social worker, health visitor, GP, community physiotherapist and community pharmacist, as well as the child's consultant and, if involved, staff from the local children's hospice.

5. Nadia's parents will probably benefit from periods of respite care, preferably at home, to enable them to have some time to themselves and give Prakash quality time while secure in the knowledge that Nadia is being well looked after (see the section below on culturally competent care and the acceptability of respite care to individual families).

Consider the different settings in which a child may receive terminal care. What might be the benefits or disadvantages of each of them?

Have you considered any of these?

1. As the parents have been in this situation before, they might wish either to have the same arrangement as previously, being cared for by staff whom they know, or to make different choices this time. This should be explored with the family, who should be reassured that whatever their choice they will be fully supported.

2. The family might wish to keep Nadia on the children's ward. They will probably know several members of staff there already, and they might find the 'high-tech' environment reassuring. However, although every effort is made to achieve continuity of care, this may be competing with other pressures on the ward.

3. The family might also be familiar with their local children's hospice, and again they might already know the staff. Within the philosophy of children's hospices it is desirable that a good rapport with families is established during the chronic stage of a child's illness, so that support can be tailored to the specific needs of families at times of crisis. This setting is more like home, and has a high staff/child/family ratio. The emphasis is on maximising quality of life for the remainder of the child's life and providing support for the family. Medical care is provided to whatever level is required, and is particularly geared to symptom control.

4. The child may be cared for at home with the support of a community service provided by either the community paediatric team/Diana nurses or the community children's hospice staff, or any combination of these. Many children prefer this option, but it does depend on the parents' ability to cope and their willingness to care for their child at home. Some parents might feel unhappy about their child actually dying at home, and subsequently move house because they cannot bear to remain there.

Which palliative care category according to ACT[6] is applicable to Nadia's situation?

> Group 3 – progressive conditions without curative treatment options, where treatment is exclusively palliative and may commonly extend over many years. Examples include Batten's disease and mucopolysaccharidosis.

What are the financial implications for the family likely to be after Nadia's death?

Have you considered any of these?

1. The disability living allowance usually stops shortly after the child's death. Many families experience real financial hardship as a result.
2. Sometimes in cases where council accommodation has been specially adapted for a disabled family member, families are required to move out, often at very short notice. All this adds greatly to the stresses that the family is experiencing at the time of bereavement.
3. Good communication between services is essential in order to avoid pre-arranged appointment letters (e.g. for outpatient appointments, equipment or vaccinations) arriving after the death of a child.
4. In the case of Nadia's family, prospective employers might not look very sympathetically at the attendance record of the father. Bereaved employees find returning even to established work quite a challenge. Russell[7] found that 42% of employees indicated that it took between 1 and 6 months to become fully effective at work. They might need to leave work early, or not to attend on 'bad' days, while others develop workaholic tendencies, burying (i.e. denying) their emotions in work. Russell[7] found that in general there is support at work, but this drops off rapidly after 2 or 3 months, by which time it is felt that the bereaved should now be able to manage/pull themselves together. In fact this is quite often the time when the full impact of the death sinks in and more rather than less support is needed.

The National Service Framework

Standard 8 is relevant in relation to the disabled child, and Standard 9 in relation to both Nadia and Prakash. Standard 10 is also relevant, as many medications for children are not yet licensed.

The ACT Care Pathway

Nadia is at the beginning of the third pathway. However, the family as a whole is in the second loop of living through the various stages with both children. Depending on how well the 'sentient' standard (end-of-life plan) was handled when the family was going through this in the terminal stages of Saleem's life, this will either help or hinder them when Nadia enters the 'end-of-life' phase. The ACT pathway requires an end-of-life plan based on the following end-of-life needs and wishes.

For Nadia:

- pain/symptom control (see section on pain assessment below); this includes convulsions and increased secretions
- quality of life/friends
- emotional safety
- spiritual issues
- cultural/religious issues
- funeral planning
- special wishes/memory box.

For family carers:

- practical support
- sibling involvement
- emotional support
- emotional safety
- spiritual issues
- cultural/religious issues
- funeral planning
- grandparents.

Needs and wishes with regard to the environment:

- place of death
- ambience
- place after death.

The Knowledge and Skills Framework

Communication

1. Communication here is the key element, particularly communication with the family, to ensure that care is negotiated. Communication with Nadia needs careful consideration, and probably the involvement of someone experienced in communication with children in Nadia's situation.
2. When caring for a child with a rare disorder, networking is vitally important to ensure that knowledge can be shared and so benefit children and their families. This helps both children and families with the same condition and healthcare professionals to avoid feeling isolated or out of their depth. The use of the Internet in this context is discussed later in this chapter.
3. Is there an agreed policy on how a 'do not resuscitate' decision should be implemented by the professionals involved? What would the position be for paramedics caring for Nadia?

Health, safety and security

1. For a child who is being cared for at home, this must include an assessment of the caregivers' ability to care for the child at home, and the stresses to which they are subject.
2. Is the environment safe? Is all equipment updated with the changing needs of the child (allowing for changes in growth and weight as well as an increasing level of disability)?
3. Is the risk assessment followed through (including the demonstration of safe moving and handling techniques by Nadia's family)?
4. Would it be possible to evacuate the child safely in an emergency?

Service improvement and quality

1. This is a question of quality control. Is the family receiving effective help? Is this reassessed at appropriate intervals?
2. How can the service be improved in the light of NSF requirements as well as new evidence?

Equality and diversity

This involves assessment of the needs in relation to equality and diversity, and seeking advice as appropriate (e.g. liaison health visitor specialising in working with families from diverse ethnic backgrounds, interpreter service).

Contemporary issues in palliative care for children in relation to neurologically degenerative illness

Pain assessment in the child with severe neurological impairment

According to the Paediatric Pain Profile website,[8] severe physical and learning impairment is a feature of many chronic and disabling conditions in children, with many potential sources of pain.

- Pain may arise from the disease process itself (e.g. neuropathic pain or muscle spasm), be secondary to the disease (e.g. musculoskeletal pain or pain from reflux oesophagitis) or be incidental (e.g. toothache or otitis media).
- However, because these children have difficulty in communicating their pain, it can go unrecognised and untreated.
- It is often the child's behaviour, rather than their verbal report, which has to be interpreted to determine whether they have pain.
- Because it can sometimes be difficult for parents and healthcare professionals to distinguish which behaviours do indicate pain and to follow the progress of pain-relieving treatments, a pain assessment scale has been developed specifically for this population of children.
- The compilers of the Paediatric Pain Profile have given their permission for pages of the profile to be photocopied and used in the care of children with severe neurological and learning impairments.

The clinical validation of this tool has been described by Hunt et al.[9] Carter et al.[10] explored the ways in which parents of children with profound special needs assess and manage their children's pain. Moffatt[11] has also presented a useful discussion on pain assessment in children with learning disability. The issue of pain is discussed further in Chapter 12.

Childhood dementia

There is a paucity of evidence about the emotional experience and needs of children with impaired/deteriorating cognitive ability. The only material that could be found was that on SeeAbility's website.[1]

This is an extremely important aspect of care delivery for children with neurologically degenerative illnesses, and further research is urgently needed. The reader is advised to consult the full article, but the salient points can be summarised as follows.

- The child will experience cognitive problems with gradual onset, which will affect performance at school, attention span and concentration as well as communication. In the early stages the child will find it difficult to learn new things as memory function, and the ability to store and retrieve information, become affected. The child may act irrationally, appear incoherent and seem to lose his or her grip on reality. Rapid deterioration may lead to irritability.
- In contrast to mental handicap, which children are born with and where development does occur, albeit at a slower rate, children with dementia are 'normal' until a certain age and then start to deteriorate – they do not develop. Dementia is gradual and irreversible, and it leads to deterioration in learning ability, social skills and emotional development. The child still has memories, but they are often vague.
- The child will experience emotional and psychological symptoms.

  - These children know what is normal and what is expected of them, but they are often unable to make their bodies act as they want them to.
  - They are growing up physically and emotionally but have to contend with deteriorating mental and bodily functions. This leads to frustration.
  - The deterioration of mental and bodily functions can lead to 'confusion, irritability, fluctuating mood change, and a loss of a grip on reality.'
  - They may suffer from fear of death and dying and anxieties caused by their continuing regression and loss of mental and bodily functions. Their experiences of hallucinations may also cause considerable anxiety.
  - Failing eyesight, epileptic fits, physical deterioration and communication problems can all lead to aggression towards parents, carers and anyone else with whom they come into contact.
  - Hallucinations in adult patients with Batten's disease seem to be related to the epileptic pattern of the individual.

No information on the link between epileptic fits and hallucinations could be identified in relation to children, and this area requires further research. When dealing with a particularly distressed child, the possibility that they are experiencing hallucinations should be explored.

Bartiméus

Bartiméus[12] is a Centre of Expertise in NCL (neuronal ceroid lipofuscinoses), a group of rare, hereditary, neurodegenerative diseases that are characterised by progressive visual loss, physical and mental deterioration, epilepsy and premature death. The centre opened in 2001, and aims to combine and further develop expertise and experience in the field of NCL, to participate in and initiate scientific research, and to stimulate innovations in the care of people with NCL.

The NCL Centre of Expertise has a national and international function. It cooperates with patients' associations, organisations for people with a visual impairment, and universities.

- It offers advice and consultations (either face to face or by telephone or email) on an individual basis.

- It refers patients and relatives to experts in the local area for guidance in the field of education, care and provision of services.
- It organises theme days for parents and relatives.
- It organises seminars for healthcare professionals.
- It provides information in the form of leaflets, books, contact addresses and websites.

An enquiry at Bartiméus as to how the centre addresses the issue of childhood dementia led to the following communication:

> The question of how much a child with Batten's disease is aware of his/her situation is very intriguing. Mostly, a child reacts to events and situations according to his (developmental) age. This also applies to the visual handicap, the epilepsy, loss of motor skills and so on that will occur in the life of a child with Batten's disease. Initially the child develops normally and will continue to do so more or less for some time, but gradually they will become multiply handicapped.
>
> It is important during the process to give the child an education and care that is as normal as possible for as long as possible. For instance, if there is a death of a grandparent in the family, the child who is 8 or 10 years old can ask questions about his own death. The parents will then be thinking of the short life expectancy of their child. It is important to be honest, but you need not give more information then the child asks for. He or she is not aware of this short life span. An answer like 'Everyone will die one day, but you never know when or how exactly you will die' will satisfy most children of that age.
>
> During the illness you will have to recognise feelings of anxiety or depression and afford support and comfort, and this is not always easy.
>
> During the declining process the perspective of the child will become smaller, because in the process their cognitive skills will also decrease. In a way this makes it easier for the child (but not for the family!) to deal with the situation.
>
> How about a child with Batten's disease who has an older sibling with the same disease? In my experience I have learned that children will ask questions like 'Will the same happen to me?' – for example, 'Will I need a wheelchair like my brother/sister?'
>
> Sometimes the child will be angry or afraid of what might happen. We tend to be honest and answer 'Well, yes, when you can't walk any more we have a wheelchair for you, so you will be able to get where you want.' On the other hand, we stress that each child is different, and say 'Your brother/sister is a different person.' Each child has their own needs, and it is important that the child experiences being treated as an individual and gets the supports they need.
>
> If a younger child experiences the death of an older sibling, it can be very hard for them. Then it is very important to have an answer, in line with the (religious) background of the family, about what happens after death. A belief in an everlasting life in heaven can be very comforting, especially when the child is told that their brother/sister no longer suffers from their illness and is no longer in pain.
>
> Janneke van Wageningen (personal communication, 2005)

Restraining children

For a small number of children and young people who are receiving palliative care, restraining is an issue. These children appear to have no insight into their behaviour and are seen to be a danger to themselves, as their behaviour results in self-harm. This can be very serious. For example, the author recalls two children who had a rare syndrome and who would bite their limbs if they could reach them with their mouth. Both children had in the past done considerable damage to their hands, and as a result they had undergone partial amputations of fingers on both hands.

The Royal College of Nursing[13] has published guidelines on restraining, holding still and containing children and young people. This document also refers to Department of Health[14] guidance on caring for people with learning disabilities. Several principles for good practice are outlined, such as using restraint as a last resort, considering the legal implications, openness about who decides what is in the child's best interest, having a clear mechanism that allows staff to be heard if they disagree with the decision, a policy that is relevant to the particular setting, adequate staffing levels, and wherever possible agreeing with the child and parent and ensuring parental presence. Sometimes children are restrained at night with the use of harnesses (e.g. in the child's own home), which might come to light during assessment when a child receives respite care. Often parents request that this practice is continued to ensure continuity or due to fear that the child might come to harm. This leaves the staff who are caring for the child with a real dilemma.

Although it focuses on care of the elderly, the Royal College of Nursing has produced further discussion and guidelines on restraint[13] that might be helpful, as they relate to a client group who might be viewed as needing protection from themselves. Aveyard *et al.*[15] warn of the risk of abusing the client by using restraint, and Watson[16] states that it should be obvious that restricting someone's movement against their wishes is entirely wrong in almost all circumstances.

Regular risk assessment here is vital, as are adequate staffing levels. A good knowledge of the range and use of available special beds can keep children and young people safe in a minimally restricted environment. These resources are expensive, and funding is difficult if such care is needed infrequently. Collaboration and sharing with other units might be an option. If there is concern about the child's management in their own home, the action required might be a risk assessment of the home and the supervision that the parents can provide for their child over a 24-hour period. If an appropriate special bed would eliminate the need for the use of harnesses, this resource should be provided for the child.

Regular risk assessment also helps to identify when a child's behaviour changes and the need for restraint no longer exists.

Because our evidence base for both childhood dementia and targeted use of complementary therapies is limited, we may not at present be utilising a comprehensive range of appropriate methods for supporting these very vulnerable children effectively. Aveyard *et al.* suggest a number of approaches for dealing with challenging behaviour (focused on adults), such as the following:

- a biographical approach to care planning
- reality orientation
- a validation approach (in which the carer acknowledges the feelings and emotions that are being experienced and accepts them without judgement)
- multi-sensory environments
- music therapy
- relaxation
- massage
- aromatherapy
- reminiscence
- occupational activities
- exercise
- counselling
- environmental awareness.

Further research is needed to evaluate and validate these approaches.

The National Study of Progressive Intellectual and Neurological Deterioration (PIND study)

Devereux *et al.*[17] have reported the findings of the PIND study. Although this study was initiated to identify children with variant Creutzfeldt–Jakob disease (vCJD) (*see* Chapter 12), information about the causes of progressive intellectual and neurological deterioration and the geographical distribution of cases is also being obtained.

- Orange surveillance cards were sent out monthly to paediatricians in the UK asking whether or not they had seen children with conditions that are currently under surveillance (for a description of the different categories, *see* Chapter 12).
- Of 1400 children who were referred, 798 were included in the study:

  - 577 children had a confirmed underlying diagnosis that was not vCJD
  - 6 children had definite or probable vCJD
  - 51 children had undiagnosed progressive intellectual and neurological deterioration, but not vCJD
  - 164 children were under investigation.

- The five most frequently diagnosed causes of progressive intellectual and neurological deterioration in the UK were found to be:

  - Sanfilippo disease
  - adrenoleukodystrophy
  - late infantile neuronal ceroid lipofusinosis
  - mitochondrial cytopathy
  - Rett syndrome.

- In some districts there were unexpectedly high numbers of cases of progressive intellectual and neurological deterioration with a mix of underlying diagnoses.
- In the five districts with the largest numbers of such cases, the children belonged to a particular ethnic group (see below).
- Geographical distribution has identified resource implications in terms of diagnostic facilities and service provision for complex needs as well as the need for genetic counselling in cases of neurological degenerative disease.

This article on the PIND study is also useful for gaining insight into how national and international studies can be set up and conducted, and the need for cooperation and keeping up the momentum, especially in longitudinal studies.

Children from different ethnic populations: culturally competent care in action

The PIND study by Devereux *et al.*[17] has identified the ethnic origin of 736 affected children. Of these, 487 children were white. The next largest group consisted of Pakistani children. The study found that the distribution of ethnic groups in some districts varied. There was a large cluster in Bradford, where 42 of the affected children came from within the Pakistani community.

Morton *et al.*[18] found that the rate of consanguinity in the Pakistani population in Bradford is 50%, whereas in their local Pakistani population the rate is 60%. Occasionally in this sample, couples are double-first cousins (i.e. they have the same four grandparents). Morton *et al.* concluded that consanguinity is therefore a likely explanation for the high incidence of autosomal-recessive diseases.

Watt and Norton[19] assert that 'race' carries a burden of historical and prejudicial connotations and is insufficiently precise for discussing how genetic factors can influence the prevalence of certain diseases within different populations. This idea is explored in the context of Leininger's statement that human beings possess cultural characteristics which shape and guide their behaviour in different ways.[20] Ryan *et al.*[21] state that in order to avoid gaps in the healthcare system, professionals need to find ways to care for individuals that do not conflict with clients' beliefs and values. Putting this in the context of the local setting, Morton *et al.*[18] listed the following action points.

- An interpreter service alone fails to meet health needs in the area of disability.
- Services need to research the specific needs of the local ethnic communities.

  - It was found that in these researchers' local community there was low uptake of respite care facilities, which could not be attributed to the presence of extended family support in Asian communities. In this particular case this has led to extra funding by the local authority for two part-time individuals who now work with the local parent support group.
  - Genetic guidance can be difficult, as individuals from ethnic minorities are proportionally under-represented in genetic clinics. This was thought to be a result of under-referral, but was found to be due to the reluctance of Pakistani families to ask for a referral, as well as non-attendance due to fear. This situation has been resolved by the appointment of a Pakistani doctor and use of a field worker.
  - Many families had been unaware that consanguinity was implicated, and if they had known about it would have wanted genetic advice earlier.
  - The authors presented the results of this study to leading members of the community, who have given a positive response and are now planning a series of sessions on the issues raised.

Clinical governance and suggestions for work-based learning and networking

Explore with your colleagues how the NSF and the ACT Care Pathway can be implemented in your working environment in relation to Nadia and her family. What are the difficulties? How can they be overcome? Departments usually have members of staff who have a designated role and/or special interest (e.g. nurse on children's ward, play specialist (some units organise siblings' weekends), schoolteacher, community nurse, member of the care team at the local children's hospice, funeral directors, bereavement centre that covers chaplaincy, patient services, mortuary, funerals, etc.).

- Discuss with colleagues who have cared for a child in the terminal stages of a chronic illness how they felt about any decisions to withhold further active treatment.
- How was such a decision communicated to the rest of the staff?
- How was the care organised?
- Were other children and their families aware that a child on the ward was dying?
- How were the staff dynamics affected?
- What are the procedures followed after the death of a child (e.g. laying out of the body)? How are junior members of staff in particular guided and supported through these?
- What are the arrangements for family members to see the child?
- Can parents participate in 'laying out' the child if they wish to do so?
- How are children transported to the mortuary?
- How easy is it to comply with parental wishes (e.g. parents wishing to take the child home)?
- What are the arrangements for collecting the death certificate, etc.? It might be useful to include colleagues from other departments in this and to visit the mortuary/patient services/social work department from the perspective of 'a patient's journey.'
- Contact bereavement/support groups such as Compassionate Friends, the Child

Bereavement Trust, etc.
- How is support organised locally for parents who have lost a child?
- How can interpreters and community leaders be accessed?
- Explore the different cultural beliefs about death and dying and find out within in your work setting you can access this information.

Draw up a workable care plan for Nadia and her family based on Pathway 3.

Now reflect on the implications for families who have more than one child affected by a life-limiting illness, and how this can be accommodated as a plan of care is formulated using Pathways 1 and 2.

Consider all of the players involved in this situation.

Nadia:
The mother:
The father:
Prakash:
Nurses on the children's ward:
Doctors on the children's ward:
Physiotherapist:
Play specialist:
Healthcare assistants:
Teacher from special needs school:
Social worker:
Family support worker:
Interpreter:

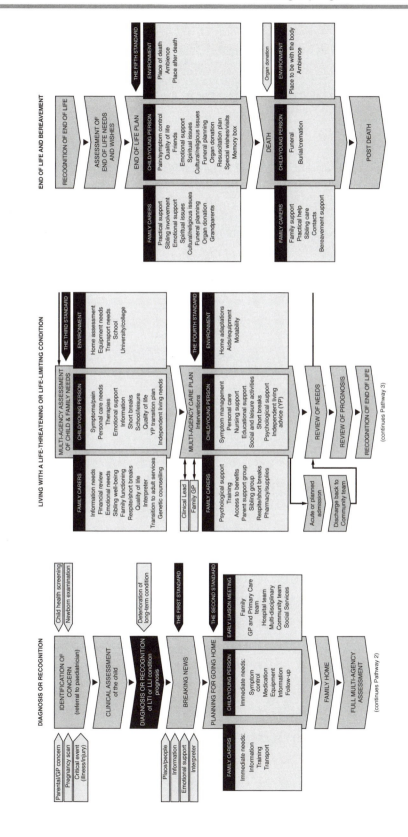

DIAGNOSIS OR RECOGNITION

Parental/GP concern
Pregnancy scan
Critical event (illness/injury)

Child health screening
Newborn examination

IDENTIFICATION OF CONCERN (referral to paediatrician)

CLINICAL ASSESSMENT of the child

Deterioration of long-term condition

DIAGNOSIS OR RECOGNITION of LTI or LLI condition prognosis

THE FIRST STANDARD

BREAKING NEWS

Place/people
Information
Emotional support
Interpreter

THE SECOND STANDARD

PLANNING FOR GOING HOME

EARLY LIAISON MEETING
Family
GP and Primary Care team
Hospital team
Multi-disciplinary team
Community team
Social Services

CHILD/YOUNG PERSON
Immediate needs:
Symptom control
Medication
Equipment
Information
Follow-up

FAMILY CARERS
Immediate needs:
Information
Training
Transport

FAMILY HOME

FULL MULTI-AGENCY ASSESSMENT

(continues Pathway 2)

LIVING WITH A LIFE-THREATENING OR LIFE-LIMITING CONDITION

MULTI-AGENCY ASSESSMENT OF CHILD & FAMILY NEEDS

THE THIRD STANDARD

ENVIRONMENT
Home assessment
Equipment needs
Transport needs
School
University/college

CHILD/YOUNG PERSON
Symptoms/pain
Personal care needs
Therapies
Emotional support
Information
Short breaks
School/leisure
Quality of life
YP transition plan
Independent living needs

FAMILY CARERS
Information needs
Financial review
Emotional needs
Sibling well-being
Family functioning
Respite/short breaks
Quality of life
Interpreter
Transition to adult services
Genetic counselling

MULTI-AGENCY CARE PLAN
Interventions

THE FOURTH STANDARD

ENVIRONMENT
Home adaptations
Aids/equipment
Motability

CHILD/YOUNG PERSON
Symptom management
Personal care
Nursing support
Educational support
Social and leisure activities
Short breaks
Psychological support
Independent living advice ('YP')

Clinical Lead
Family GP

FAMILY CARERS
Psychological support
Training
Access to benefits
Parent support group
Sibling group
Respite/short breaks
Pharmacy/supplies

Acute or planned admission

Discharge back to Community team

REVIEW OF NEEDS

REVIEW OF PROGNOSIS

RECOGNITION OF END OF LIFE

(continues Pathway 3)

END OF LIFE AND BEREAVEMENT

RECOGNITION OF END OF LIFE

ASSESSMENT OF END OF LIFE NEEDS AND WISHES

THE FIFTH STANDARD

ENVIRONMENT
Place of death
Ambience
Place after death

END OF LIFE PLAN

CHILD/YOUNG PERSON
Pain/symptom control
Quality of life
Friends
Emotional support
Spiritual issues
Cultural/religious issues
Funeral planning
Organ donation
Resuscitation plan
Special wishes/visits
Memory box

FAMILY CARERS
Practical support
Sibling involvement
Emotional support
Spiritual issues
Cultural/religious issues
Funeral planning
Organ donation
Grandparents

Organ donation

ENVIRONMENT
Place to be with the body
Ambience

DEATH

CHILD/YOUNG PERSON
Funeral
Burial/cremation

FAMILY CARERS
Family support
Practical help
Sibling care
Contacts
Bereavement support

POST DEATH

Summary

This chapter has considered the needs of the child with a neurological degenerative disease and their family. While aspects of care for technology-dependent children are discussed further in Chapters 4, 5, 6, 7 and 11, contemporary issues in this chapter have focused on childhood dementia, pain assessment, exploring further topics pertaining to ethnicity, and the PIND study.

SWOT

It might be useful to revisit the SWOT analysis at this point in order to determine any further learning needs in relation to this chapter and the Knowledge and Skills Framework (KSF) requirements, namely:

1. communication
2. personal and people development
3. health, safety and security
4. service improvement
5. quality
6. equality and diversity.

Strengths	Weaknesses
Opportunities	Threats

Action plan for further learning

References

1. SeeAbility; www.seeability.org/research/ssjb02/ss_jbatdoc.htm
2. Yoos H (1994) Children's illness concepts: old and new paradigms. *Pediatr Nurs.* **20:** 134–40.
3. Brown E (1999) *Loss, Change and Grief: an educational perspective.* David Fulton Publishers, London.
4. Hockenberry M, Wilson D, Winkelstein M *et al.* (2003) *Wong's Nursing Care of Infants and Children.* Mosby, St Louis, MO.
5. Elston S (2003) *Assessment of Children with Life-Limiting Conditions and their Families: a guide to effective care planning.* ACT, Bristol.
6. Association for Children with Life-Threatening or Terminal Conditions and their Families (ACT) and the Royal College of Paediatrics and Child Health (2003) *A Guide to the Development of Children's Palliative Care Services.* ACT, Bristol.
7. Russel K (1998) Returning to work after a bereavement. *Bereavement Care.* **17:** 11–13.
8. Paediatric Pain Profile; www.ppprofile.org.uk/index.htm
9. Hunt A, Mastroyannopoulou K, Goldman A *et al.* (2003) Not knowing – the problem of pain in children with severe neurological impairment. *Int J Nurs Stud.* **40:** 171–83.
10. Carter B, McArthur E and Cunliffe M (2002) Dealing with uncertainty: parental assessment of pain in their children with profound special needs. *J Adv Nurs.* **38:** 449–57.
11. Moffat V (2000) *Pain Assessment in Children with Learning Disabilities. Focus on update 7.* National Board for Nursing, Midwifery and Health Visiting for Scotland, Edinburgh.
12. Bartiméus; www.bartimeus.nl/NCL
13. Royal College of Nursing (2003) *Restraining, Holding Still and Containing Children and Young People. Guidance for nursing staff;* www.rcn.org.uk
14. Department of Health (2002) *Guidance for Restrictive Physical Intervention: how to provide safe services for people with learning disabilities and spectrum disorder.* The Stationery Office, London.
15. Aveyard B, Naldrett T, Moore S *et al.* (2004) *Restraint Revisited: rights, risks and responsibility. Guidance for nursing staff.* Royal College of Nursing, London; www.rcn.org.uk
16. Watson R (2002) Assessing the need for restraint in older people. *Nurs Older People.* **14:** 31–2.
17. Devereux G, Stellitano L, Verity C *et al.* (2004) Variations in neurodegenerative disease across the UK: findings from the national study of progressive intellectual and neurological deterioration (PIND). *Arch Dis Child.* **89:** 8–12.
18. Morton R, Sharma V, Nicholson J *et al.* (2002) Disability in children from different ethnic populations. *Child Care Health Dev.* **28:** 87–93.
19. Watt S and Norton D (2004) Culture, ethnicity, race: what's the difference? *Paediatr Nurs.* **16:** 37–42.
20. Leininger M (1978) *Transcultural Nursing: concepts, theories, research and practices.* John Wiley & Sons, New York.
21. Ryan M, Hodson Carlton K and Ali N (2000) Transcultural nursing concepts and experiences in nursing curricula. *J Transcult Nurs.* **11:** 300–7.

Chapter 9

A cognate child with end-stage renal disease

This chapter covers

Content	Relevant to other areas of palliative care for children and young people
Scenario	
• Relevant features of cystinosis • Setting the scene • The National Service Framework • The ACT Care Pathway • The Knowledge and Skills Framework	• This chapter: all of the contemporary issues explored here have relevance to other chapters
Contemporary issues	**Relevant topics in other chapters**
• Facilitating communication with a life-limited child • Young people as healthcare consumers • The minefield of compliance • Health and wellbeing of carers • Body image and sexuality in childhood	• Chapter 2: emotional safety during adverse events • Chapter 4: place of care • Chapter 4: sudden serious illness – organ transplants • Chapter 5: the adolescent with cancer • Chapter 6: the transition to early adulthood – genetic disease • Chapter 8: financial and workplace issues
Related to cognate children experiencing degenerative disease	• Chapter 10: technology-dependent children • Chapter 11: congenital complex disability – respite care
• Contemporary issues in palliative care for children and young people in relation to the cognate young person • Clinical governance and suggestions for work-based learning and networking • Summary	• Chapter 11: social care and schooling • Chapter 12: coping and being present • Chapter 12: treatment decisions • Chapter 13: 'letting go'

Relevant features of cystinosis

Cystinosis is an autosomal-recessive disease that affects 1 in 100,000–200,000 live births. It is caused by the abnormal accumulation of cystine within various tissues. The nephropathic forms of cystinosis are associated with multi-organ damage, particularly progressive renal failure leading to dialysis and/or renal transplantation. To date, the only specific treatment for the nephropathic forms of cystinosis is cysteamine, which lowers intracellular cystine levels, thereby reducing the rate of progression of renal failure and significantly diminishing damage to other organs.[1,2] Early complications include corneal crystals, poor growth, hypothyroidism and nephrocalcinosis. Late complications include myopathy, swallowing difficulties, pancreatic endocrine and exocrine insufficiency, retinal blindness, male hypogonadism, decreased pulmonary function and neurological deterioration.[3] Cysteamine is unpleasant to take and causes gastrointestinal upset in many patients, but must be taken every 6 hours to have maximal effect. Despite its availability in capsule form for older children and the use of gastric acid inhibitors, there is a major problem with compliance, especially in adolescence.[4] Further information can be obtained from the websites of the Cystinosis Foundation UK[5] and the National Organization for Rare Disorders.[6]

Setting the scene

Luke is 9 years old and suffers from cystinosis. He has had two failed renal transplants and is currently on peritoneal dialysis. His 6-year-old sister Maika also suffers from the disease and is awaiting her first renal transplant, and at present she too is on peritoneal dialysis.

Luke's diagnosis followed a nearly fatal attack of diarrhoea and vomiting as an infant. Since then he has had a very difficult time. Cysteamine was commenced soon after diagnosis, but Luke has never been able to tolerate the drug and was soon vomiting in anticipation of his 6-hourly cysteamine treatment. Despite the fact that his parents were very motivated, the amount of medication that Luke received was haphazard, and the treatment was discontinued after he developed an ulcer despite taking acid-inhibiting medication. He is now in the terminal stages of renal failure, and dialysis is no longer considered to be an option, due to complications.

Maika has not had quite such serious problems as her brother, as she was diagnosed and commenced treatment soon after birth. She is coping remarkably well on cysteamine, so long as it is given in copious amounts of chocolate syrup – which then has to be incorporated as a 'trade-off' when she has her peritoneal dialysis. However, a urinary tract infection at the age of 4 years has also resulted in renal failure.

Both Luke and Maika and their parents regularly visit the local children's hospice to give the parents respite from eight daily cycles of peritoneal dialysis. When the children are at home the paediatric community nurse visits on a daily basis, and the local church community has a roster to help out with daily chores. The family derive great comfort from their Christian faith. The parents were both in their forties when they met, and considered it a blessing when Luke and Maika came along at that stage in their lives.

The parents are well aware that many cystinosis sufferers can live well into adulthood and might even have children. They are aware that this is not a likely outcome for Luke, and that despite the better prognosis she has now, Maika also faces an uncertain future.

Luke is a very intelligent and thoughtful child, and is fully aware that he is not very well. He has recently started to ask questions pertaining to his prognosis, such as 'I know I have bad kidneys and the doctors can give me new kidneys. But what will happen when the cystinosis is going to affect my brain?'

Jot down your initial reaction to this situation.

<table>
<tr><td></td></tr>
<tr><td></td></tr>
<tr><td></td></tr>
</table>

Does this bring back memories of a situation you have encountered?

Does this help or hinder?

All these reactions are normal.

SWOT

What are your personal learning needs when considering this scenario? They could look similar to those in the chart opposite.

There might be issues that you wish to explore, in which case feel free to do so, but also think about the following.

The National Service Framework

All of the following sections of the Children's NSF are relevant: Standard 8: Disabled and young people and those with complex needs; Standard 9: The mental health and psychological well-being of children and young people; Standard 4: Growing up into adulthood.

The NSF for Renal Services

Part One[7] focuses on dialysis and transplantation, and Part Two[8] focuses on chronic kidney disease, acute renal failure and end-of-life care for both children and adults.

Each standard stipulates the outcomes for children, young people and adults, and cites markers of good practice, highlighting where these differ for children and young people compared with adult provision.

The ACT Care Pathway

The various sections of the NSF can easily be applied to and incorporated in the ACT Care Pathway.

Strengths	Weaknesses
• We have a well-established multi-disciplinary team with regular multi-disciplinary meetings between inpatient, transplant and outreach and psychology services. • This means that on the whole we have an excellent rapport with the families we support, as there is effective communication all round.	• I have always expected that it would be the psychologist who had 'deep' conversations with a child. I tend to shy away from encouraging a child to talk about the eventual outcome of their disease. • I find it very hard to understand why some children do not get their medication regularly, especially when the family is aware of the consequences of non-compliance.
Opportunities	Threats
• I can utilise clinical supervision to explore with an experienced member of staff how to deal with children's questions. • I have negotiated to spend some time with the psychology services and the play specialist so that I can become more alert to cues that children might give about their fears, and how to deal with them.	• In a way I feel as a children's nurse it is expected that I would have this knowledge already, and I feel vulnerable. • Although I can prepare in theory, I still dread having to deal with reality.

The Knowledge and Skills Framework

The requirements are as follows:

1. communication
2. personal and people development
3. health, safety and security
4. service improvement
5. quality
6. equality and diversity.

These can be mapped against NSF requirements within the concept of multi-disciplinary teamwork. The emphasis must be on clear communication and coordination via a key worker.

There might be issues that you wish to explore, in which case feel free to do so, but also think about the following.

What are the issues that each family member is likely to be grappling with at this time?

Have you considered any of these?

1. The parents have had to live with their children's situation for a very long time. They might find it increasingly difficult to deal with the physical restrictions on their daily life as well as answering the children's questions.

2. As Maika becomes older, she is also becoming increasingly aware of her situation and the fact that her illness is likely to take a similar course to that of her older brother. She is not only preparing for the loss of her brother, but also in many ways experiencing what is likely to happen to her.

3. Both children are experiencing serious challenges to their development. Life-limited children usually have the same wishes and aspirations as their healthy peers. The challenge for effective care is to facilitate children's fulfilment of their ambitions. This can range from leading a fairly normal life, doing well at school and finishing their exams to rather more 'special' dreams of a trip with their family, etc.

4. Luke has reached the 'formal operational' stage of his cognitive development (for further information on cognitive development, the reader is referred to a developmental text such as that by Bee and Boyd[9]) and has the ability to think through issues at an adult level of comprehension, although he lacks the level of experience that an adult brings to thinking through a situation. Both children are fortunate in the sense that their parents have always been completely open about their situation and have been totally supportive of them.

What are the children likely to understand about their illness at the ages of 9 and 6 years? Is this likely to differ from the understanding of their peers at school?

Have you considered the following?

Luke is at the 'formal operational' stage, as mentioned above. Maika has reached the 'concrete operational' stage.[9] Both children will have considerable knowledge of illness and might discuss illness and death, and cystinosis in particular, in quite a matter-of-fact way. Both of them will be aware of and have made friends with children in hospital who have subsequently died. It is important to remember that although both children will be wise beyond their years with regard to illness, they cannot be expected to be equally advanced in other aspects of their lives.

How can both children be assisted in exploring and coming to terms with their likely disease progress and inevitable death?

Have you considered any of these?

1. The most important principle here is honesty. Hockenberry *et al.*[10] assert that although giving truthful answers is usually the most difficult option, it lessens many conflicts that would arise later from lies, half-truths or conspiracies. Although this approach will lead to more questions being asked in the future, it also fosters trust.
2. Hockenberry *et al.* warn that being told the truth might prompt other distressing questions, such as 'Am I going to die?', and they stress the need to leave room for hope. Hope is redirected from care to comfort.
3. Honesty leaves room for negotiation, letting the child determine how much they want to know (e.g. 'Do you want us to tell you everything, even if the news is not good?').
4. Edwards and Davis[11] suggest that negotiation takes place both with the child and with the carer with regard to what information is given, how and by whom. This is updated and revised as necessary over time to meet the changing needs of the child.

What are the priorities in providing palliative care for this family unit?

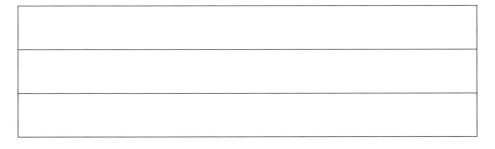

Have you considered any of these?

1. This can probably be best addressed by the 11 recommendations of the Association for Children with Life-Threatening or Terminal Conditions and their Families (ACT) and the Royal College of Paediatrics and Child Health.[12]

    Every child and family should expect to:

    1. Receive a flexible service according to a care plan which is based on individual assessment of their needs, with reviews at appropriate intervals. Children and families should be included in the process of care planning.
    2. Be provided with appropriate and timely information.
    3. Have their own named key worker to coordinate their holistic care and provide access to appropriate professionals across the network.

4. Have access to a local paediatrician in their home area and have access to a local multi-disciplinary children's palliative care team with knowledge about the whole range of relevant services.
5. Be in the care of an identified lead consultant paediatrician expert in the child's condition.
6. Be supported in the day-by-day management of the child's physical and emotional symptoms and have access to 24-hour care in the terminal stage.
7. Receive help in meeting the needs of parents and siblings, both during the child's illness and during death and bereavement.
8. Be offered a range of regular respite, both in the home and away from home and over varying periods of time. This should include nursing care and symptom management.
9. Have available appropriate supplies of medications, oxygen and specialised feeds, and have all disposable items such as feeding tubes, suction catheters and stoma products supplied regularly, effectively and preferably through a single source.
10. Have access to housing adaptations and specialised equipment for use at home and school, in an efficient and timely manner without recourse to several agencies.
11. Be given assistance in procuring benefits, grants and other financial help.

What palliative care category according to ACT and the Royal College of Paediatrics and Child Health[12] is applicable to both Luke and Maika?

Group 3

Although a successful renal transplant resolves renal problems, children and young people with cystinosis will suffer some neurological impairment which cannot be resolved by a renal transplant. Otherwise cystinosis could be considered to fit into group 1, on the basis that if a renal transplant is successful the person is 'cured.'

Luke is very likely to stay alert to the end of his life. How can a cognate child best be supported through the final stages of life?

Have you considered any of these?

1. Sources[13] describes how as a child confronts impending death, he or she may show signs of preparation. Anticipatory grief is palpable as the child experiences the intensity of separation in its ultimate form. Sadness permeates many departures.

> Thank you for giving me aliveness.
> Six-year-old child quoted by Sources[13]

2. The parents need to know how the child is likely to die. Many adults have never seen anyone die and are terrified by the prospect. They need reassurance that the death will be peaceful, with the symptoms under control. This is discussed in more detail in Chapter 12.

3. Hockenberry *et al.*[10] have provided a very comprehensive care plan for the child who is terminally ill or dying. The following elements are helpful in this scenario:

- nearness of all family members
- answering questions as honestly as possible while maintaining a positive, hopeful approach
- as Luke becomes less able to interact, anticipating questions and providing explanations and reassurance pre-emptively
- encouraging Luke to talk about his feelings as well as providing an outlet for aggression
- structuring the environment to allow for maximum self-control and independence within the limitations of Luke's condition
- ensuring that care is geared to conserving energy (i.e. limiting interventions to essential care and comfort)
- respecting the need for privacy without neglecting the child
- appreciating that symptom control is an essential component of physical and emotional care during the terminal stage
- implementing measures to avoid Luke experiencing loneliness in the terminal stages when he might be unable to communicate (e.g. offering calm reassurance, talking to him even though he might not appear to be awake, avoiding discussing his condition in his presence, orienting him to his surroundings when he is awake, and playing his favourite music and reading him stories).

What extra support is Maika likely to need as her brother deteriorates and dies?

Have you considered any of these?

1. Possibly the most important aspect is to be aware of her needs and alert to cues that

she might give. Children are usually very perceptive of their parents' distress, and Maika might hold back her needs in order to protect her parents.

2. Her fears must be addressed and she should be involved as much as possible with Luke's care. Well-managed terminal care for Luke and a 'good death' will provide Maika with a framework within which she will eventually be able to understand her own situation.

3. She will experience grief for the brother she is losing, and is likely to experience similar feelings that are common in sibling bereavement, such as jealousy of the attention that Luke is getting, and guilt about being alive when her brother is not. She will have to deal with the stress of having a grieving family while knowing that she will suffer the same fate.

4. Her questions should be answered honestly, reinforcing her perception of comforting elements, and ideas that cause her distress must be reality tested.

5. Maika's 'need to know' can be challenging for parents and significant others who are grappling with their own emotions.

6. Edwards and Davis[11] provide a particularly helpful discussion on the needs of the sick child's siblings, although the emphasis is on healthy siblings.

Contemporary issues in palliative care for children and young people in relation to the cognate young person

In children with diseases in this category the disease tends to have an uncertain course. Although the above scenario involves a child who is likely to face death in childhood, many children and young people experience long periods of comparative well-being, allowing them to participate in normal childhood activities. It is therefore pertinent to examine both issues relating to the cognate terminally ill child, and issues that affect families with a child on a long illness trajectory.

Facilitating communication with a life-limited child

Band Aides and Blackboards[14] is a useful website that deals with various aspects of chronic illness.

Rollins[15] studied the stressors of everyday life and disease, the coping strategies that children use to manage the stressors, and the use of drawing to enhance communication. Although this study was conducted on children with cancer, many of the issues identified are likely to affect any child with a chronic life-threatening or life-limiting illness. The participants had little difficulty expressing through drawing what was stressful. Rollins found that more than one child expressed the view that they had never really thought through the experience until they were drawing and talking about it in the interview. Although the children were asked to reflect on their previous experiences, the findings of the study led Rollins to suspect that the opportunity to draw offers children with cancer a chance to appraise a current stressor and the coping resources available to them. The process would therefore help the child to sort out his or her thoughts. The reader is strongly recommended to consult the article, as it depicts and discusses many of the actual drawings made by the children, and the interpretation of these.

With regard to talking to dying children about death, Faulkner[16] has made the following recommendations.

•   Any approach to communication needs to be flexible. Straightforward approaches don't always work with children.

•   Many children communicate best through non-verbal means such as favourite toys, artwork or music. Faulkner cites as an example a 5-year-old who was withdrawn, had been refusing his pain medication and would not let her assess him. The child was happy for his teddy to be examined, but stopped the nurse from palpating teddy's abdomen, asserting 'that hurts him, don't touch it!'

- It was thus possible to establish that teddy would benefit from more painkiller medication, and that the bubble-gum-flavoured one was agreeable to teddy.
- Children might wish to be alone or to share their thoughts. Allow conversation without forcing it.
- Be receptive when a child initiates conversation. There is a need to respond immediately.
- Be specific in your explanations about death. Euphemisms that equate death with sleep or going on a long journey can be very confusing to children.
- A child's life can be complete, even if it is brief. Dying children need to know that they will always be loved and remembered.
- Help the child to find a sense of accomplishment in his or her life.
- Empower the child as much as possible in circumstances concerning their own death.
- The child needs to be reassured that they will experience continued love and physical closeness, adequate symptom relief and involvement in their care.

Young people as healthcare consumers

Research on children as healthcare consumers is addressed in the literature and is beyond the scope of this chapter. Rollins[15] states that there has been a growing awareness and acknowledgement that children have strong feelings about, reactions to, and the right to full participation in events in their lives. Thus, according to Rollins, health-related research on children is shifting from seeking information about children to seeking information directly from them. The Department for Education and Skills[17] has published guidelines for involving children and young people in healthcare policy, service planning, delivery and evaluation. Sloper and Lightfoot[18] investigated the involvement of disabled and chronically ill children and young people in health service development and found that it is at an early stage. These children are likely to be long-term and heavy users of health services, and therefore according to the authors have considerable knowledge and experience of NHS services and much to contribute to service development. A total of 27 initiatives that involved consulting children and young people were reviewed. The processes involved are discussed extensively in Sloper and Lightfoot's article, but can be summarised as follows.

- Consultation resulted in changes to the following services:
  - the hospital environment, including ward decor and recreational facilities (in 7 initiatives)
  - food (4 initiatives)
  - clinic times (2 initiatives)
  - ward routine (4 initiatives).
- The involvement process itself was said to have changed services in four cases by providing increased social contact and peer support for children, and ongoing mechanisms for listening to young patients.
- Changes in service commissioning or priorities included commissioning a home care programme for intravenous drug administration for young people with cystic fibrosis.
- Other changes included the following:
  - better provision of information for children
  - achieving a permanent commitment to involving children
  - extending methods of obtaining children's views
  - setting up a youth club for children with autistic spectrum disorder.
- A total of 13 initiatives reported no change to service provision.

The minefield of compliance

Reading around the subject of cystinosis and the need for treatment that is very unpleasant highlights the issue of compliance. According to Schneider,[4] some preparations of cysteamine smell of rotten eggs and cause gastrointestinal symptoms, and this becomes a cause for teasing in school because the smell affects the child taking the medication. In addition, El-Mekresh[19] estimates that two-thirds of young people over the age of 12 years who have undergone transplantation do not comply with anti-rejection treatment, mainly due to concerns about the effects of the medication on their appearance, such as facial oedema, obesity, acne, short stature and excessive body hair. According to El-Mekresh, non-compliance is more likely among adolescents with disrupted families and minimal family support.

Chapter 5 has explored the demands made on parents to manage their child's treatment, and these demands affect parents across all areas of caring for sick children. Eliciting a young person's feelings about stressors in their lives and empowering them to make informed choices, explaining that it is in their best interest to comply with treatment, and what the consequences will be if they do not comply, logically follow on from the points discussed above.

Hockenberry et al.[10] have suggested a range of useful strategies to improve compliance. These include the following.

- Organisational strategies – adopting treatment schedules that incorporate the treatment plan into daily routine (e.g. physiotherapy or daily bath).
- Educational strategies – recognising that the more knowledge patients have about their disease, the more likely they are to comply with treatment.
- Treatment strategies – assessing whether the timing or the preparation of the treatment can be adjusted so that it suits the family better. Gordon[20] describes 'trade-offs' for children who are sodium and potassium restricted due to poor renal function. For example, to help them to cope with these restrictions, the child may be allowed to have chocolate or a packet of crisps during the first hour of dialysis. What can and cannot be 'traded' will obviously depend on the individual child's electrolyte status and the type of dialysis used.
- Behavioural strategies – these might vary from positive reinforcement to 'time out' and formal contracting with an older child. This might include, for example, agreement that the young person takes their medication before going to school without needing to be reminded, but also agreement that the parents stop nagging the young person!

In the case of families who have lived with the child's illness for a long time, these strategies may have been tried very often, and a stalemate may have been reached. The child and their parents might reach a point where they feel that insistence on treatment is doing more harm than good. These issues need to be addressed in a sympathetic environment, and it is impossible to generalise about the likely outcomes for individual children and families.

For all the scenarios described in this text the outcomes are likely to vary, and regardless of what the outcome is likely to be, everyone involved in the decisions will have to live with it.

So far in this scenario, Luke, Maika and their parents have had to come to terms with the fact that Luke is unable to benefit from what is considered to be the 'gold-standard' treatment for his condition. Meanwhile Maika is following a treatment regime that is demanding both for her and for her parents, and the challenges may increase during the adolescent years ahead.

In the scenario described in Chapter 6, Stuart and his family had a very clear idea of what the outcome of refusal of available treatment would mean for his situation, and Stuart was in a good position to make an informed decision if appropriately supported.

In contrast to this, it has been established that treatment for children with HIV (*see* Chapter 7) is likely to considerably improve both quality and length of life, and that non-compliance with treatment for a young child is likely to result in child protection proceedings. On a practical level, this is not just a matter of personal preference, nor can these issues be resolved by purely legal or ethical reasoning. It is unlikely that heavy-handed decisions will be imposed on families, but rather a careful review of all the different perspectives must be undertaken to establish whether the issue, which might result from total mental and physical exhaustion or depression on the part of either the parent or the young person, can be resolved.

It might become necessary to re-evaluate goals. If a young person's quality of life could be good, but is spoilt by their having a difficult time at school, or struggling with the demands of puberty in addition to everything else, then the goal remains to help them to come through this and to grow into adulthood. The interventions might need to be changed. In this case the goal needs to be set with the young person, the way in which it can be achieved needs to be negotiated, and the factors that hinder this (the experience of schooling and the negative body image) need to be addressed. Ways in which information can be given in a manner that is acceptable to young people have been discussed in Chapter 5.

Gordon[20] states that it is essential to desensitise the condition of a chronically ill child or young person if he or she is to integrate into school. This can be achieved by liaison nurses or community nurses going into the school and educating the child or young person's peers and teachers about the condition and its management. The teachers can then meet the specific requirements that the child or young person might have while at school. For example, Gordon[20] describes how teachers had managed to keep a child in school by putting a beanbag in the library so that the child could have a sleep if they wished to do so. Russell[21] states that the National Service Framework[22] clearly identifies partnership between different agencies as crucial to the improvement of children's life chances and essential for maximising social and educational inclusion for children with disabilities or special healthcare needs. Such cooperation according to Russell can function at different levels, but will offer new opportunities to community nursing services to work in partnership with families and schools.

The health and well-being of the carers: mothers and fathers

Lenton *et al.*[23] examined how non-malignant life-threatening illness in childhood affected families, and found that 54% of mothers and 30% of fathers had mental health problems, while 24% of healthy siblings displayed significant emotional and behavioural problems. Ironically, however, health promotion is not a subject commonly associated with either paediatric or adult palliative care in the literature. Yet according to Porock and Parker Oliver[24] an unspoken assumption of the health service system is that the family caregivers themselves are healthy and able to provide the necessary care. These authors examined the average age of caregivers for adults and found it to be between 50 and 62 years, an age range in which many caregivers are likely to have their own diagnosis of chronic illness and consequently some related fatigue. This age range is likely to correspond to that of many caregivers for children and young people, as many parents now start their families later in life, or may be the main carers for young people with chronic life-limiting illnesses who are well into their twenties and thirties.

Penson *et al.*[25] suggest a comprehensive assessment of caregivers which includes screening of the psychosocial domains with a view to optimising control of symptoms, maintaining psychological integrity and finding meaning in the chaos. The assessment can be summarised as follows.

- What did the illness mean to the caregivers?
- What are their coping styles?

- What is the extent of their social network?
- What are the strengths and weaknesses of their major relationships with healthcare providers?
- What are the major stressors?
- What spiritual resources are available?
- Are there psychiatric vulnerabilities, such as depression, anxiety or drug dependence?

According to Penson et al.,[25] bereavement is associated with a decline in health, inappropriate health service use, increased risk of depression, sleep disruption, increased consumption of tobacco, alcohol and tranquillisers, and increased suicide and death rates. Despite this, Penson et al. found that many individuals received little or no support from healthcare professionals during the bereavement period. Laakso and Paunonen-Ilmonen[26] conducted a study of bereaved mothers in Finland and found that although these women attempted to relieve their grief with alcohol and drugs, they gradually gave these up when their life situation had stabilised. Reading, writing about their feelings, painting and listening to music were also used to help with grief work. Their partners' ability to deal with the child's illness and death was central to the bereavement process of mothers in this study, with relationships being affected both positively and negatively. The father's perspective was only examined through the opinion of the mother, and the fact that fathers generally resumed work sooner than the mothers made the mothers feel lonely.

Wood and Milo[27] examined grief in fathers. Fathers experience a double loss, first when they learn the diagnosis, and then, after months or years of difficult parenting, at the time of death. Although these authors studied fathers whose children had developmental disability, there are many parallels to children with any life-limiting illness. Fathers used greater emotional stoicism and activity, rather than talking or social support, as their primary coping strategy. Many relevant points were raised, and the reader is urged to consult the full text. The four themes that the authors identified can be summarised as follows.

- Fathers use an action orientation for coping with painful feelings and to prevent these feelings from overwhelming them.
- Fathers experience deep feelings of isolation, based first on the child's disability, and then on loss of the child when he or she dies.
- Fathers reported that the source of their grief was often seeing their wives in pain, and they acknowledged significant differences in grieving which they perceived to be based on gender differences.
- Fathers reported a consistent self-identity and world view that influenced their ways of grieving and healing, in contrast to the mothers, who reported significant changes in identity and world view.

Wood and Milo[27] drew the following conclusions.

- Professionals need to dispel the myth that men grieve less for their children by inviting men to participate in conversations about their child's disability and death and their own subsequent bereavement period.
- Professionals need to facilitate and maintain a connection to the father by providing straightforward information, inviting questions and discussion, and acknowledging the difficulty of the situation.
- As these fathers felt that their grief and isolation differed from that experienced by other fathers who had lost a child, discussion groups that specifically target this population may be helpful, especially in view of the fact that the fathers in the study reported that they had found the opportunity to meet each other helpful.
- Fathers had used their workplace for respite both before and after the death. Granting equitable opportunities for mothers and fathers to make use of family medical leave and bereavement leave is an important part of allowing time for healing, and also pro-

tects marriages. Relevant social policy should reflect the needs of fathers.

- Several questions for future research have been identified, including further examination of gender differences, particularly as men are increasingly becoming equal partners or even the primary caregivers in parenting. A cross-generational investigation of men's emotional experience is suggested in the light of social changes towards increased tolerance of disability and also greater willingness by men to articulate their stories of pain as an aspect of their lives. The authors suggest that the concept of 'grieving for my wife' also warrants further illumination.

Penson et al.[25] have identified that skilled end-of-life care includes both the ability to give skilled care and relationship building. It has been demonstrated in Chapter 5 in the section on examining 'place of care' that consideration of these aspects should not be confined to the end of life.

Body image and sexuality in childhood

This topic has been addressed in relation to young people in Chapters 5 and 6. Finnegan[28] explains that socialisation about the topic begins with the baby, continues throughout childhood, and often relies on non-verbal, incidental communication. Interactions with other children (e.g. at nursery) reinforce appropriate and inappropriate behaviours with regard to dress, touch and respect for others. According to Finnegan, intentional socialisation and verbal information often begin in children between the ages of 6 and 9 years, with parents providing much-needed factual information about puberty and reproduction. Black[29] found that definitions of sexuality included concepts such as self-awareness, self-esteem and body image, feelings and emotions, intimacy and relationships. Although it is well recognised that chronic illness influences the development of identity in relation to sexuality, it also affects the younger child, where the effects of treatment or illness may result in the child being seen as different from his or her peers (e.g. the child on cysteamine, who may have a lingering smell from the medication, or the child who may have a puffy appearance due to fluid retention or steroid treatment). Even young children are aware that 'physical perfection and beauty' are valued and defined in society, and Finnegan[28] states that individuals who perceive that their appearance and abilities may be derided or dismissed as undesirable may hesitate to initiate or respond to friendship and attraction. Similarly, peers might shy away from a friendship with a chronically ill child because this might affect their own popularity.

Finnegan[28] explores further aspects of sexuality in relation to disabled teenagers, and this article is relevant reading. A theme that is discussed by both Finnegan[28] and Black[29] is the extent to which parents' wishes not to discuss information relating to sexual matters with their adolescent child can be honoured. There is evidence of sexual behaviour among young people with chronic health problems which suggests that young people do need this information in order to avert negative consequences for their health.

An important point raised by Black[29] is the fact that disabled people are more likely to experience physical, sexual and emotional abuse than individuals from other groups, and the author believes that withholding basic education on the subject makes disabled children and young people more vulnerable to exploitation.

Clinical governance and suggestions for work-based learning and networking

Explore with your colleagues how the NSF and the ACT Care Pathway can be implemented in your working environment in relation to Luke, Maika and their family. What are the challenges? How can they be overcome?

Departments usually have members of staff who have a designated role and/or special inter-

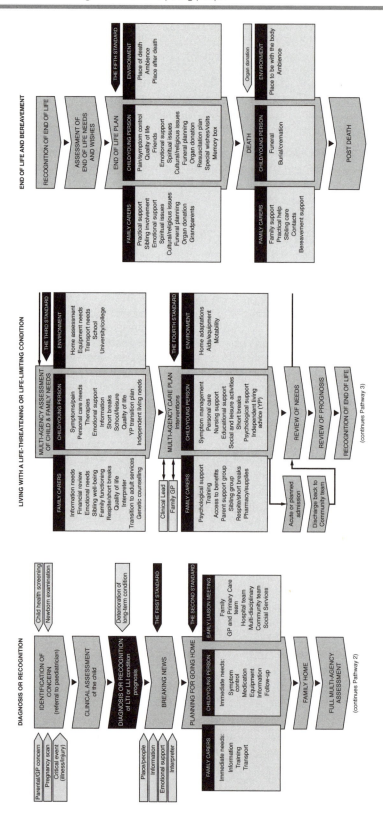

est (e.g. transplant coordinator, renal outreach nurse, member of staff experienced in supporting children and families through organ transplantation, family bereavement counsellor, play specialist (some units organise siblings' weekends), schoolteacher, therapists, chaplaincy, patient services, mortuary, funerals, etc.).

Consider how you could best utilise the ACT Care Pathways here.

Would it be easier to use one set of pathways and mark each member of the family, as well as healthcare professionals and helpers, in relation to each child, or to use one set of pathways for each child? Please make a note on the pathway, using either option, to indicate the point that you believe each player in this scenario has reached.

Luke:
Maika:
Mother (perspective in relation to each child):
Father (perspective in relation to each child):
Community nurse:
Hospital doctors:
Hospital nurses:
Organ transplant coordinator:
Staff at children's hospice:
Local church community:
Luke's peers at school:
Maika's peers at school:
Fellow peers in hospital:

Draw up a workable care plan for both children based on ACT Care Pathway 2.

- To what extent would her experience of Luke's illness require interventions for Maika and her family travelling through Pathway 2?
- To what extent does this pave the way for Pathway 3?

Now look back at Pathway 1.

What would the unique issues have been for this family? Consider this pathway in terms of commissioning services required from the point of diagnosis for both children and their family to facilitate advance planning.

Draw up a workable care plan for Luke based on ACT Care Pathway 3.

Summary

This chapter has considered the needs of a family with two cognate children experiencing degenerative disease who are also heavily dependent on technology. The specific needs of cognate children with life-limiting illness have been discussed in relation to the child experiencing the terminal stage of the illness. Particular consideration has also been given to the sibling who has to deal with the loss of a brother or sister, but who is witnessing a fate that he or she will also eventually have to experience. Contemporary issues identified in this chapter have focused on the long-term consequences for the mental and physical health of the carers, children's involvement in service planning, the use of communicating tools with children, and the ongoing physical and psychosocial/sexual development of young people with long-term health problems.

SWOT

It might be useful to revisit the SWOT analysis at this point (*see* chart opposite) in order to determine any further learning needs in relation to this chapter and the Knowledge and Skills Framework (KSF) requirements, namely:

1. communication
2. personal and people development
3. health, safety and security
4. service improvement
5. quality
6. equality and diversity.

'Presence' exercise

An exercise relating to 'being present with' a person is introduced in Chapter 12 (*see* page 206). It might be useful to consider the issues raised in the context of supporting a family that is experiencing such a complex situation. Reflect on the points raised by Rushton (2006) in relation to picking up on and dealing with issues each family member might be struggling with:

- Am I present in my work?
- When am I most present in my work?
- How does it make me feel?
- What keeps me from being present in my work?

Strengths	Weaknesses
Opportunities	Threats

- How does it make me feel when I am not present in my work?
- What can I do to be more present? Personally? Professionally?
- How can I contribute to making my practice environment more healing?

Action plan for further learning

References

1. Dohil R, Newbury R, Sellers Z *et al.* (2003) The evaluation and treatment of gastrointestinal disease in children with cystinosis receiving cysteamine. *J Pediatr.* **143:** 224–30.
2. Gahl W, Thoene J and Schneider J (2002) Cystinosis. *NEJM.* **347:** 111–21.
3. Kleta R, Bernardini I, Ueda M *et al.* (2004) Long-term follow-up of well-treated nephropathic cystinosis patients. *J Pediatr.* **145:** 555–60.
4. Schneider J (2004) Treatment of cystinosis: simple in principle, difficult in practice. *J Pediatr.* **145:** 436–8.
5. The Cystinosis Foundation UK; www.cystinosis.org.uk
6. National Organization for Rare Disorders; www.rarediseases.org
7. Department of Health (2004) *National Service Framework for Renal Services Part One: dialysis and transplantation.* Department of Health, London.
8. Department of Health (2005) *National Service Framework for Renal Services Part Two: chronic kidney disease, acute renal failure and end-of-life care.* Department of Health, London.
9. Bee H and Boyd D (2005) *Lifespan Development.* Addison-Wesley, Menlo Park, CA.
10. Hockenberry M, Wilson D, Winkelstein M *et al.* (2003) *Wong's Nursing Care of Infants*

and Children. Mosby, St Louis, MO.

11. Edwards M and Davis H (1997) *Counselling Children with Chronic Medical Conditions.* British Psychological Society, Leicester.

12. Association for Children with Life-Threatening or Terminal Conditions and their Families (ACT) and the Royal College of Paediatrics and Child Health (2003) *A Guide to the Development of Children's Palliative Care Services.* ACT, Bristol.

13. Sources B (1996) The broken heart: anticipatory grief in the child facing death. *J Palliat Care.* **12**: 56–9.

14. Band Aides and Blackboards; www.lehman.cuny.edu/faculty/jfleitas/bandaides/

15. Rollins J (2005) Tell me about it: drawing as a communication tool for children with cancer. *J Pediatr Oncol Nurs.* **22**: 203–21.

16. Faulkner K (1997) Talking about death with a dying child. *Am J Nurs.* **97**: 64, 66, 68–9.

17. Kirby P, Lanyon C, Cronin K *et al.* (2003) *Building a Culture of Participation: involving children and young people in policy, service planning, delivery and evaluation.* Department for Education and Skills, Annesley.

18. Sloper P and Lightfoot J (2003) Involving disabled and chronically ill children and young people in health service development. *Child Care Health Dev.* **29**: 15–20.

19. El-Mekresh M (2000) Renal transplantation in children. *British J Urology.* **85**: 979–86.

20. Gordon P (1999) Helping children cope: chronic renal failure. *J Child Health Care.* **3**: 24–6.

21. Russell P (2005) Working in partnership with education. In: A Sidey and D Widdas (eds) *Textbook of Community Children's Nursing* (2e). Elsevier, Edinburgh.

22. Department of Health (2003) *Getting the Right Start: National Service Framework for Children. Standard for hospital services;* www.doh.uk/nsf/children/gettingtherightstart

23. Lenton S, Stallard P, Lewis M *et al.* (2001) Prevalence and morbidity associated with non-malignant, life-threatening conditions in childhood. *Child Care Health Dev.* **27**: 389–98.

24. Porock D and Parker Oliver D (2005) Commentary on Schneider RA (2004) Assessing the fatigue severity scale for use among caregivers of chronic renal failure patients. *J Clin Nurs.* **14**: 1153–4.

25. Penson R, Green K, Chabner B *et al.* (2002) When does the responsibility of our care end? Bereavement. *Oncologist.* **7**: 251–8.

26. Laakso H and Paunonen-Ilmonen M (2001) Mothers' grief following the death of a child. *J Adv Nurs.* **36**: 69–77.

27. Wood J and Milo E (2001) Fathers' grief when a disabled child dies. *Death Stud.* **25**: 635–61.

28. Finnigan A (2004) Sexual health and chronic illness in childhood. *Paediatr Nurs.* **16**: 32–6.

29. Black K (2005) Disability and sexuality. *Paediatr Nurs.* **17**: 34–8.

Chapter 10

Technology-dependent children

This chapter covers

Content	Relevant to other areas of palliative care for children and young people
Scenario	*Relevant to other areas of palliative care for children and young people*

• Relevant information for the scenario
• Setting the scene:
  – Long-term emotional implications
  – Long-term practical implications
  – Safety issues
  – Transporting very sick children
  – 'Normality'
  – Long-term needs of the family
• NSF
• KSF
• ACT Care Pathway
	• Chapter 8: financial consequences
	• Chapter 11: schooling for children with complex needs

	Relevant topics in other chapters
	• Chapter 2: siblings • Chapter 11: respite, social care and schooling
Related to technology-dependent children	
• Contemporary issues in children's palliative care in relation to technology dependence • The National Service Framework pathway • Home versus hospital • *Which* pathway? • A new meaning of 'home' • Respite care • Educational provision for the technology-dependent child • Stem-cell research • Technological interventions for children with Werdnig–Hoffman disease: an ethical dilemma • Clinical governance and suggestions for work-based learning and networking • Summary	

Relevant information for the scenario

The following resources are relevant to this chapter:

*   UK Children on Long-Term Ventilation website[1]
*   *From Hospital to Home* by Noyes and Lewis.[2]

Setting the scene

Vicky had been a normal healthy child, the eldest of four, until 18 months ago at the age of 8 years she was run over on the way home from Brownies. A van had careered out of control and knocked her down on the pavement. Three of her friends were also injured, and the baby sister of one of her friends died at the scene.

Vicky sustained serious head and spinal injuries and was airlifted to the nearest neuro-surgical unit. She suffered a number of intracranial bleeds over the next few months and has now stabilised but is making no real progress. Over the last 6 months it has become obvious that Vicky is going to be ventilator dependent for the rest of her life. She is blind and is paralysed from the neck down (C4). She is attempting to communicate by facial expression, but this is made difficult by a left-sided facial weakness. She has been fed through a gastrostomy tube for many months and is re-learning to take oral food, but it is a struggle as she seems to have lost all sensation of hunger. She is doubly incontinent and has a tendency to suffer from constipation, which triggers urinary retention and has on four previous occasions led to persistent urinary tract infections, so she is now on pro-phylactic antibiotics. Vicky has also had a number of severe chest infections and requires frequent and meticulous physiotherapy.

Vicky's parents have found it very difficult to come to terms with their daughter's situation. They have followed with great interest the progress of actor Christopher Reeve and were hoping – almost expecting – that a breakthrough with research in which he was involved was imminent and that Vicky at some point would have the chance to come off her ventilator and – who knows – maybe walk again. Christopher Reeve's death has had a different effect on each of Vicky's parents. Although Vicky's mother at first reacted with feelings of devastation at having her hopes dashed, Vicky's father has expressed the view that this has helped him to realise that this is how things are for Vicky from now on, and he has thrown his energies into working out the practicalities in preparation for Vicky's homecoming.

The other three children in the family are all under the age of 5 years. Timmy is nearly five and will be starting school next term, and the twins, Tilly and Stevie, are 2 years old.

Jot down your initial reaction to this situation.

Does this bring back memories of a situation you have encountered?

Does this help or hinder?

SWOT

Strengths	Weaknesses
• I enjoy the challenge of caring for highly dependent children and their families.	• I do not know what the arrangements are locally for transporting children in this situation by the ambulance services. • I have not cared for a ventilator-dependent child and have only had opportunities to observe during my training.
Opportunities	Threats
• It gives our team a new challenge. • We can make a big difference to this family. • We can gain and utilise new skills.	• There is a lot to learn in terms of caring for a ventilated child, moving and handling, electric wheelchairs, transporting and creating a 'normal routine' for Vicky. • It will be a big responsibility to care for a child in her own home without being able to just call for assistance.

What are your learning needs when considering this scenario? They could look similar to those in the chart above.

There might be issues that you wish to explore, in which case feel free to do so, but also think about the following.

What are the long-term emotional implications when planning home care for a technology-dependent child?

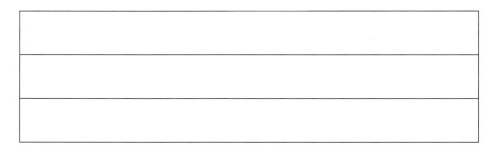

Have you considered any of these?

1. This family has had an extremely disrupted life over the last 18 months. They have been through the emotional roller-coaster of having a critically ill child and being uncertain for a long time whether Vicky would survive. Progress since then has been slow, with the gradual realisation that Vicky will never return to her previous normal self, and in fact will never be able to breathe unaided.

2. The family will have gone through a bereavement process as a result of losing the normal, healthy child they once knew.

3. There will have been considerable strain on this family in terms of the following:

   • the relationship between the parents
   • finances
   • emotional resources
   • logistics.

4. Effective family networks are crucial, and in this family have been put to the test. Members of the extended family might have their own views about the feasibility of Vicky's family taking on her home care and continuing professional support.

5. Life for the siblings will have had to continue as normally as possible, with all of the children requiring quality parental attention and time.

6. The family will now need to plan for a shift in the amount of time and attention that is given to Vicky. She herself probably has only a hazy memory of what home was like and needs careful preparation, hopefully with visits before a permanent transition is made. Units that care for ventilator-dependent young people resist the expression 'home from home', as they feel such a unit can never be a child's home in the same way as their familiar home environment (Perks, personal communication, 2005).

7. The family need to be aware that the initial period after Vicky returns home is likely to be quite difficult, with adjustments being made by the family, Vicky settling back in and the other children adjusting to yet another change in their routine. There will also be 'strangers' in the house 24 hours a day caring for Vicky on her ventilator, which is a major intrusion on the family.

What are the long-term practical implications when planning home care for a technology-dependent child?

Have you considered any of these?

1. Although discharge planning begins at the point of admission, in this situation the end goal will not have been clear 18 months ago when Vicky was admitted to hospital. Uncertainties pertain to the child's medical condition and the effect that this type of life event might have on the family. It is not unheard of for families to break up under

the strain imposed by caring for a critically ill child. Some families feel unable to care for a technology-dependent child at home, and planning for discharge might aim for a residential unit or a foster home. There is a possibility that neither of these options may be available in the foreseeable future.

2. For Vicky, home care is an option. However, if the existing accommodation is unsuitable the family home will need adaptations or the family may need to move house. This in itself is a stressful process, whether it involves selling the present house and buying a new family home, or being rehoused in disabled-adapted council accommodation.

3. According to Widdas *et al.*,[3] there are four principles that underpin the assessment process:

   • the parents are the experts and primary carers
   • the home is the centre of caring
   • assessment should be carried out within the context of family life and the community and culture in which the family lives
   • coordination is needed to produce a single and multi-agency assessment.[4]

4. There are most definitely financial implications. Few families come through a child's critical illness without major financial fallout, which may have implications for mortgages, employment, etc. Chapter 11 explores some of the issues, and more detail can be found in publications by Joy[5] and Langerman and Worrall.[6]

5. Close multi-professional teamwork between Vicky's referral unit and her care group team will be required. A team of carers will need to be trained to become competent in the management of Vicky's ventilator if appropriate, and this is based on a risk assessment and other aspects of her care. It can take several months for a carer to become competent in the management of a ventilator-dependent child. Some carers might be involved on a part-time basis, which will result in much longer lead-in times. Recruitment will take around 3 months, and retention of carers might also be an issue. Support through the GP services can be difficult, as in reality this draws on skills that are not usually required of GPs! Local children's community nursing services need to be secured. These do not operate to a standardised format across the country, and according to Widdas *et al.*[3] this has resulted in individual service models that have evolved around isolated children with complex care needs, and enormous differences in the level of support. For example, Noyes *et al.*[7] have found that this can vary from one night a week to 24-hour nursing care for children with central hyperventilation syndrome.

6. Widdas *et al.*[3] provide an interesting discussion on the legal implications of employing non-nursing support workers.[3] A competency framework is suggested that can be adapted and expanded for individual application according to the individual patient, family and carer, based on principles encompassing areas of concern, required skills and knowledge, and levels of competency. In a cyclical process based on the Kennedy Report,[8] application, maintenance and audit of the system is suggested. Dimond[9] asserts that a National Service Framework for the community care of the sick child should assist professionals in pressing for the necessary resources to ensure high standards. According to Dimond,[9] the legal implications of these statutory changes are that where national evidence of research and standards are not implemented by local providers, parents who claim that their child has suffered harm as a result of this can point to published league tables.

What are the particular safety issues that arise when planning for Vicky's discharge?

Have you considered any of these?

The website of UK Children on Long-Term Ventilation[1] has a comprehensive checklist of factors that need to be considered when making arrangements for discharge. Some of these are listed below as an example of the range of considerations that are needed.

- All-important systems must have a back-up.
- Maintenance contracts.
- Competencies/training.
- Equipment levels.
- Readmission criteria.
- Staffing levels.
- Back-up lighting.
- Power-cut procedures.
- Ambulance procedures.
- Communication systems.
- On-call support.

The risk assessment must then consider the particular circumstances in Vicky's home.

- Is it possible to evacuate Vicky safely from the house in the event of an emergency?
- Can safe levels of supplies such as oxygen and other equipment be stored on the premises?
- Can Vicky be safely transported both in her wheelchair and by car? Are ramps, etc., adequate for her to be able to leave the building safely?
- Are the facilities at Vicky's school adequate with regard to safety?

Widdas et al.[3] cite as good practice an ongoing principle used by the Avon Life-time Service. If there is a chance of a risk being greater than 10%, that event should be actively planned for (e.g. the interruption of the electric power supply, which would cause loss of oxygen flow from an oxygen concentrator and inability to monitor the child visually).

What issues need to be considered when transporting very sick children?

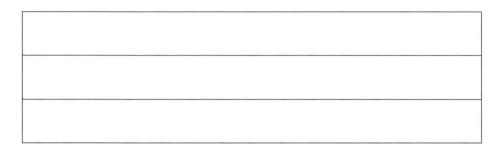

Have you considered any of these?

1. Paramedic staff are obliged to take the child to the nearest hospital in an emergency. The way in which individual arrangements are communicated in different areas varies.
2. At present the same applies to 'do not resuscitate' (DNR) decisions. For example, in one area the possibility of a 'gold card' is under discussion. It is envisaged that families will have a document that contains details such as DNR decisions and where to take the child in an emergency, negotiated between the child's hospital consultant, the family and, for example, the local children's hospice, and agreed with the ambulance service. Sidey and Bean[10] explain that within home care the following points need to be considered.

    - Who makes and reviews the decision?
    - Have the wishes of the dying child been ascertained?
    - Where is the decision most appropriately documented?
    - Who assumes responsibility for the decision?
    - What is the format of information about the decision and where is that information located?
    - Which service providers are covered by the decision (e.g. GP, community children's nurse, school staff, paramedics, parents, siblings, hospice staff, ward staff)?
    - Are there criteria for treatment, ventilation, resuscitation, use of antibiotics, etc.?

3. When children are being transported, all equipment must be fit for its purpose and batteries suitably charged, with emergency back-up.
4. The distance that has to be travelled is a consideration not just in terms of equipment failure, but also in terms of geographical boundaries and the possibility that agreements forged with the local health authority and ambulance service cannot be honoured outside the authority.

How can a degree of 'normality' be achieved for Vicky and her family?

Have you considered any of these?

1. Vicky is of school age and has missed out not just on the schooling appropriate for her age, but also on normal experiences such as going to school, playing with friends, going on holidays, and gradually and age-appropriately becoming more independent.
2. Before discharge, schooling needs to be arranged with a view to integrating Vicky back into mainstream schooling (see below).
3. For the last 18 months Vicky's life has been dominated by medical and nursing procedures, and unfortunately these will continue to play a significant part in her daily routine as she is so prone to chest infections and urinary and bowel problems.
4. In order not to overwhelm the family, realistic goals need to be set, with respite care being one of the main considerations. The amount of support provided by carers is likely to be up to 17 hours per day, depending on the assessment of need as discussed above. The aim of respite care needs to be negotiated with the family, whether it is in the home or whether the family would benefit from residential respite care for Vicky. The need for respite care may require regular reassessment as all of the family members adjust to the new situation. The availability of respite care might dictate what Vicky and her family receive, and it might even be that she receives foster care in her own home.

What are the likely long-term needs of a family with a technology-dependent child?

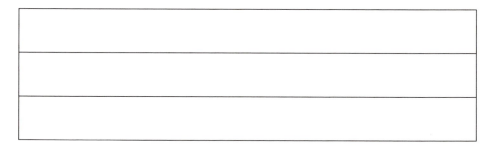

Have you considered any of these?

1. Discharging a child from a tertiary centre in this situation does not represent the end, but rather a new beginning with very different challenges for the family.
2. The child's condition might improve or deteriorate, requiring regular reassessment of the situation. Monitoring of a child's physical condition as well as developmental milestones can give a good indication of how things are going, but it also provides an insight into the following.

   - How are the parents coping? Caring for a child with such major needs will take its toll on the parents. They might be too preoccupied to follow up concerns about their own health. Are there any concerns about their physical and mental health?
   - How are the siblings coping? Are there any concerns about their physical or mental health? How are they developing?
   - Health and safety issues need to be revisited on a regular basis. For example, are moving and handling aids adequate? Are hoists, wheelchairs, bathing aids, seating, etc. appropriate for Vicky's needs?

How can we achieve realistic goals for the family and not dash their hopes about the possibility of a cure for Vicky?

<table>
<tr><td></td></tr>
<tr><td></td></tr>
<tr><td></td></tr>
</table>

Have you considered any of these?

1. This is a challenge for any family that is going through the bereavement process for the healthy child they no longer have. Counselling, whether informal or formal, is a key component of helping families to cope. Each of the parents may be at different stages of this process and may have different ideas about how to take things forward.
2. Professionals need to be aware of current developments in their specialties. Often parents go to great lengths to find information about their child's condition, and sometimes they do find information that is new. In the author's own experience a family in England found, via the Internet, a family in India with a child suffering from the same rare disorder as their own child. The two families have been able to offer each other mutual support.

Contemporary issues in children's palliative care in relation to technology dependence

Children who require long-term ventilation

This chapter proved to be an area where it is difficult to make a judgement as to whether a child is in a palliative care situation or not. The situation for Vicky in the scenario in this chapter should be clear. However, there is a wide range of children who are labelled as 'technology dependent', and many children with tracheostomies and night-time continuous positive airway pressure (CPAP) ventilation are not routinely considered within a palliative care category. According to Boosfield and O'Toole,[11] children may require ventilation for any of the following reasons.

- They were born prematurely and have developed severe, chronic lung disease.
- Their primary problem relates to instability of the upper airway.
- They have survived acute illness or trauma.
- They have neuromuscular disease.
- They are children with complex long-term needs who have survived deterioration within a chronic or acute life-threatening illness, such as trauma or major surgery.

The uncertainty of whether a child is life-limited or not

No statistics could be found on the mortality rates for long-term ventilated children. Carron *et al.*[12] reviewed the long-term outcomes for 204 children who had tracheostomies between 1988 and 1998. The children were divided into six categories according to the indications for tracheostomy, namely craniofacial abnormalities (13%), upper airway obstruction (19%), prolonged intubation (26%), neurological impairment (including chronic ventilator dependency as a result of neuromuscular illness) (27%), trauma (7%) and vocal fold paralysis (7%).

The overall mortality rate was 19% (31 children), with 3.6% of deaths (6 children) directly related to the tracheostomy. The authors concluded that tracheostomy is a procedure that is performed relatively frequently at tertiary care children's hospitals. Although children who have undergone tracheostomies have a high overall mortality rate, deaths are usually related to the underlying disease, not to the tracheostomy itself.

The National Service Framework exemplar

The Department of Health and the Department for Education and Skills[13] have published a pathway for the ventilator-dependent child suffering from congenital central hypoventilation syndrome (CCHS). Three stages of the pathway are described, namely:

- the discharge process
- living at home
- growing up and transition.

The pathway follows clearly from neonatal intensive care to children's intensive care, directly to the community, to holidays, nursery, primary school, secondary school, transition to adult services and independent living at university. It is mapped consistently against all relevant NSF standards and therefore makes excellent reading on how we can work with the NSF standards. It clearly lays out how care packages need to be developed from the point of diagnosis and can be projected in the light of the 10-year plan suggested for the children's NSF.

Fortunately for the family in the Department of Health and Department for Education and Skills[13] scenario, when it came to planning discharge into the community for a child on a ventilator, there was local expertise (as opposed to a tertiary transitional care unit dealing with a care environment often a considerable distance away), and expertise in home-ventilated children within the community team, with trained carers. Discharge planning therefore went without a hitch, and even re-housing took place swiftly. The parents were married (there was no divorce due to the strain put on the relationship), and there was even a supportive grandmother and a family friend to hand. Nursery and schooling were positive and able to accommodate a technology-dependent child and, amazingly, at the point of transfer the adult services had the expertise to care for a home-ventilated 15-year-old.

Palliative care was not an issue here. Two chest infections in the first year of life passed uneventfully.

Although this scenario is very optimistic, one must not overlook the fact that in many ways the outcomes for both the child and their family are excellent. Even if for many families it is not quite such plain sailing, there will still be benefits for both the child and the family.

Home versus hospital

Home care for technology-dependent children is the gold standard, with plenty of evidence to support the view that hospital is not a suitable long-term environment. According to Ludvigsen and Morrison,[14] an extended stay in hospital:

- reduces (and can cause loss of) contact with the child's family
- can cause children to become 'institutionalised'
- makes children vulnerable to hospital infections.

In contrast, with home care:

- there are social and emotional benefits
- 'normalisation' can be achieved in terms of play and education.

However, home care also has a number of drawbacks.

- The requirement for a carer always to be present can be an intrusion.
- It is difficult to maintain a 'normal' home environment, due to lack of privacy, choice and independence.
- The provision of short breaks is vital.
- There are issues pertaining to the commissioning of services.

  - A survey of 25 units in 1997 showed that 18 out of 152 paediatric intensive-care beds were occupied by long-term ventilated children. During the same period 143 children were refused admission, and 120 could have been admitted if the beds had not been needed for long-term ventilated children.
  - In 1998 the cost was £160,000–180,000 per year for home ventilation, £258,429 for a bed in the Transitional Care Unit at Great Ormond Street Hospital and £438,000–657,000 for a paediatric intensive-care bed (a figure considered to be nearer to £750,000 in 2005).

- The main barriers to rapid discharge are the difficulties in recruiting home care staff, incomplete funding and unsuitable housing.
- A number of changes have been proposed by Ludvigsen and Morrison,[14] which have been addressed in recent reports, but as yet still need to filter through to grass-roots level. They include the following:

  - access to an identified and effective key worker system
  - multi-agency plans for children on long-term ventilation that acknowledge their educational needs and clearly state how these are to be met
  - a balance between children's ongoing nursing needs and their right to a normal life. According to Ludvigsen and Morrison,[14] this will require a shift in culture concerning what are acceptable and manageable levels of risk.

Which pathway?

There might be a temptation to expect all families with technology-dependent children to fit into this pathway described by the Department of Health and the Department for Education and Skills.[13] Using this pathway as intended in conjunction with the Barnados report by Noyes and Lewis,[2] the complexity of children with palliative care issues is fully considered, and it will therefore be appropriate to include the ACT Care Pathway when end-of-life issues arise. This requires the multi-disciplinary team to be conversant with a number of pathways and to integrate them imaginatively. There is no mention in the NSF pathway of the ACT Pathway, yet the ACT Pathway is considered to be a companion publication to Standard 8 of the NSF.

Bearing in mind how comparatively few children are affected and consequently how infrequently local services are involved in setting up services for technology-dependent children, it is important that services draw from the full range of options that are available to them. This issue is further explored in Chapter 6 (on the transition to adulthood).

A further pathway for acquired brain injury[15] lays out a pathway for the child who has sustained serious head injuries. Again this very clearly describes the child's journey against the children's NSF theme and evidence/links for best practice. Both the Expert Patients Programme[16] and Connexions[17] are suggested as evidence/links. Following up the 'expert patients' link suggested in the document, it would appear that at present it is of limited use to this client group.

Townsley[18] cites significant concerns experienced by the Connexions service relating to the understanding of the wider role of Connexions by families and healthcare professionals. Personal advisers themselves have highlighted the fact that they lack knowledge, information and training in certain areas, such as mental health issues, adult protection and more general support services.

As new services and pathways evolve there needs to be clear guidance on which path to take in order to avoid getting lost or following inappropriate protocols. As the ACT Care Pathway is designed to be used to develop local pathways, this should help to bridge the gap when planning care provision for children like Vicky.

A new meaning of 'home'

Wang[19] states that the introduction of medical technology into a home has social and ethical consequences, as the home is often transformed into a miniature intensive-care unit. Although 'home' is usually a place where a person feels 'at home', surrounded by familiar faces, furniture, sounds, smells, tastes and comforting rituals, according to Wang the development of a high-tech home care industry has resulted in blurring of the boundary between hospital and home. There is also a blurring of roles between the parent who nurses and the nurse who parents. Kirk *et al.*[20] found that parents redefined their role by differentiating parental caregiving and its underpinning knowledge from caregiving by professionals, particularly nurses. Conflicts about caregiving can easily arise, and the authors highlight parental concerns about the competency of nursing staff supporting them at home as one factor implicated in the problematic parent–professional relationship.

Widdas and Sidey[3] highlight the fact that intensive home care is invariably accompanied by an array of complex social boundary issues which may include care of siblings, domestic tasks and maintenance of the parental role. They explain that early complex packages did not include planning for such considerations, and then could not prevent conflict and misunderstanding between family and non-family carers. These authors provide an example of an agreement of care.

According to Noyes and Lewis,[2] there is much research evidence to suggest that the care and services provided for children on long-term ventilation do not bring about the stated improved outcomes, and children and their families do not always experience positive benefits.[21] These authors state that recent studies have found that many parents experience services as an additional stress as opposed to an added benefit. When parents complain about low-quality or inappropriate services that do not bring about the desired outcome, the response has frequently been to provide additional services which in turn contribute to an already complex care package, when 'less can be more.'

It is not unheard of for families of children with complex needs to have up to 22 professionals involved (Brown, personal communication, 2005). However, some areas have addressed this problem by establishing highly developed key-worker roles within the community children's nursing teams.

Although no information is provided on how long the children in this study had been technology dependent, Heaton *et al.*[22] report that the following problems are experienced by families:

- lack of availability of appropriate respite care
- difficulty in combining caring and working
- sleep disruption
- social isolation, particularly for single parents and mothers from minority ethnic groups
- the relatively limited or disrupted participation of the child and their siblings at school and in social activities.

Wang[19] points out that lack of evidence can also result in difficulties in establishing efficient and effective social, legal, clinical and fiscal policies to help technology-dependent children to return to the community, and to improve and sustain quality of life for them and their families.

Respite care

Kirk *et al.*[20,23] have indicated that the most frequent unmet need for children with palliative care needs and their families is for respite care. This is where the 'label' that indicates whether children or young people are in a palliative care situation matters.

Families with ventilator-dependent children also require respite care (despite often complicated care packages). The reasons for this will vary, and may include the chance to spend some quality time with siblings or without resident professional carers in the home. Heaton *et al.*[22] have studied respite care in the home as a service which was not always found to be dependable or adequate. Respite care away from the home was provided either through a children's hospice, which was greatly valued by the families, or by a family placement where just the child stayed. This was also valued, but is unsuitable for families who do not want to be parted from their child.

Miller (personal communication, 2005) believes that due to the technical skills required, the setting in which a ventilator-dependent child is most likely to receive respite care is a children's hospice. Anecdotal evidence suggests that where there is no previous expertise in working with ventilator-dependent children, even hospices might be reluctant to take these children due to the extensive training that staff require to make the care safe. It might therefore be more practicable for staff who are caring for the child at home to accompany them to the respite facility. However, a child who is not identified as having palliative care needs might be unlikely to be referred for, and therefore benefit from, this option.

Educational provision for the technology-dependent child

Rehm[24] undertook a small study of schooling for medically fragile/technology-dependent children. The main points of the study were as follows.

- Children with serious and/or life-threatening genetic, congenital or postnatally acquired conditions such as cystic fibrosis, organ failure, cancer, HIV or severe prematurity were studied.
- Technological support included oxygen, ventilators, tube feeding, intravenous medication, and nappy changing during school hours.
- There was a lack of relevant statistics (estimates in the USA in 1987 ranged from 11,000 to 68,000 children).
- There is a need to prepare students, classmates, educators and families in order to minimise stigma and facilitate inclusion.
- Individual planning is necessary to ensure academic and social success.
- Provision of support and healthcare is needed during the school day.
- School personnel often felt inadequately prepared to understand the nature of the child's problems or to handle medical emergencies in the classroom. School staff often wanted to limit their knowledge of particular care skills (commonly including resuscitation procedures) in order to limit their own responsibility or liability in situations in which they are vulnerable.
- There is a need to clarify legal ambiguities with regard to training and care provision. DNR orders were a cause for particular concern. This initially led to the school insisting that any child would be resuscitated, due to the trauma caused to onlookers if they were not. This situation has now been rectified so that DNR decisions are honoured. No child with a DNR order has died at school, and staff are confident that parents would be extremely unlikely to send a child who was close to death to school.

Stem-cell research

Information available from the Christopher and Dana Reeve Paralysis Resource Center[25] makes informative and inspiring reading. One of the areas supported by the Resource Center is stem-cell research. Juengst and Fossel[26] have explained how embryonic stem cells are early 'universal' cells with the potential to form virtually any somatic cell in the human body. They state that if research can overcome substantial technical hurdles, these cells would allow for the growth of transplantable organs. To eliminate the rejection risks currently experienced in mismatched organ transplantation, in theory a perfect genetic match could be achieved by the following process. The nucleus (i.e. the genetic material) would be transferred from a patient's somatic cell into an enucleated human ovum, stimulating it to divide. The resulting embryonic stem cells would then be harvested, from which new organs could be grown. Henningson *et al.*[27] have highlighted the potential of both embryonic stem cells and adult stem cells (which have more recently also been found to be capable of differentiation) to cure diseases by repairing or replacing damaged cells or tissue – for example, in Parkinson's disease, diabetes, injury of the spinal cord, Purkinje cell degeneration, Duchenne muscular dystrophy, liver and heart failure and osteogenesis imperfecta.

There are huge ethical hurdles to be overcome. According to Juengst and Fossel[26] these include the following.

- Producing human embryos that have been created solely in order to obtain embryonic stem cells requires greater justification than the use of donated cells or organs.
- Although there are clear physiological milestones in the development of the embryo, each appropriate to the biological venue, the moral status of the early human embryo remains firmly a matter for religious conviction and social values, tempered by clear philosophical thinking.
- Equally, a competent ethical discussion cannot ignore the cost (in terms of missed opportunities) of not using stem cells.
- Many of the current discussions will be abandoned as non-embryonic cell sources are developed.
- Meanwhile, Henningson *et al.*[27] state that in principle these cells can proliferate indefinitely, so it should be possible for medical research to be conducted on the relatively few human stem cells that have been derived so far.
- Stem-cell research has also revealed promising indicators for the management of young people with Duchenne muscular dystrophy (*see* Chapter 6). So far the technology has been found to work in mice, and is being prepared for use in humans.[28,29]

It might be realistic to observe that genetic treatments are not expected for several years and are therefore unlikely to benefit young people who are currently in their teens or early twenties. Knebel and Hudgings[30] stress the need for accurate information so that families can make informed choices, and also so that patients' hope is not completely crushed and they will therefore continue to take the best possible care of themselves and not give in to despair.

Technological interventions for children with Werdnig–Hoffman disease: an ethical dilemma

Chapter 6 explores the issues relating to failing respiration in older teenagers with muscular degenerative illness who are receiving technological intervention. According to Knebel and Hudgings,[30] the possibility of technological intervention can also lead to complicated decision making for children with Werdnig–Hoffman disease, the infantile type of spinal muscular atrophy. These children die of complications of this disease by the age of 2 years. According to Knebel and Hudgings, although withholding and withdrawing life-sustaining treatment is standard practice, in Japan ventilator care is provided if families express a strong wish for this treatment. The authors highlight the need for guidance in ethical decision making. Their argument for the use of different approaches when giving treatment, in the light of futility of treatment in patients with Werdnig–Hoffman disease, as opposed to the situation of patients with, for example, muscular dystrophy, can be summarised as follows.

- Patients with muscular dystrophy are usually able to express their desire for treatment, supporting the ethical principle of patient autonomy.
- In contrast, patients with Werdnig–Hoffman disease are usually unable to express their wishes.

Chapter 12 explores the guidelines on withdrawing and withholding treatment issued by the Royal College of Paediatrics and Child Health.[31] Further ethical decisions in the context of neuromuscular disease are explored in Chapter 6.

Clinical governance and suggestions for work-based learning and networking

Explore with your colleagues how the NSF and the ACT Care Pathway as well as the Knowledge and Skills Framework standards can be implemented in your working environment in relation to Vicky and her family.

Draw up a workable care plan for Vicky and her parents based on Pathway 2.

What are the challenges? How can they be overcome? It might be helpful to include colleagues from other departments who have a designated role and/or special interest (e.g. nurse based in the children's intensive-care unit, play specialist, schoolteacher, community team, social services department, ambulance service, dietitian, physiotherapist).

Now reflect on Pathway 1.

- To what extent was the pathway followed in the case of Vicky and her family?
- To what extent does this pave the way for Pathway 2?

Now turn your attention to Pathway 3.

Although it is unlikely that Vicky will enter Pathway 3 for a long time, what considerations of this pathway will be useful for advance planning for Vicky and her family?

Summary

This chapter has examined the needs of the technology-dependent child in the context of a ventilator-dependent child who is being cared for at home. The issues that have been examined pertain to the range of exemplars that are being developed. The reality of caring for a highly dependent child at home has been explored, and the need for respite care and the associated difficulties have been discussed.

SWOT

It might be useful to revisit the SWOT analysis at this point in order to determine any further learning needs in relation to this chapter and the Knowledge and Skills Framework (KSF) requirements, namely:

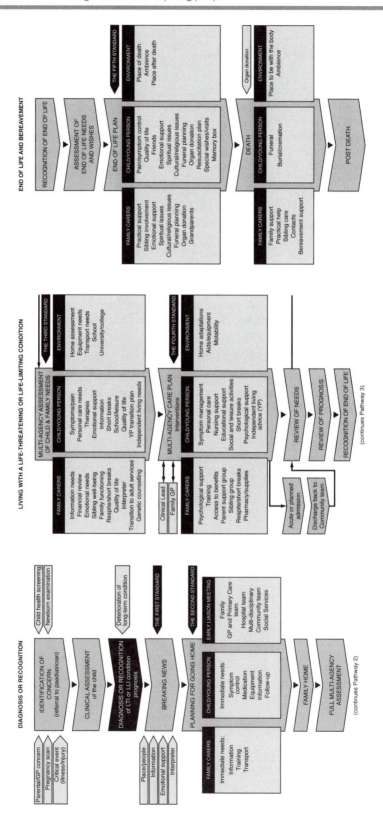

1. communication
2. personal and people development
3. health, safety and security
4. service improvement
5. quality
6. equality and diversity.

Strengths	Weaknesses
Opportunities	Threats

Action plan for further learning

References

1. UK Children on Long-Term Ventilation; www.longtermventilation.nhs.uk
2. Noyes J and Lewis M (2005) *From Hospital to Home: guidance on discharge management and community support needs of children using long-term ventilation.* Barnados, Ilford; www.longtermventilation.nhs.uk
3. Widdas D, Sidey A and Dryden S (2005) Delivering and funding care for children with complex needs. In: A Sidey and D Widdas (eds) *Textbook of Community Children's Nursing* (2e). Elsevier, Edinburgh.
4. Association for Children with Life-Threatening or Terminal Conditions and their Families (ACT) and the Royal College of Paediatrics and Child Health (2003) *A Guide to the Development of Children's Palliative Care Services.* ACT, Bristol.
5. Joy I (2005) *Valuing Short Lives: children with terminal conditions.* New Philanthropy Capital, London.
6. Langerman C and Worrall E (2005) *Ordinary Lives: disabled children and their families.*

New Philanthropy Capital, London.

7. Noyes J, Hartmann H, Samuels M *et al.* (1999) The experience and views of parents who care for ventilator-dependent children. *J Clin Nurs.* **8:** 440–50.

8. Kennedy I (2001) *Learning lessons from Bristol. The report of the public inquiry into children's heart surgery at the Bristol Royal Infirmary, 1984–1995;* www.bristol-inquiry.org.uk

9. Dimond B (2005) Legal aspects of the community care of the sick child. In: A Sidey and D Widdas (eds) *Textbook of Community Children's Nursing* (2e). Elsevier, Edinburgh.

10. Sidey A and Bean D (2005) Meeting the palliative care needs of children in the community. In: A Sidey and D Widdas (eds) *Textbook of Community Children's Nursing* (2e). Elsevier, Edinburgh.

11. Boosfeld B and O'Toole M (2000) Technology-dependent children: transition from hospital to home. *Paediatr Nurs.* **12:** 20–2.

12. Carron J, Derkay C, Strope G *et al.* (2000) Pediatric tracheostomies: changing indications and outcomes. *Laryngoscope.* **110:** 1099–104.

13. Exemplar ventilated child; www.dh.gov.uk/AdvancedSearch/SearchResults/fs/ en?NP =1&PO1=C&PI1=W&PF1=A&PG=1&RP=20&PT1=national+service+framework&SC= dh_site&Z=1

14. Ludvigsen A and Morrison J (2003) *Breathing Space: community support of children on long-term ventilation.* Barnados, Ilford.

15. www.dh.gov.uk/AdvancedSearch/SearchResults/fs/en?NP=1&PO1=C&PI1=W&PF1= A&PG=1&RP=20&PT1=national+service+framework&SC= dh_site&Z=1

16. Expert Patients Programme; www.expertpatients.nhs.uk

17. Connexions (2003) APIR (assessment, planning, implementation and review framework); www.connexions.gov.uk

18. Townsley R (2004) *The Road Ahead?* Norah Fry Research Centre, University of Bristol, Bristol.

19. Wang K and Barnard A (2004) Technology-dependent children and their families: a review. *J Adv Nurs.* **45:** 36–46.

20. Kirk S (1998) Families' experiences of caring at home for a technology-dependent child: a review of the literature. *Child Care Health Dev.* **24:** 101–14.

21. Sudbury J and Noyes J (1999) *Ventilator-Dependent Children: bibliography and analysis of the literature;* www.longtermventilation.nhs.uk

22. Heaton J, Noyes J, Sloper P *et al.* (2003) *Technology-Dependent Children and Family Life. Research works, 2002–03.* Social Policy Research Unit, University of York, York.

23. Kirk S, Glendinning C and Callery P (2005) Parent or nurse? The experience of being the parent of a technology-dependent child. *J Adv Nurs.* **51:** 456–64.

24. Rehm R (2002) Creating a context of safety and achievement at school for children who are medically fragile/technology dependent. *Adv Nurs Sci.* **24:** 71–84.

25. Christopher and Dana Reeve Paralysis Resource Center; www.paralysis.org

26. Juengst E and Fossel M (2000) The ethics of embryonic stem cells – now and forever, cells without end. *JAMA.* **284:** 3180–4.

27. Henningson C, Stanislaus M and Gerwirtz A (2003) Embryonic and adult stem cell therapy. *J Allergy Clin Immunol.* **111:** S745–53.

28. Biggar W, Klamut H, Demacio P *et al.* (2002) Duchenne muscular dystrophy: current knowledge, treatment and future prospects. *Clin Orthop.* **401:** 88–106.

29. Metules T (2002) A new age for childhood diseases: Duchenne muscular dystrophy. *Registered Nurse.* **65:** 39–44, 47–8.

30. Knebel A and Hudgings C (2002) End-of-life issues in genetic disorders: summary of workshop held at the National Institutes of Health on September 26, 2001. *Genet Med.* **4:** 373–8.

31. Royal College of Paediatrics and Child Health (2004) *Withholding and Withdrawing Life-Saving Treatment in Children: a framework of practice.* Royal College of Paediatrics and Child Health, London.

Chapter 11

Congenital complex disability

This chapter covers

Content	*Relevant to other areas of palliative care for children and young people*
Scenario	
• Setting the scene:	• This chapter: the role of school and social care
– NSF	• This chapter: child protection/ children in need
– KSF	
– ACT Care Pathway	• This chapter: families with disabled children and the Internet
	• This chapter: financial implications for the family
Related to children with complex needs	• This chapter: selection of websites that have been found to be particularly helpful
• Contemporary issues in palliative care for children with complex disability	• This chapter: implementing NSF principles – deciding on 'place of care' for the child with a poor prognosis
• Funding issues and finances	
• Families with disabled children and the Internet	• Chapter 6: transition
• Complementary therapies	• Chapter 8: financial and workplace issues
• Facing the future: young adulthood with complex disability	• Chapter 11: going home for terminal care
• Clinical governance and suggestions for work-based learning and networking	*Relevant topics in other chapters*
• Summary	• Chapter 4: place of care
	• Chapters 8 and 12: pain assessment in the child with severe neurological impairment/neurological deterioration (PIND study)
	• Chapter 9: the health and well-being of the carers: mothers and fathers
	• Chapter 4: implementing NSF principles – deciding on 'place of care' at the point of death
	• Chapter 6: transition

Setting the scene

Jasmine was a much wanted baby. Born after extensive infertility treatment at 24 weeks' gestation, she required intubation, surfactant and ventilation within 2 hours of birth. After a ventricular haemorrhage during her first week of life, Jasmine's prognosis was considered to be bleak. Although the parents were deeply traumatised, there was a good rapport between the neonatal team and the parents. There was mutual agreement between the multi-disciplinary team and the family to withdraw ventilatory support. Against all the odds Jasmine started breathing on her own and was weaned on to low-level oxygen via nasal spectacles. She required a ventriculo-peritoneal shunt and has developed severe cerebral palsy.

Initially, after Jasmine had been discharged from the neonatal intensive-care unit, the family was visited by the neonatal outreach nurse, but as Jasmine came off the oxygen treatment quickly and the family was coping exceptionally well, the 'extra' community input was quickly reduced and the parents now only receive standard health visitor input. Jasmine's progress is monitored 6-monthly at the local child development centre. Her parents have been reassured that Jasmine has been assessed as not having any palliative care needs, but in the light of the amount of care and supervision she needs she is on the waiting list for respite care.

Jasmine's hospital admissions are infrequent, but although the parents are never resident with her, they can be highly critical of the care she is receiving. The staff in turn feel that the parents should be resident with their child, as most parents with non-disabled children are.

Jasmine is now aged 3 years and is breathing unaided, but has severe asthma. She has never gained her swallowing reflex and is fed via gastrostomy tubes. She has severe, poorly controlled convulsions, which seem to be triggered by constipation. This means that on days when her bowels have not moved by 3 p.m., she has a series of convulsions, which if not treated promptly by administration of rectal diazepam in turn trigger a severe asthma attack, and the family is well used to initiating home nebulisation.

Today Jasmine has been admitted directly from her special nursery at 4 p.m., and she is twitching continuously. Within the space of 30 minutes she has had three salbutamol nebulisers given through oxygen, and a second dose of 5 mg rectal diazepam. She is maintaining her oxygen saturations at 89%. Her mother has just arrived and demands that Jasmine is administered an enema. The house officer and staff nurse who are attending to Jasmine tell the mother that this is inappropriate and in fact the locum registrar is on his way to evaluate whether it is necessary to intubate Jasmine in order to manage her respiratory distress and fitting. A second staff nurse is overheard to say 'I've heard it all now – enemas for respiratory distress and status!'

Jot down your initial reaction to this situation.

| |
| |
| |
| |

Does this bring back memories of a situation you have encountered?

Does this help or hinder?

SWOT

What are your learning needs when considering this scenario? They could look similar to the following:

Strengths	Weaknesses
• I enjoy the challenge of caring for highly dependent children and their families. • A couple of our healthcare assistants have been here for many years and know the children with complex needs quite well. They often focus on their care, and know the peculiarities of many of the children.	• I have not cared for a child with complex needs since my initial nurse training. • This is a very busy unit and we simply do not have the time to give care above meeting basic needs of children with complex needs. • This can be very stressful for the staff, as we would like to be able to do so much more for these children, but their care is very time consuming. • I know there is an NSF standard for children with disabilities, but as we are an acute unit, we did not realise that this is relevant for us.
Opportunities	**Threats**
• To explore multi-professional working as required in the 'Complex disability' exemplar.	• There is a lot to learn in terms of care of a child with complex needs – moving and handling, electric wheelchairs, transporting and creating a 'normal' routine for Jasmine. • It will be a big responsibility to care for a child in her own home without being able to just call for assistance.

This could include the Knowledge and Skills Framework, which has the following requirements:[1]

1. communication
2. personal and people development
3. health, safety and security
4. service improvement
5. quality
6. equality and diversity.

There might be issues that you wish to explore, in which case feel free to do so, but also think about the following.

Where on the ACT Care Pathway[2] would you locate Jasmine, her family and the hospital staff in their thinking?

Jasmine:
Parents:
Health visitor:
Nursery:
Social worker:
Paediatrician at the child development centre:
Hospital staff:

ACT[3] describes four categories of palliative care needs for children and young people. Which group is applicable to Jasmine?

> Group 4
>
> Services often have great difficulty in deciding whether a child or young person meets the criteria for their service. Although there is often little doubt that the quality of life of a child and their family can be improved, decisions might have to be made to only accept children with the most serious needs. In Jasmine's situation it can be argued that her life is limited, both in quality and length (there is a high risk that she will not survive beyond early adulthood).

Draw up a workable care plan for Jasmine and her parents based on Pathway 2.

Examine the role that school and social care could play in the multi-disciplinary care Jasmine should be receiving in the context of NSF guidance.

Have you considered any of these?

The NSF Exemplar for Complex Disability[4] is relevant here. It explains clearly how health, social care and education need to work together to meet the overall needs of children with complex needs and their families. The exemplar extends from the pregnancy and prema-

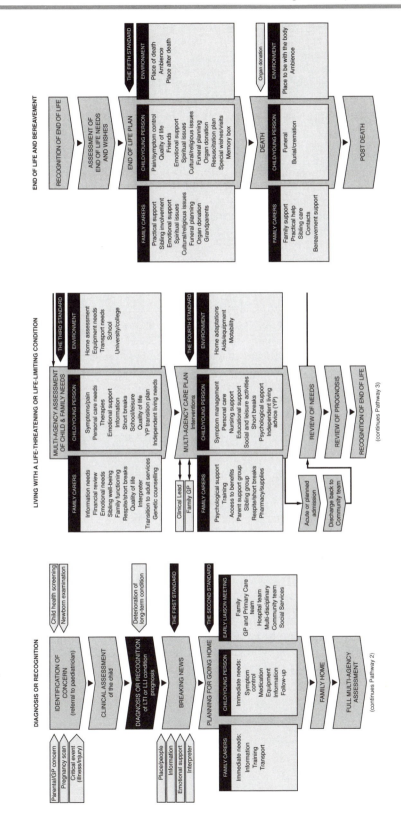

DIAGNOSIS OR RECOGNITION

Parental/GP concern
Pregnancy scan
Critical event (illness/injury)

Child health screening
Newborn examination

IDENTIFICATION OF CONCERN
(referral to paediatrician)

CLINICAL ASSESSMENT of the child

Deterioration of long-term condition

DIAGNOSIS OR RECOGNITION of LTI or LLI condition prognosis

THE FIRST STANDARD

BREAKING NEWS

Place/people
Information
Emotional support
Interpreter

THE SECOND STANDARD

PLANNING FOR GOING HOME

EARLY LIAISON MEETING
Family
GP and Primary Care team
Hospital team
Multi-disciplinary
Community team
Social Services

CHILD/YOUNG PERSON
Immediate needs:
Symptom control
Medication
Equipment
Information
Follow-up

FAMILY CARERS
Immediate needs:
Information
Training
Transport

FAMILY HOME

FULL MULTI-AGENCY ASSESSMENT

(continues Pathway 2)

LIVING WITH A LIFE-THREATENING OR LIFE-LIMITING CONDITION

THE THIRD STANDARD

MULTI-AGENCY ASSESSMENT OF CHILD & FAMILY NEEDS

ENVIRONMENT
Home assessment
Equipment needs
Transport needs
School
University/college

CHILD/YOUNG PERSON
Symptoms/pain
Personal care needs
Therapies
Emotional support
Information
Short breaks
School/leisure
Quality of life
YP transition plan
Independent living needs

FAMILY CARERS
Information needs
Financial review
Emotional needs
Sibling well-being
Family functioning
Respite/short breaks
Quality of life
Interpreter
Transition to adult services
Genetic counselling

THE FOURTH STANDARD

MULTI-AGENCY CARE PLAN
Interventions

ENVIRONMENT
Home adaptations
Aids/equipment
Motability

CHILD/YOUNG PERSON
Symptom management
Personal care
Nursing support
Educational support
Social and leisure activities
Psychological support
Independent living advice (YP)

Clinical Lead
Family GP

FAMILY CARERS
Psychological support
Training
Access to benefits
Parent support group
Sibling group
Respite/short breaks
Pharmacy/supplies

Acute or planned admission

Discharge back to Community team

REVIEW OF NEEDS

REVIEW OF PROGNOSIS

RECOGNITION OF END OF LIFE

(continues Pathway 3)

END OF LIFE AND BEREAVEMENT

RECOGNITION OF END OF LIFE

ASSESSMENT OF END OF LIFE NEEDS AND WISHES

THE FIFTH STANDARD

ENVIRONMENT
Place of death
Ambience
Place after death

END OF LIFE PLAN

CHILD/YOUNG PERSON
Pain/symptom control
Quality of life
Friends
Emotional support
Spiritual issues
Cultural/religious issues
Funeral planning
Organ donation
Resuscitation plan
Special wishes/visits
Memory box

FAMILY CARERS
Practical support
Sibling involvement
Emotional support
Spiritual issues
Cultural/religious issues
Funeral planning
Organ donation
Grandparents

DEATH

Organ donation

ENVIRONMENT
Place to be with the body
Ambience

CHILD/YOUNG PERSON
Funeral
Burial/cremation

FAMILY CARERS
Family support
Practical help
Sibling care
Contacts
Bereavement support

POST DEATH

ture birth of the child through to the early years, school and transition to adult services. The document maps suggested care and interventions against relevant services and agencies, all of which are clearly referenced.

A child with severe disabilities like Jasmine is unlikely to gain many academic skills. However, the roles played by school for this group of children are manifold. It gives the child a routine that is as normal as possible.[5] Langerman and Worrall[6] state that all children deserve and need to make friends, play and take part in leisure activities and hobbies. Whereas for the young child play is part of learning and development, for the older disabled child school attendance reduces social isolation. Although nursery or school attendance offers respite to the family, one must not underestimate the major milestone that this signifies for the family. Noyes and Lewis[5] explain that parents still worry about matters such as whether the child will eat at lunchtime or develop friendships. Useful documents for the reader to refer to include the Department for Education and Skills Special Needs Action Programme,[7] the Government Strategy for Special Needs Education[8] and the Code of Practice for Schools.[9] Usually there is good communication between the school and the family, and staff at the school might well be able to assist in building better communication channels between hospital services and the family.

Noyes and Lewis[5] have elaborated on multi-agency working as follows.

- The Special Educational Needs (SEN) Code of Practice[10] provides guidance to local authorities, early education settings and schools on carrying out their statutory duties to identify, assess and make provision for children with special educational needs.
- The code puts strong emphasis on education, health and social services working together to assess children's needs and develop packages to support children with SEN and enable them to access education.
- The Early Support Programme[11] promotes multi-agency working with disabled children from birth to 3 years of age and their families. A good practice guide on supporting pupils with special medical needs can be downloaded from this website.

Sidey and Bean[12] have studied the benefits of a 'named' social worker who is allocated specifically to a child and their family, and who may be:

- a generic social worker from local social services
- based within local authority children's or disability social work teams
- part of a multi-disciplinary team (e.g. a Diana team)
- based within a hospital social work department.

According to Sidey and Bean, assessment is central to the social worker role and is driven by the Framework for the Assessment of Children in Need and their Families.[13]

The role of social workers is manifold. The support that they offer includes the following:[12]

- liaison between social services and healthcare services
- multi-professional assessments
- giving social work advice to team members
- individual work with children and their families to offer support or to advocate for their needs
- facilitation of parents' groups
- bereavement support
- facilitation of respite care
- psychological care
- creating family support services
- addressing the emotional, social and financial impact of illness
- helping families to deal with practical problems
- childcare

- travel and accommodation
- giving advice about employment, financial concerns, the impact of the illness, benefits and financial assistance to meet the child's needs.

Now reflect on Pathway 1.

- To what extent was this pathway followed in the case of Jasmine and her family?
- What should have been done differently in order to pave the way for Pathway 2?

Now turn your attention to Pathway 3.

Although it is unlikely that Jasmine will enter Pathway 3 during this admission, what considerations of this pathway will be useful for advance planning for Jasmine and her family?

Contemporary issues in palliative care for children with complex disability

Child protection issues: 'It doesn't happen to disabled children'[14]

It would appear that disabled children are more likely to be looked after by local authorities than non-disabled children. The National Society for the Prevention of Cruelty to Children (NSPCC) report, 'It doesn't happen to disabled children',[14] identifies both the potential risk of abuse of a child who might not be able to express what is happening, and the context of the 'child in need.'

There are many additional stressors that are encountered by families with disabled children.

- Lack of appropriate or coordinated support services can leave disabled children and their families unsupported and physically and socially isolated. Isolation is widely recognised as being a risk factor for abuse.[14]
- A lack of comprehensive and multi-agency assessment and planning leads to both failure to promote a child's welfare and failure to identify early indications of possible abuse.[14]

Social services are required to provide services under Section 17 of the Children Act[15] following an assessment under the Framework for the Assessment of Children in Need and their Families[13] and the associated 'Practice Guidance.'[16]

The NSF Exemplar for Complex Disability[4] addresses the issue of regularly reviewing the 'child in need' plan.

Entrusting others with your child

Ford and Turner[17] studied paediatric nurses' experiences of caring for hospitalised children with special needs and their families. Four themes were identified, namely special relationships, multiple dimensions causing conflict as to who is expert, developing trust between nurses and families, and feelings of frustration and guilt.

Respite care

Some families appear to be rejecting the idea of respite care. Anecdotal evidence reveals a variety of reasons for this, and the ones highlighted in the example below involved failure to demonstrate clear communication and re-evaluation of need:

> A mother was told that her child had weeks, at the most months, to live. When offered respite care, on discussion with the social worker she emphatically rejected any offers of help – she needed to be with her child every waking moment she had left with him. It was not until eight years later that the offer was repeated. By then the child's parents were divorced, the mother was taking antidepressants, and the 12-year-old sibling was seeing a child psychiatrist.

The following example also pertains to poor communication and attributing different meanings:

> A mother was asked whether she wanted her child to go to 'Rainbows.' Again, the mother emphatically refused. This was duly recorded as 'refuses respite.' When this was explored further by a different member of staff, it transpired that the mother assumed that 'Rainbows' were the junior Brownies. The mother in fact was quite incensed at the apparent lack of insight by the professional into her child's needs.

Sidey and Bean[12] have explained that the strain of caring for a sick child in the home is immense, with possible consequences of physical, psychological and emotional exhaustion, as well as isolation. Olsen and Maslin-Prothero[18] evaluated the kind of respite support that parents valued, and found that they often expressed different ideas of how they would benefit from a home respite service. Parents hoped that respite would enable them to fulfil other family responsibilities, such as supporting healthy siblings, allowing parents to go out, and having time to sleep, recover some emotional strength, have a bath, go to the shops or have a driving lesson. Other parents in this study needed to have time together with their partners and to 'recharge their batteries.' Some parents valued having some time away from the sick child, and help such as the outreach nurse taking the child for hospital appointments was appreciated.

According to Sidey and Bean,[12] provision of respite varies widely between service providers. They argue that introduction to a provider at an early stage of palliative care avoids the possible need for unknown carers to be introduced to the child and their family at a time of crisis.

They cite the following examples of respite care providers:

- health-service-funded nursing teams
- Diana community children's nursing teams
- NOF (New Opportunity Funding) teams
- continuing care funding
- charitably funded teams
- hospices
- hospice outreach services
- social services home care
- social services residential care
- learning disabilities residential and outreach care
- short-term fostering (family link)
- family and friends.

The Social Care Institute for Excellence (SCIE) Research Briefing[19] investigated short breaks (respite) for children with learning disabilities. They state it is vital that disabled children are consulted about the services they receive. So far research indicates that children value the opportunity to meet and make friends, to engage in a variety of activities, to develop independence and to have a break from their family. Parents identified continuity of carer, consistency of service, concerns about what will happen as the child grows older or grows up, and appropriateness of the placement as the most important issues. Outcome indicators included the child appearing happy, a reduction in carer stress, respite breaks being given when needed and not cancelled, the continued use of known and trusted carers, and the child being offered a variety of experiences.

Funding issues and finances

The Irish Department of Health and Children and the Irish Hospice Foundation[20] have identified that parents have a lack of choice regarding the place of their child's death. Important factors include lack of facilities and resources, lack of information, parents' fears, and lack of experience in paediatric palliative care. Echoing the comments made by Langerman and Worrall,[6] there might be fears that if children with complex needs are identified as having palliative care needs and are referred appropriately, this could drain already limited resources. Harrington Jacob[21] has examined the principle of justice in terms of 'giving to each his due.' Different theories emerge about 'what is due' and 'to whom it is due' when issues arise concerning the allocation of scarce resources. The NSF Exemplar for Complex Disability[4] maps out clearly what the family in this example is entitled to and it is recommended that readers look at the document for an appreciation on the dynamic nature of this process throughout the child's life. The family's benefits and allowances are reviewed at various points, as their eligibility may have changed since the child was younger and they might be missing out on some entitlements. It is also pointed out that at the age of 16 years direct payments in the young person's own right can be arranged. This provides useful ammunition when advocating for individual families.

To illustrate the reality of the comments by Harrington Jacob,[21] Langerman and Worrall[6] made the following points.

- Adaptations to housing are subject to means testing, with a maximum state contribution of £25,000. Families are expected to pay the remainder of the sum. If the existing accommodation is deemed unsuitable, state funding is not available, and the family will have to fund the full amount. Keeping a technology-dependent child in intensive care for 3 years while a housing solution is found could, according to Ludvigsen and Morrison,[22] cost £438,000–£657,000 per year, which could mount to up to £2 million over 3 years.
- The average cost of bringing up a severely disabled child is £8300 per year, or £143,000 by the age of 17 years.[6] Most of this is spent on transport, with the rest being spent on hospital trips, heating, housing, clothing, bedding, laundry, equipment and housing adaptation.
- The authors have put forward the following sobering equation:

extra cost (three times the cost of raising a non-disabled child)

\+

inability to work (only 16% of mothers are in full- or part-time employment)

=

poverty (55% of families with a disabled child live in poverty)

\+

debt (84% of families with a disabled child are in debt).

Families with disabled children and the Internet

Blackburn and Read[23] found that the Internet has become a mainstream method of delivering a wide range of public and private information and services for the population as a whole. Their paper draws on a subset of data from the 'Carers Online' project, which reports on the experiences of carers. Of these, 788 carers were parents of disabled children aged 0–17 years. The main points can be summarised as follows.

- The field of community informatics analyses developments which may be relevant to

the specific needs that families might have as a result of their caring role, and the health and social care needs of children as well as many parents.
- The Internet is already a well-developed source of social and healthcare-related information.
- It offers opportunities for computer-mediated social support, self-help, chat rooms and exchange of lay knowledge.
- Of the respondents in this study:[23]

  - 91% had access to the Internet from their own home
  - 63% used the Internet once a week or more and 37% used it less than once a week
  - 72% used the Internet to obtain information on benefits, services and medical conditions
  - 36% used it to make contact with organisations relevant to their disabled children or their own parental and caring responsibilities
  - the Internet was also used for ordering equipment for the child, shopping, work or education, obtaining information on leisure activities, keeping up with the news and playing games or listening to music
  - problems or barriers were experienced in terms of technical problems related to equipment and systems, as well as parents' circumstances
  - 86% of respondents commented on the time it took to find the information they required, 85% reported having made unsuccessful searches for specific information; 79% found some websites difficult to locate and 73% were on slow computer connections
  - there was a significant number of non-users. These tended to be from socially disadvantaged families. Low-income families have already been identified as having unmet needs for information and other services. If the Internet is to service this group of families well, the barriers of cost and lack of equipment and skill need to be addressed. Otherwise mainstream systems for delivering services and information will be even further beyond their reach
  - using the Internet was regarded as time consuming, with respondents having only limited time available due to their caring commitments
  - although the Internet might offer a fast track to some information and services, this might not be the case for someone attempting to obtain information about a range of complex matters and with only limited time in which to do so
  - 25% of parents had never used the Internet, lack of skill and interest being the main factors responsible for this. Although flexible training programmes can be developed, parents and children still have needs for and rights to services and information. Information delivery systems need to be sensitive to the diverse needs of individuals.

The following is just a small selection of websites that have been found to be particularly geared towards empowering parents.

Association for Children with Life-Threatening or Terminal Conditions and their Families (ACT)[24]

Most readers will be familiar with ACT as the umbrella organisation for children with life-threatening or terminal conditions and their families. ACT offers a wide range of information for both healthcare professionals and parents, as well as links to other organisations. A number of ACT publications can be accessed directly from the website, as can PaedPalLit, which is a regularly published literature search of pertinent topics in children's and young people's palliative care. The section 'For professionals' allows an easy search of the ACT library. 'ACT NOW' is a newsletter that can be accessed via the website and which gives updates on national policy and guidance as well as conferences and courses.

Contact a Family[25]

The website for Contact a Family offers information ranging from descriptions of conditions to advice about help that might be available and details of support groups. A huge range of links can be accessed from this site. There is an excellent section for fathers, tackling anything from peer support to financial responsibilities for estranged families. A useful report, 'Debt and Disability', jointly published with The Family Fund,[26] can be downloaded from this website.

The Family Fund[26]

The Family Fund provides aid for low-income families with disabled or seriously ill children, and can help with anything from a washing machine to a grant towards a holiday, but only if there is no statutory responsibility for the requested item. A useful report, 'Expenditure of Families with Severely Disabled Children', can be downloaded from this website.

Philanthropy Capital[27]

This organisation has published two research papers contextualising the care provision for families, both of which are highly relevant to anyone working within palliative care for children and young people:

- 'Ordinary Lives: Disabled Children and their Families', by Langerman and Worrall[6]
- 'Valuing Short Lives: Children with Terminal Conditions', by Joy.[28]

Complementary therapies

Fearon[29] offers a useful overview of the use of complementary therapies in community children's nursing. She asserts that the term 'complementary therapies' implies that they are an adjunct to mainstream care rather than an alternative to it. This distinction between 'complementary' and 'alternative' is particularly important in situations where parents might make a desperate attempt to re-establish the control they have lost over their child's illness,[30] or try to find a cure for their child and in the process possibly reject mainstream medicine, which might be viewed as having failed their child. Lee and Kemper[31] have voiced concern about the approach of some therapists who reject the continuation of conventional medicine or fail to recognise potentially serious illness. Steinhorn and Rogers[32] give a number of case histories relating to palliative care for children and young people which illustrate that complementary and alternative medicine (CAM) can encourage a sense of well-being, a reduction in distressing symptoms, and feelings of being cared for and nurtured, resulting in exactly the improvement in quality of life that is the aim of palliative care. In addition to much anecdotal evidence of the benefit of many complementary therapies, there is an increasing number of small studies that all point to the benefit of many of the therapies that are used, such as aromatherapy and massage.[33] The value of music therapy is increasingly recognised in different settings (e.g. for children with complex needs, or as a tool for communication and self-expression in palliative care for children and young people[34,35]).

Studies that can evaluate benefit and which are not based on anecdotal evidence are hard to find. A cost-effectiveness analysis has been undertaken by De Loach and Walworth[36] in the context of procedural support. A powerful example is given of how a 13-year-old could be successfully extubated with the use of music, despite two previous failed attempts. This involved obtaining information about the young person's favourite music from the parents. Two sessions were conducted in order to establish rapport before extubation was attempted. According to De Loach and Walworth,[36] the music therapist began live guitar playing and singing before the procedure began, during the procedure, and after it until the patient fell asleep. Using the isoprinciple, the therapist matched the music to the patient's current behavioural state in order to achieve the desired outcome. Practically this meant that the tempo and intensity of the music changed in line with changes in heart and respiratory rate until the patient fell asleep. Another study, by Lee *et al.*,[37] also describes the effect of music on physiological responses. *Bandolier*[38] has evaluated complementary therapies at the end of life and draws the following conclusions.

> Most of the studies reviewed could show some benefit of treatment with some outcome. The problems, though, are manifest. Firstly, most were too small to tell anything, even if their conduct was immaculate. Secondly, their conduct was not immaculate. Few were blinded, and most had…major structural flaws. There is really no solid evidence that complementary and alternative therapies have any value for treating pain, dyspnoea or nausea and vomiting at the end of life.

According to Steinhorn and Rogers,[32] absence of proof may not represent the absence of efficacy, but rather it may simply reflect imperfect tools of inquiry.

Facing the future: young adulthood with complex disability

The NSF Exemplar for Complex Disability[4] suggests that preparations for transfer to adult services should commence at the age of 13 years. Read[39] highlights the growing number of children and young people with complex and multiple disabilities who are now surviving into adulthood, and with this the growing concern that although they may be diagnosed with palliative conditions they could have difficulty accessing appropriate assessment. Read discusses how adult palliative care services can respond to the very special needs presented by clients with learning disabilities. In contrast, Todd[40] has reported prejudices whereby staff in learning disability services viewed palliative care as just another expression of medical or hospital care within which learning-disabled people would be overlooked and neglected. Read[39] describes an educational programme which will bring together two independent and somewhat diverse disciplines to learn and work alongside to promote best practice.

As implementation of the Children's NSF and the Knowledge and Skills Framework gain momentum, a further section of the Children's NSF, 'Transition: getting it right for young people', highlights the knowledge and skills required by professionals relating to communication and consultation skills, a holistic approach to transition planning, children in special circumstances, and person-centred planning.[41]

Read cites a number of useful websites, and further information can be obtained via Living with Cancer – Learning Disability,[42] the Northern Cancer Network,[43] and the coordinator of the National Network for the Palliative Care of People with Learning Disabilities.[44]

Clinical governance and suggestions for work-based learning and networking

Explore with your colleagues how the NSF Exemplar for Complex Disability and the ACT Care Pathway, as well as the Knowledge and Skills Framework standards, can be implemented in your working environment in relation to Jasmine and her family. What are the challenges? How can they be overcome? It might be helpful to include colleagues from other departments who have a designated role and/or special interest (e.g. nurse on the child development unit, play specialist, schoolteacher, special school or nursery, community team, social services department (in relation to the 'child in need'), dietitian, speech therapist, paediatrician, physiotherapist).

Summary

This chapter has examined the needs of the child with complex disability in the context of the NSF Exemplar for Complex Disability and the ACT Care Pathway. Contemporary issues relating to child protection and the child in need have been highlighted, as well as financial issues that affect families. The way in which families access information has been examined with regard to use of the Internet, and a selection of relevant websites has been described.

SWOT

It might be useful to revisit the SWOT analysis at this point in order to determine any further learning needs in relation to this chapter and the Knowledge and Skills Framework (KSF) requirements, namely:

1. communication
2. personal and people development
3. health, safety and security
4. service improvement
5. quality
6. equality and diversity.

Strengths	Weaknesses
Opportunities	Threats

Action plan for further learning

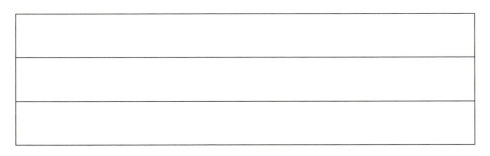

References

1. Department of Health (2004) *The NHS Knowledge and Skills Framework (NHS KSF) and the Development Review Process*. Department of Health, London.
2. Elston S (ed.) (2004) *Integrated Multi-Agency Care Pathways for Children with Life-Threatening and Life-Limiting Conditions*. ACT, Bristol.
3. Association for Children with Life-Threatening or Terminal Conditions and their Families (ACT) and the Royal College of Paediatrics and Child Health (2003) *A Guide to the Development of Children's Palliative Care Services*. ACT, Bristol.
4. Department of Health and Department for Education and Skills (2005) *National Service Framework for Children, Young People and Maternity Services: complex disability*; www.dh.gov.uk/policyAndGuidance/HealthAndSocialCareTopics/ChildrenServices/fs/en
5. Noyes J and Lewis M (2005) *From Hospital to Home: guidance on discharge management and community support needs of children using long-term ventilation*. Barnados, Ilford; www.longtermventilation.nhs.uk
6. Langerman C and Worrall E (2005) *Ordinary Lives: disabled children and their families*. New Philanthropy Capital, London.
7. Department of Health and Department for Education and Skills (2003) *Special Needs Action Programme*; www.teachernet.gov.uk
8. Department for Education and Skills (2004) *Removing Barriers to Achievement: the Government strategy for special needs education*; www.teachernet.gov.uk/wholoschool/sen/senstrategy
9. Disability Rights Commission (2002) *Code of Practice for Schools*; www.drc-gb.org/thelaw/practice.asp
10. Special Educational Needs (SEN) Code of Practice; www.teachernet.gov.uk/ doc/3724/SENCodeOfPractice.pdf
11. Department for Education and Skills (2002) *The Early Support Programme*; www.early-support.org.uk
12. Sidey S and Bean D (2005) Meeting the palliative care needs of children in the community. In: A Sidey and D Widdas (eds) *Textbook of Community Children's Nursing* (2e). Elsevier, Edinburgh.
13. Department of Health and Department for Education and Employment (2000) *Framework for the Assessment of Children in Need and their Families*. Department of Health, London.
14. National Society for the Prevention of Cruelty to Children (NSPCC) (2003) *It Doesn't Happen to Disabled Children*. NSPCC, London.
15. Children Act 1989; www.opsi.gov.uk/acts/acts1989/Ukpga_19890041_en_1.htm
16. Department of Health and Department for Education and Skills (2004) *Practice Guidance*. Department of Health, London.
17. Ford K and Turner DS (2001) Stories seldom told: paediatric nurses' experiences of caring for hospitalised children and their families. *J Adv Nurs*. **33**: 288–95.
18. Olsen R and Maslin-Prothero P (2001) Dilemmas in the provision of own-home respite support for parents of young children with complex health care needs: evidence from an evaluation. *J Adv Nurs*. **34**: 603–10.
19. Social Care Institute for Excellence (SCIE) Research Briefing 5 on short breaks (respite care) for children with learning disabilities; www.scie.org.uk/publications/ briefings/briefing05/index.asp
20. Irish Department of Health and Children and the Irish Hospice Foundation (2005) *Palliative Care Needs Assessment for Children*; www.dohc.ie/publications/needs_assessment_palliative.html
21. Harrington Jacobs H (2005) Ethics in pediatric end-of-life care: a nursing perspective. *J Pediatr Nurs*. **20**: 360–9.
22. Ludvigsen A and Morrison J (2003) *Breathing Space: community support of children on long-term ventilation*. Barnados, Ilford.

23. Blackburn C and Read J (2005) Using the Internet? The experiences of parents of disabled children. *Child Care Health Dev.* **31:** 507–15.
24. Association for Children with Life-Threatening or Terminal Conditions and their Families (ACT); www.act.org.uk/
25. Contact a Family; www.cafamily.org.uk/
26. The Family Fund; www.familyfund.org.uk
27. Philanthropy Capital, London; www.philanthropycapital.org
28. Joy I (2005) *Valuing Short Lives: children with terminal conditions.* New Philanthropy Capital, London.
29. Fearon J (2005) Complementary therapies in community children's nursing. In: A Sidey and D Widdas (eds) *Textbook of Community Children's Nursing* (2e). Elsevier, Edinburgh.
30. Rosen L (2004) Complementary and alternative medicine use in children is underestimated. *Arch Pediatr Adolesc Med.* **158:** 291.
31. Lee A and Kemper K (2000) Homeopathy and naturopathy. *Arch Pediatr Adolesc Med.* **154:** 75–80.
32. Steinhorn D and Rogers M (2006) Complementary and alternative medicine. In: A Goldman, R Hain and S Liben (eds) *The Oxford Textbook of Paediatric Palliative Care.* Oxford University Press, Oxford.
33. McNeilly P (2004) Complementary therapies for children: aromatherapy. *Paediatr Nurs.* **16:** 28–30.
34. An introduction to music therapy can be found on the website of Martin House (Yorkshire's first hospice for children); www.martinhouse.org.uk/Care/What%20 we%20offer/Team/music.htm
35. Pavlicevic M (2005) *Music Therapy in Children's Hospices.* Jessica Kingsley Publishers, London.
36. De Loach D and Walworth M (2005) Procedural support music therapy in the health care setting: a cost-effectiveness analysis. *J Pediatr Nurs.* **20:** 276–84.
37. Lee O, Chung Y, Chan M *et al.* (2005) Music and its effect on the physiological responses and anxiety levels of patients receiving mechanical ventilation: a pilot study. *J Clin Nurs.* **14:** 609–20.
38. *Bandolier* (complementary therapy at the end of life); www.jr2.ox.ac.uk/bandolier/ booth/palliative/CATeol.html
39. Read S (2005) Learning disabilities and palliative care: recognizing pitfalls and exploring potential. *Int J Palliat Nurs.* **11:** 15–20.
40. Todd S (2005) Surprised endings: the dying of people with learning disabilities in residential services. *Int J Palliat Nurs.* **11:** 80–2.
41. Department of Education and Skills and Department of Health (2006) *National Service Framework for Children, Young People and Maternity Services Transition: getting it right for young people.* DES and DoH, London; www.dh.gov.uk/childrensnsf
42. Living with Cancer – Learning Disability; www.learningdisabilitycancer.nhs.uk
43. Northern Cancer Network; www.cancernorth.nhs.uk
44. Coordinator of the National Network for the Palliative Care of People with Learning Disabilities; Linda.mcenhill@st-nicholas-hospice.org.uk

Part Three

Safe practice in expanding boundaries

Chapter 12

Underpinning safe practice

This chapter covers

Content Scenario	Relevant to other areas of palliative care for children and young people
• Introduction • Coping • Being present • Symptom control • Pain assessment • To feed or not to feed • Witnessing resuscitation • 'Do not resuscitate' decisions • Withholding or withdrawing life-sustaining treatment in children • Advance directives • Limited knowledge base to draw upon: Creutzfeldt–Jakob disease • Preserving evidence • Summary	• This chapter is relevant to all chapters in this book

Introduction

This chapter will consider the skills and knowledge that are required for the safe care of children and young people in areas that can be difficult or controversial or where the evidence base might be just developing. It therefore seems prudent to begin with two aspects of caring that are central to care delivery to children and their families, namely coping and being present.

Coping

According to Boyle and Carter,[1] the way in which an individual copes is related to their perception of the situation as threatening or non-threatening and how they manage these demands. This is helped by drawing on past experiences of coping strategies that were used successfully, personality, skills and knowledge, which are blended together in a way that is unique to the individual. The authors point out that personal perception of a demand may change over time, so that a particular situation that was once seen as threatening may no longer hold the same threat for an individual.

A model based on a balance weighing scale using the principle of 'demands' and 'resources' has been found immensely helpful, although the original reference has been lost over the years and no plagiarism is intended!

This model requires the carer to take stock of their personal and practical resources. Like on an old-fashioned weighing scale, the other side of the scale balances the demands. It could look like this:

Resources	Demands
• I feel happy as a person, in my private and work life.	• It can be difficult juggling work and family.
• I have a good knowledge base.	• Caring for a very sick child can be very intense and consumes a lot of energy, especially when extra demands are made, such as emergency calls at night.
• I work in a supportive environment.	
• My partner understands the pressures of my work and is supportive.	• Often we are understaffed, which means many unscheduled 'on calls.'
• We make time to talk to each other and share our concerns.	• Recently I have cared for a family whose dying son was the same age as my son. I found this very upsetting and arrived home in tears many times.
• We enjoy many activities to balance our work and private life.	
• As a family we have a healthy lifestyle, including a healthy diet and plenty of exercise.	• This has caused a fair amount of friction at home.
• We have many friends whom we see regularly.	• Although my partner is very supportive, he often feels the burden that I carry at work, which is not fair on him.
• We try to have some 'us time' a couple of times a year.	

On a day-to-day basis we are able to maintain a balance between resources and demands. At times when increased demands are made on our coping abilities there are ways of increasing our resources, which help to maintain the balance. If the balance tips heavily towards the demands, stress occurs. If resources at this point cannot be increased and high demands lead to unrelieved stress, ways need to be found to relieve the burden of the demands. Otherwise 'burnout' may occur.

Being present

Benner[2] defines the concept of 'presence' as 'being with' rather than 'doing for', and identifies it as one of the eight competencies demonstrated by expert nurses. Rushton[3] explores this concept further.

- Being present involves the capacity to engage with and take action on behalf of another person within the tension of unknowing.
- A prerequisite for full presence is accepting the situation as it is, letting go of personal agendas or views about what others ought to do, and resisting the inclination to retreat when difficulties arise.
- Authentic presence involves the capacity to stay with the child and family until the end of the journey, experiencing whatever feelings are expressed, from loss to love, and from awkwardness to anger.
- By being fully present, healthcare workers can reassure children and their families that they are safe and cared for. However, a nurse can be physically present for

patients without being fully available to and engaged with them.

- Presence is not traditionally factored into time and cost analyses of nursing services because it is not easily quantifiable.

Rushton[3] offers the following self-assessment of the capacity to be present with dying children and their families.

- Am I present in my work?
- When am I most present in my work?
- How does it make me feel?
- What keeps me from being present in my work?
- How does it make me feel when I am not present in my work?
- What can I do both personally and professionally to be more present?
- How can I contribute to making my practice environment more healing?

Symptom control

There are a number of very good publications on symptom management, and they are easily accessible. For example, the symptom control manual developed at Rainbows children's hospice is available both from the Rainbows website (www.rainbows.eazytiger.net/index.asp) and on the ACT website. The *Oxford Textbook of Children's Palliative Care*[4] also includes a substantial section on symptom control, and the recently published *British National Formulary for Children*[5] has a section on children's palliative care.

Children and young people who are being cared for in any area, ranging from neonatal intensive care to receiving palliative care for a neurologically degenerative disease in their own home, require symptom control. The way in which this is assessed and implemented is not always suited to a 'blanket' approach. This has been highlighted, for example, in Chapter 4 with regard to the child who is paralysed by their medication and can express neither physical nor emotional distress.

Pain assessment[6]

There is a more detailed discussion of pain assessment in children with severe neurological impairment in Chapter 8. Issues relating to the administration of pain medication to the dying child are examined in Chapter 13.

Fowler-Kerry[7] states that there are 268 paediatric pain scales, yet there is a reluctance to use them. Anecdotal evidence suggests that there is a great deal of scepticism about the value of these scales, especially in children who have complex needs or are terminally ill. Although pain may have been the trigger, the distress that escalates around the initial trigger often also needs to be addressed. Loving attention and care alongside pain management will soothe and relieve the distress of feeling lonely, a drink will help to moisten a throat which is getting sore from crying, etc. Even where pain medication is given, a child is not left unattended until he or she has settled again. What makes pain scales invaluable is the fact that they require reassessment. This makes it necessary to check whether the action taken has worked and the pain and distress have been relieved, and if not, to enter a second loop of assessment and action.

Fowler-Kerry[7] suggests that we do have the technology to deal with this reluctance to use pain scales. Some countries utilise IT for care planning, and one option could be to prevent staff from logging out of a child's records until there is input of data on pain assessment, and evidence of how this was treated.

To feed or not to feed

The Royal College of Paediatrics and Child Health[8] identifies feeding as a particularly emotive area for parents and staff, and opinions about this vary. The College recommends that assisted feeding by nasogastric tube or gastrostomy should be considered very carefully and discussed fully with the family. It provides the following guidance to clarify the appropriateness of artificial feeding.

* It may be entirely appropriate for the child with a swallowing disorder due to a slowly progressive neurodegenerative disease.
* It would rarely be introduced for a child with a rapidly progressive, disseminated malignant disease.
* In other circumstances, its withdrawal can be accepted if it is well managed.

A very helpful discussion is provided by Zerwekh,[9] and although it is a little dated and focuses on adult hospice patients, the points raised might help to clarify and guide our decision making.

* Zerwekh highlights our role in sharing nursing expertise and our unique understanding of the patient so that informed decisions about hydration can be made and misconceptions about dehydration that may cause emotional distress to both patients and families can be challenged.
* There is a distinction between dehydration that is experienced when a patient is acutely ill and 'terminal dehydration.'

Miller suggests that terminal dehydration is a painless part of the dying process (personal communication, 2006). As the body 'winds down', perceptions are dulled and dehydration is not a major issue. Attempts to correct dehydration can be counterproductive, as nasogastric feeds are likely to cause vomiting and the siting of intravenous infusions may in itself cause distress.

This is one of the areas where staff using the Liverpool Care Pathways in research by Jack et al.[10] have reported greater confidence in managing care.

Witnessing resuscitation

Leveton et al.[11] state that bereavement is less complicated for families who have witnessed their child's resuscitation attempt than for those who wanted to be present but were barred from entering the room.

The Royal College of Nursing[12] has examined the wider issues of relatives witnessing resuscitation and has identified their needs, whether witnessing or being removed from the scene, as follows:

* to be with the dying person
* to be kept informed
* to know that the dying family member was not in pain.

Reasons for not allowing relatives in the room pertain mainly to the possibility that a family member's expression of uncontrolled grief or becoming physically involved in the resuscitation attempt could be disruptive. Furthermore, actions or remarks made by a team member might offend a relative or increase legal risks. Witnessing resuscitation is an experience that is non-therapeutic and traumatic. A final point pertains to the availability of trained staff to support the family. According to the Royal College of Nursing,[12] the benefits are as follows.

* The relative is able to see for him- or herself rather than just be told that everything possible is being done. It is believed that the reality of the resuscitation is far less hor-

rifying than what many relatives may imagine.

- The relative is able to touch the patient while their body is still warm.
- The relative can speak to the dying patient while there is still a chance that they can hear.
- The grieving process is hard enough without removing any processes that may help adjustment.

'Do not resuscitate' decisions

Simpson[13] describes an incident in a residential setting in which a child with profound learning disabilities was suffering an apnoeic episode. This responded to suctioning, and oxygen was administered until vital signs returned to normal, when further comfort measures were implemented.

This is where it becomes difficult. Is this resuscitation or is it part and parcel of the care according to an individual child's care plan? According to the *Concise Oxford Dictionary*,[14] the term 'resuscitate' means 'revive from unconsciousness or apparent death' or 'return or restore to…vividness.'

In Simpson's scenario, resuscitation never extended beyond airway management, the first step in the ABC of resuscitation, although for convenience a suction unit was used. In a palliative care context this does not conflict with the philosophy of palliative care where, for example, the use of suction is a standard intervention to alleviate distress.

Brykczynska[15] affirms that the needs of children who live with severe, often multiple disabilities should never be abandoned, reminds us of the intrinsic worth of all children with incurable diseases or non-treatable conditions, and urges us to ensure that they receive appropriate care. Resuscitation should be considered if this is likely to maintain the quality of life. Fertleman and Fox[16] have cited useful examples of cases where decisions to withhold or withdraw treatment have been clarified by a court of law. The current high-profile decision made on behalf of Charlotte Wyatt, now aged 2 years, is an example where a 'do not resuscitate' decision has been challenged by the child's parents. Charlotte was born at 26 weeks' gestation and has severe problems due to prematurity. The Hospital Trust believes that Charlotte has a poor quality of life, is unlikely to survive beyond infancy due to lung damage, and in the event of cardiopulmonary arrest should not be resuscitated. There have now been a number of court rulings. The current ruling is to resuscitate her if this is considered to be in her best interest. This has been reported amidst much media hype and speculation.[17]

> Mr Wyatt, 33, told the judge: 'When you get to the stage when you grow to love someone, you can't just throw them away like a bad egg and say you will get a different egg.'

Saunders *et al.*[18] state that in terminally ill patients it is not only quality of life that is important, but also the concept of a good death. They cite the following factors as being important for a good death:

- control of symptoms
- preparation for death
- opportunities for closure or a 'sense of completion of the life'
- a good relationship with healthcare professionals.

Boland[19] comments on the death of her 19-year-old son. During the terminal phase of cancer he developed a life-threatening haemorrhage which required embolisation and transfer to a different hospital for the procedure. The son insisted on having this treatment, despite being told that it was uncertain whether it would be successful. He survived this acute emergency for a span of time that gave both him and his parents time to come to terms with his impending death, and to achieve closure. Reflecting on the decision that was taken at the time, the mother concedes that it wasn't until the following day that she realised there was an element of doubt about the value of such an intervention – she did not think about the futility of the situation until later. She does not know how she would have felt if the procedure had not gone well.

In relation to Mr Wyatt's statement quoted above, it could also be argued from a philosophical perspective that it can be appropriate to let someone die out of love for that person. According to Saunders et al.,[18] although doctors have to consider what is best emotionally and psychologically for the family, and in particular how and where the patient should die, the doctor's responsibility is still in the first instance to consider the best interest of the child. Saunders et al. state that physiological quantitative measures such as survival to discharge after cardiopulmonary arrest can only be part of the assessment of whether treatment is futile. However, Neuberger[20] urges us to recognise the health that lies in dying well. An understanding that people differ in how they think about death and dying, and respect for those differences, goes a long way towards making people whole.

Withholding or withdrawing life-sustaining treatment in children

The Royal College of Paediatrics and Child Health[8] has updated and expanded the 1997 edition of *Withholding or Withdrawing Life-Sustaining Treatment in Children: a framework for practice* to take into account changes and advances that have occurred since the first edition was published. This document is available from the RCPCH website,[8] and it is strongly recommended that practitioners access the complete text. The main points are summarised below.

- The subject of withholding or withdrawing life-sustaining treatment in children is contentious, difficult and at times emotive.
- The framework is not a prescriptive formula to be applied in a rigid way in all cases, but an attempt to guide management in individual cases with the fundamental aim of considering and serving the best interest of the child.
- All members of the child health team, in partnership with the parents, have a duty to act in the best interest of the child.
- This includes sustaining life, and restoring health to an acceptable standard. However, there are circumstances in which treatments that merely sustain 'life' neither restore health nor confer any other benefit, and are therefore no longer in the child's best interest.
- There are five situations in which it may be ethical and legal to consider withholding or withdrawing treatment:

  - the brain-dead child
  - the child who is in a permanent vegetative state
  - the 'no chance situation'
  - the 'no purpose situation'
  - the 'unbearable situation.'

- In situations where there is uncertainty or disagreement about the degree of future impairment, the child's life should always be safeguarded in the best way possible.
- Decisions must never be rushed, and must always be made on the basis of all the evidence available, avoiding rigid rules even for conditions that seem hopeless.
- The decision to withhold or withdraw life-sustaining therapy should always be associated with consideration of the child's overall palliative or terminal care needs, including symptom alleviation and care that maintains human dignity and comfort.

Ethical principles

A number of ethical principles apply.

1. There is a duty of care with the primary intention of sustaining life and restoring the child's health. Whether or not a child can be restored to health, there is an absolute duty to comfort and cherish them and to prevent pain and suffering.
2. In fulfilling the duty of care, the healthcare team and the parents will enter a partnership of care to serve the best interests of the child.
3. This duty of care also involves respecting the ascertainable wishes and views of the child in the light of their knowledge, understanding and experience (for a discussion of advance directives, see below).

Legal principles

The following legal principles apply.

1. According to the Children Act 2004:[21]

   - the child's welfare is paramount
   - particular interest is paid to the wishes and feelings of the child
   - a child who is able to fully understand the nature of the proposed treatment can consent to that treatment
   - the person with parental responsibility can override a competent child's refusal to treatment.

2. The United Nations Convention on the Rights of the Child[22] enshrines the right of the child to enjoyment of the highest attainable standard of health, and to facilities for the treatment of illness and the rehabilitation of health, subject to the resources available.
3. However, a number of judgements on withholding or withdrawing life-sustaining treatment have established that:

   - there is no obligation to give treatment which is futile and burdensome – indeed this could be regarded as an assault on the child
   - treatment goals may be changed in the case of children who are dying
   - feeding and other medical treatment may be withdrawn in patients in whom the vegetative state is thought to be permanent (but in each case it is suggested that legal advice should be taken)
   - treatment may be withdrawn from patients if continuation is not in their best interest. Such treatments include:
     - experimental therapies which are not currently validated by research evidence
     - cardiopulmonary resuscitation
     - mechanical ventilation
     - intravenous inotropic agents
     - antibiotics
     - artificial nutrition (see above)
     - intravenous hydration.

Axioms on which to base practice

The Royal College of Paediatrics and Child Health[8] has presented the following axioms on which to base practice.

- There is no significant ethical difference between withdrawing (stopping) and withholding treatments.

- Optimal decision making about children's care requires open and timely communication between members of the healthcare team and the child and family, respecting their values and beliefs and the fundamental principles of ethics and human rights.
- Parents may ethically and legally decide for children who are unable to do so, unless the parents are clearly acting against the child's best interest, or are unable, unwilling or persistently unavailable to make decisions on behalf of their child.
- The wishes of the child who has sufficient understanding and experience in the evaluation of treatment options should be given substantial consideration in the decision-making process.
- Resolution of disagreement should be by discussion, consultation and consensus.
- The duty of care is not an absolute duty to preserve life by all means available. There is no obligation to provide life-sustaining treatment if:
  - its use is inconsistent with the aims and objectives of an appropriate treatment plan
  - the benefits of the treatment no longer outweigh the burden to the patient
  - redirection of management from life-sustaining treatment to palliation represents a change in beneficial aims and objectives and does not constitute withdrawal of care.
- It is never permissible to withdraw procedures that are designed to alleviate pain or promote comfort.

Disability

- The Royal College of Paediatrics and Child Health[8] states that the Court of Appeal accepts that it is lawful to withdraw life-prolonging treatment when the quality of life that the child would have to endure, given the treatment, would be so impaired as to be intolerable to the child. However, the court recognised that what could be considered intolerable to an able-bodied person would not necessarily be unacceptable to a child who has been born disabled.
- Many people with severe impairment describe a life that is of a high quality and say they are happy to be living it. Impairment is not incompatible with a life of quality.

Euthanasia

- Withdrawal of life-sustaining treatment in appropriate circumstances is *not* regarded by the courts as active killing, nor is it viewed as a breach of the right of life under Article 2 of the European Convention on Human Rights.
- Where withdrawal of ventilator support does not lead to death, it is made clear that euthanasia is *not* appropriate and that palliative care should be offered. The lives of unexpected survivors, even when they are badly disabled, should be respected and they should be cared for appropriately.
- Giving a medicine with the primary intention of hastening death is unlawful. Giving a medicine to relieve suffering which may, as a side-effect, hasten death is lawful and can be appropriate.
- It is recognised in English and Scottish law that increasing doses of analgesia necessary for the control of pain or distress may shorten life. The giving of opioids is for the benefit of the patient during life, not in order to cause or hasten death.

Clinical responsibilities of the healthcare team

The Royal College of Paediatrics and Child Health[8] has made it clear that treatment must not be inflicted on children just because a treatment has become available. It must be introduced for the benefit of the child and withdrawn when it is no longer of benefit.

The clinical team will almost always have to start from a premise of uncertainty. It is crucial to wait until enough information is available to decide on individual outcome. It is recognised that such delay may become a source of tension within the team. This information must include a clear diagnosis where possible and an awareness of the likely prognosis, given an appraisal of the possible therapeutic options. Decisions to stop or withhold certain treatments will almost always be based on probabilities rather than certainties. Some children whose medical treatment is withdrawn go on to survive, and it is not a wrong decision if this is the outcome. Treatment is withdrawn because it is futile, but not with the intention that to do so will bring about death. Continuing support, respect and palliative care are required for the unexpected survivor. In the situation where treatment is being withheld, the team need to be flexible in the face of changing circumstances.

pp. 29–30[8]

Advance directives

Gillick[23] describes advance directives as the cornerstone of advance planning, encompassing instructions both about what kind of care should be provided (living wills) and about who should make decisions if the patient cannot do so (proxy destinations). Although specific issues can be identified, such as the use of feeding tubes or ventilators, it is unlikely that all the potential situations in which patients might find themselves could ever be covered. Gillick warns that the precision of advance directives makes them inflexible, as whether or not a given procedure is acceptable may depend on what the intervention is expected to achieve and what alternatives are available.

With regard to the literature on advance directives in the context of competent adults, this is applicable to young people over the age of 16 years according to the Family Law Reform Act 1969.[24] It is apparent that a very similar terminology is used in the Mental Capacity Act 2005[25] to that in the Royal College of Paediatrics and Child Health document[8] for ascertaining competence both in a child and in a vulnerable adult. In the case of a dissenting child of any age the decision can be overruled by the person who holds parental responsibility or by the court.

According to the factsheet published by the Department for Constitutional Affairs,[25] the key principles of the Mental Capacity Act 2005 are as follows.

- An assumption of capacity.
- Capacity is decision specific. (In the case of a young child this might mean that the child has a very good understanding of their own disease, what it is like to have another transplant or more chemotherapy, and they also know from experience of other children in hospital that they might die and further treatment might or might not help. The same child would still have the cognitive abilities corresponding to their age and stage of development in every other respect.)
- Participation in decision making – everyone should be encouraged and enabled to make their own decisions, or to participate as fully as possible in decision making, by being given the help and support necessary to make and express a choice.
- Individuals must retain the right to make what might be seen as eccentric or unwise decisions. (This might apply to a young adult – as discussed, for example, in Chapter 6 – and in the case of a child is subject to agreement by the person with parental responsibility or the courts.)
- All decisions must be in the person's best interest. Decisions that are made on behalf of people without capacity should be made in their best interest, giving weight to the decision that is what they themselves would have wanted.
- Designated decision makers can be appointed, known as 'lasting powers of attorney' (LPAs).

- There will also be two new statutory bodies, namely a court of protection and a public guardian.

The Royal College of Paediatrics and Child Health[8] states that the antecedent wishes and preferences of the child, if known, should also carry considerable weight, given that conditions at the time for action closely match those envisaged in advance. This implies that children can be helped to formulate 'living wills' or advance directives within the context of their understanding of their situation and possible interventions.

Gillick[23] asserts that advance care planning is a process that begins with the physician helping their patient to articulate and prioritise their goals of care before a crisis develops.

According to the Royal College of Paediatrics and Child Health,[8] good practice involves informing children, listening to them, taking into account their views so that these can influence decisions, and respecting the competent child as the main decision maker about proposed healthcare interventions. Although decisions are ultimately likely to be made by the person with parental responsibility, these clear channels of communication ensure that a parent can be guided and will hopefully endorse the wishes of the child.

Lo and Steinbrook[26] consider that advance directives have not fulfilled their promise of facilitating decisions about end-of-life care for incompetent (adult) patients. They suggest that they would be more useful if they emphasised discussion of end-of-life care with physicians rather than completion of a legal document. This might be particularly relevant to older children and young adults, for whom the transition to adult services might be in progress. It is probable that young adults would nominate their parents as proxies.

A practical example of an advance declaration can be found on the website of the Guild of Catholic Doctors.[27] The authors regard the strength of the document as the fact that it sees medical care as a partnership between patient, family and healthcare personnel seeking to act in the best interest of the patient.

However, Lo and Steinbrook[26] found that proxies cannot accurately state patients' wishes in specific scenarios. Gillick[23] highlights the dilemma concerning Terry Schaivo, who died in 2005 in a persistent vegetative state. Since 1990 she had been caught up in a bitter argument between her husband and her parents as to whether feeding should be stopped. This eventually involved the US senate and the president, and made international headlines.

Discussion of end-of-life decisions should include the topic of palliative care (while discussion of disease-oriented care is continued), spiritual and religious concerns, and the importance of not undermining hope. [26]

Limited knowledge base to draw upon: Creutzfeldt–Jakob disease

In the last few years there have been several cases particularly of young people who have contracted the human form of 'mad cow disease', which has resulted in rapid deterioration of neurological function and death in these individuals. Very little information could be identified in relation to variant Creutzfeldt–Jakob disease (vCJD) in children.

According to the British Paediatric Surveillance Unit:[28]

- the presentation of vCJD is not typical of classical CJD, making the clinical presentation of any cases in children difficult to predict
- the strategy employed by the surveillance unit is to detect suspected vCJD cases by looking at a broader group of conditions that cause progressive intellectual and neurological deterioration in children (the PIND study; *see also* Chapter 8)
- children who present with the following symptoms are included in the study:

  – progressive deterioration for more than 3 months, with loss of already attained intel-

lectual/developmental abilities and development of abnormal neurological signs
  - children who meet the above definition even if specific neurological diagnoses have been made
  - metabolic disorders leading to neurological deterioration
  - seizure disorders if associated with progressive deterioration
  - children who have been diagnosed as having neurodegenerative conditions but who have not yet developed symptoms.

- Using this approach, not only are vCJD cases detected, but also unique epidemiological data are collected on a variety of PIND conditions.
- In June 2006, the National Creutzfeldt–Jakob Disease Surveillance Unit (http//:cjd.ed.ac.uk) gave the total number across all age groups as 161. This breaks down into different age groups for young people under 40 years of age (personal communication, Ian Mackenzie, 2006).

	Age at death	Current age (alive cases) at 15 June 2006
10–14	1	–
15–19	20	–
20–24	30	5
25–29	36	–
30–34	32	–
35–39	18	–

Stewart and Ironside[29] have affirmed the link between bovine spongiform encephalopathy (BSE or 'mad cow disease') and vCJD. Although it is impossible to estimate how many people are likely to become ill as a consequence of this, Coulthart and Cashman[30] state that due to the widespread distribution of foodstuff containing bovine products, one infected animal could expose 500,000 consumers to BSE.

Horby[31] describes vCJD as follows.

- It is one of a family of neurological diseases known as either 'prion disease' or transmissible spongiform encephalopathies (TSE).
- It is characterised by the deposition of an abnormal protein in the central nervous system and vacuolation of the grey matter.
- CJD can be sporadic, inherited or acquired (vCJD is acquired).
- The age range of affected patients by 2002 was 12–74 years.
- More than 115 people are known to have died from vCJD.
- Diagnosis is based on clinical presentation, characteristic appearance of magnetic resonance imaging (MRI) and the exclusion of other causes. A distinctive feature of vCJD is the widespread distribution of the abnormal protein in peripheral tissues, such as lymphoid tissue, spleen, lymph nodes, tonsils, optic nerve and retina. Although pre-mortem diagnosis is possible by brain or tonsil biopsy, the clinical diagnostic criteria seem to be sufficiently reliable to allow definitive diagnosis to wait until after death.
- The early and predominant symptoms are psychiatric (e.g. depression, anxiety and apathy), sometimes accompanied by painful sensory symptoms, which helps to distinguish vCJD from sporadic CJD.

Allroggen *et al.*[32] also describe other neurological signs such as ataxia and involuntary movements later in the course of the disease, and patients succumbing in a state of akinetic mutism and myoclonus.

As with all medical problems that are encountered for the first time, symptoms are dealt with as they present, guided by the evolving picture and knowledge of the disease. Mallucci and Collinge[33] warn that clinicians need to be alert for behavioural and psychiatric abnormalities in young people in association with cerebellar or cognitive abnormalities. They stress that the psychiatric presentation of CJD is not specific, and that diagnosis relies on the development of progressive neurodegenerative features.

We know that vCJD is a transmissible disease, which has implications for the prevention of infection. This is guided by so-called 'universal precautions', which have been adopted universally since the early 1980s. Madeo[34] highlights the fact that studies have shown that compliance with hand hygiene is only adhered to in about 40% of situations.

Policies are in place across health authorities to offer guidance and advice through a well-established network of a multi-disciplinary team within the specialty of infection control.

In the case of prion disease the agent is extremely resistant to current methods of decontamination. Horby[31] states that current processes cannot guarantee complete inactivation of infectivity, and recommends the tracking and quarantining or destruction of instruments used on people who are subsequently diagnosed with CJD. Jackson et al.[35] state that inactivation on surfaces requires autoclaving at high temperatures or treating with sodium hypochlorite for an extended period. It follows that wherever possible disposable equipment should be used and non-disposables destroyed according to relevant local guidelines. It is therefore prudent to explore how likely a patient is to shed infective material on an individual basis in order to adhere to health and safety guidelines. Fishman et al.[36] provide a sobering account of a situation where either a patient with CJD or his infected tissue passed through a number of departments, and was handled or dealt with using reusable equipment which was then decontaminated using standard methods that do not inactivate prion-infected material. As a result, the unit was unable to identify used equipment, thus potentially putting both staff and patients at risk. After the patient's death, communication with the funeral directors also proved to be ineffective. This resulted in the patient being embalmed, again using reusable equipment which therefore could not be adequately decontaminated, posing a potential risk to personnel handling infectious body fluids and tissues.

However, there is a need to be clear about the overall infection risk and management in order to prevent the kind of hysteria that was sometimes encountered in the early 1980s with regard to patients with HIV/AIDS, although it was quickly discovered that normal social contact with people infected with HIV/AIDS posed no risk to either healthcare workers or the general public.

Health authorities have guidelines in place on dealing with patients who are infected with prion disease. The Paediatric Intensive Care Society[37] gives guidelines for handling bodies with infections, which for CJD and vCJD requires the use of body bags and does not permit the bereaved to touch and spend time with the body.

Stringent guidelines have been introduced to reduce the risk of transmission posed by blood and blood products.[32] However, there have been 55 reported cases of transmission of CJD in France through the use of human growth hormone.[38] Fishman et al.[36] identify the following body tissues as infectious:

- corneal transplants
- cadaveric human growth hormones
- cadaveric dura mater grafts
- cerebrospinal fluid
- human pituitary extract.

Kidney, liver and lung are potentially infectious, and lymph tissue as well as the other items on this particular list has since been identified as infectious, illustrating the need to regularly review practices in the light of new evidence.

Coulthart and Cashman[30] warn that the unsettling nature of the available evidence warrants prudence with regard to public health policy and regulation, as well as a for-ward-looking approach to research. Knight[39] states that there has been media coverage of some potential treatments (e.g. quinacrine, pentosan polysulphate and flupirtine), and the Medical Research Council is funding a trial (PRION 1) designed to study the possible effects of quinacrine. Knight stresses that to date no treatment has been shown conclu-sively to slow or halt the disease process of vCJD. This is also the advice from the CJD Advisory Group.[40] At the time of writing this book it was announced that a blood test to identify vCJD might be available soon.[41]

Preserving evidence

Looking at the symptoms investigated by the British Paediatric Surveillance Unit,[28] the need to preserve 'evidence' as discussed in the Introduction becomes clear. There might be conditions that are coming to light for the first time, they might not have a 'label' and they might be considered to be 'one-offs'. Being able to retrospectively identify and diag-nose diseases might give vital clues to how a disease evolves over the longer term. It might well turn out that some undiagnosed 'one-off' neurological diseases have been around much longer than was thought to be the case, but that the technology necessary to iden-tify them was not available when they first presented.

Summary

This chapter has considered issues relating to caring for the dying child or young person and their family. Issues that have been explored include feeding and hydration, 'do not resuscitate' decisions and decisions about withdrawal or withholding of treatment. Advance directives have been considered and found to be of value in encouraging dia-logue between parents, the child or young person and medical personnel. Establishing and respecting the wishes of a child or young person as far as possible needs to be seen first and foremost as good practice, rather than just as a legal issue.

Creutzfeldt–Jakob disease has been examined as a new disease in children and young people in terms of the learning process of applying new evidence as it evolves.

SWOT

It might be useful to revisit the SWOT analysis at this point in order to determine any fur-ther learning needs in relation to this chapter.

Strengths	Weaknesses
Opportunities	Threats

Resources and demands exercise

At this point the reader might wish to examine the resources and demands in their own personal and professional life and reflect how their personal coping strategies could be bolstered before determining any further learning needs in relation to this chapter.

Resources	*Demands*
1.	1.
2.	2.
3.	3.
4.	4.
5.	5.
6.	6.

Action plan for further learning

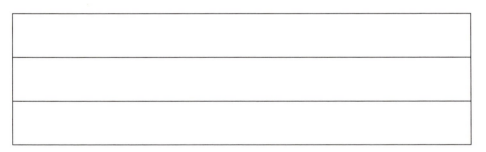

References

1. Boyle M and Carter D (1998) Death anxiety amongst nurses. *Int J Palliat Care.* **4**: 37–43.
2. Benner P (1984) *From Novice to Expert: excellence and power in clinical nursing practice.* Addison-Wesley, Menlo Park, CA.
3. Rushton C (2005) A framework for integrated paediatric palliative care: being with dying. *J Pediatr Nurs.* **20**: 311–25.
4. Goldman A, Hain R and Liben S (2006) *The Oxford Textbook of Paediatric Palliative Care.* Oxford University Press, Oxford.
5. British Medical Association (BMA) (2006) *British National Formulary for Children (BNFC).* BMA, London; www.bnfc.org
6. Paediatric Pain Profile; www.ppprofile.org.uk/index.htm
7. Fowler-Kerry S (2004) A working model. Second International Paediatric Palliative Care Conference, Evidence: who needs it? Cardiff, December 2004.
8. Royal College of Paediatrics and Child Health (RCPCH) (2004) *Withholding or Withdrawing Life-Saving Treatment in Children: a framework of practice.* RCPCH, London; www.rcpch.ac.uk

9. Zervekh J (1997) Do dying patients really need IV fluids? *Am J Nurs.* **97:** 26–30.
10. Jack B, Gambles M, Murphy D *et al.* (2003) Nurses' perceptions of the Liverpool Care Pathway for the dying patient in the acute hospital setting. *Int J Palliat Nurs.* **9:** 375–81.
11. Leverton M, Liben S and Audet M (2004) Palliative care in the intensive-care unit. In: B Carter and M Leveton (eds) *Palliative Care for Infants, Children and Adolescents.* The Johns Hopkins University Press, Baltimore, MD.
12. Royal College of Nursing (2002) *Witnessing Resuscitation: guidance for nursing staff.* Royal College of Nursing, London.
13. Simpson R (2000) Do not resuscitate: critical incident reflection. *Paediatr Nurs.* **12:** 23–6.
14. Fowler H and Fowler F (1992) *Concise Oxford Dictionary.* Clarendon Press, Oxford.
15. Brykczynska G (1998) When life-saving treatment is futile. *Paediatr Nurs.* **10:** 6–7.
16. Fertleman M and Fox A (2003) The law of consent in England as applied to the sick neonate. *Internet J Pediatr Neonatol.* **3;** www.ispub.com/ostia/index.php?xml FilePath=journals/ijp/vol3nl/consent.xml
17. http://news.bbc.co.uk/1/hi/health/3723656.stm
18. Saunders Y, Ross J and Riley J (2003) Planning a good death: responding to unexpected events. *BMJ.* **327:** 204–6.
19. Boland L and Laverty D (2003) Commentary: mother's response. *BMJ.* **327:** 206–7.
20. Neuberger J (2003) A healthy view of dying. *BMJ.* **327:** 207–8.
21. Children Act 2004; www.opsi.gov.uk/acts/acts2004/20040031.htm
22. Joint Committee on Human Rights (1991) *The UN Convention on the Rights of the Child.* The Stationery Office, London.
23. Gillick M (2004) Advance care planning. *NEJM.* **350:** 7–8.
24. Family Reform Act 1969; www.opsi.gov.uk/acts/acts1990
25. Mental Capacity Act 2005; www.opsi.gov.uk/acts/acts2005/20050009.htm
26. Lo B and Steinbrook R (2004) Resuscitation advance directives. *Arch Intern Med.* **164:** 1501–6.
27. Guild of Catholic Doctors; www.catholicdoctors.org.uk/books/livwill_book.htm
28. British Paediatric Surveillance Unit; http://bpsu.com/current.htm
29. Steward G and Ironside J (1998) New variant Creutzfeldt–Jakob disease. *Curr Opin Neurol.* **11:** 259–62.
30. Coulthart M and Cashman N (2001) Variant Creutzfeldt–Jakob disease: a summary of current scientific knowledge in relation to public health. *Can Med Assoc J.* **165:** 51–8.
31. Horby P (2002) Variant Creutzfeldt–Jakob disease: an unfolding epidemic of misfolded proteins. *J Paediatr Child Health.* **38**: 539–42.
32. Allroggen H, Dennis G, Abbott R *et al.* (2000) New variant Creutzfeldt–Jakob disease: three case reports from Leicester. *J Neurol Neurosurg Psychiatry.* **68:** 375–8.
33. Mallucci G and Collinge J (1997) Neuropsychiatric presentation of prion disease. *Curr Opin Psychiatry.* **10:** 59–62.
34. Madeo M (2004) Commentary on Bennett G and Mansell I (2004) Universal precautions: a survey of community nurses' experience and practice. *J Clin Nurs.* **13:** 1017–19.
35. Jackson M, Rickman L and Pugliese G (2000) Emerging infectious diseases. *Am J Nurs.* **100:** 66–71.
36. Fishman M, Fort G and Mikolich D (1998) Prevention of Creutzfeldt–Jakob disease in health care workers: a case study. *Am J Infect Control.* **26:** 74–9.
37. Paediatric Intensive Care Society (2002) *Standards for Bereavement Care.* Paediatric Intensive Care Society, London.
38. D'Aignaux H, Costagliola D, Maccario J *et al.* (1999) Incubation period of Creutzfeldt–Jacob disease in human growth hormone recipients in France. *Neurology.* **53:** 1197–201.
39. Knight R (2005) Potential treatments for Creutzfeldt–Jacob disease; www.cjd.ed.ac.uk/TREAT.htm

40. CJD Advisory Group; www.dh.gov.uk/PolicyAndGuidance/HealthAndSocialCare Topics/CJD/CJDGe

41. BBC News item on progress towards a blood test for variant Creutzfeldt–Jakob disease, broadcast on 29 August 2005 at 10 p.m. on BBC1.

Chapter 13

End-of-life care

This chapter covers

Content	Relevant to other areas of palliative care for children and young people
<ul><li>Introduction</li><li>Recognition of end of life</li><li>The Knowledge and Skills Framework</li><li>The National Service Framework</li><li>The ACT Care Pathway</li><li>The setting</li><li>The journey towards 'letting go'</li><li>Death anxiety among healthcare professionals</li><li>The process of death and dying</li><li>The biological processes of death</li><li>When death has occurred</li><li>Time-of-death arrangements</li><li>Post-mortems</li><li>Self-reflection</li><li>Summary</li></ul>	<ul><li>This chapter is relevant to all other chapters</li></ul> ***Relevant topics in other chapters***<ul><li>Chapter 4: funerals</li><li>Chapter 4: helping siblings</li><li>Chapter 2: emotional safety in adverse events</li><li>Chapter 3: emergency baptism</li></ul>

Introduction

This chapter will consider the skills and knowledge that are required for the safe care of children and young people and their families as they enter the final stage of life. Neuberger[1] has observed that nothing can prepare a young doctor, nurse or rabbi for facing people whose death is imminent and their families, and realising that it is in their power to make a huge difference. Harrington Jacobs[2] states that nursing at the end of life combines the science of nursing with ethics, philosophy, the humanities, diverse world views, and individual and family life experiences in order to provide holistic care to families who are experiencing life-limiting illness. This is where it becomes obvious how the ACT Care Pathway, the Knowledge and Skills Framework and Evidence Based Practice work in action!

Recognition of end of life

So far in this book much consideration has been given to whether or not a child or young person is perceived as being 'palliative.' In terms of the ACT Care Pathway, children and their families might have come through Pathways 1 and 2, and some families will have gone through several loops of Pathway 2. This is the point at which they enter Pathway 3.

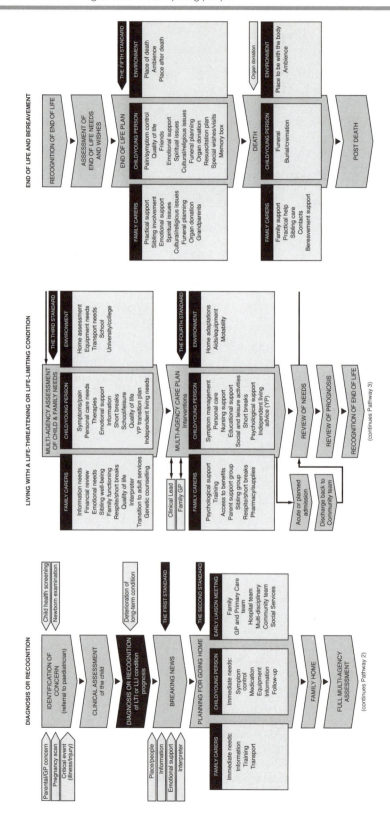

The Knowledge and Skills Framework[3]

This has the following requirements:

1. communication
2. personal and people development
3. health, safety and security
4. service improvement
5. quality
6. equality and diversity.

The National Service Framework[4]

Although the Core Standards, Disabled Child and Mental Health are helpful, the detail will be found in the ACT Care Pathway.

The ACT Care Pathway[5]

Throughout this book the reader has been encouraged to consider where the child, their family and the carers are on the pathways.

On reflection it might have been found that individuals in a scenario did not find themselves in the same place at the same time, due to a variety of reasons (e.g. denial on the part of one of the parents, or a consultant already a step ahead). Hynson *et al.*[6] assert that a holistic approach to palliative care requires a multi-disciplinary team approach to ensure meticulous attention to planning, coordination and communication. Ellershaw and Ward[7] found that the most important element in diagnosing dying is that the members of the multi-disciplinary team who are caring for the patient agree that the patient is likely to die. If this agreement is not reached, then mixed messages with opposed goals of care can lead to poor patient management and confused communication. In addition, according to Rushton,[8] too often assumptions are made about parental intentions and understanding without examining their perspectives and experiences. It is important that all involved use the same terminology and regularly touch base to avoid conflict. Browne (personal communication, 2005) would like the 'end-of-life' plan to be considered at regular intervals throughout a child's life. According to Browne this does not have to be a long conversation, but maybe just involves asking 'Is there anything you would like to discuss in relation to this part of the pathway today?' Even in cases where this is still many years away, it allows an evaluation of the stage that a family has reached – at a time of no crisis. This ensures that when a child does enter this final part of the pathway it is more likely that the plan for this part of the journey can be reviewed and implemented smoothly.

Harrington Jacob[2] confirms that proactive planning reduces tension in decision making, specifically with regard to withdrawal of medical therapies. Rather than focusing on what will not be done, the emphasis will be on aggressive palliative interventions that *will* be done! Jack *et al.*[9] evaluated the Liverpool Care Pathway for the dying patient and found that the pathway had an extremely positive impact, resulting in increased confidence and knowledge about care for dying patients.

There are a number of common ethical dilemmas in caring for terminally ill children. These might include 'do not resuscitate' decisions, withdrawal of treatment (which might range from ventilator support to nutritional support) and deciding whether a child should be sedated or allowed to be lucid. These have been considered in more detail in Chapter 12, but are also relevant to the content of this chapter.

The terminal phase of a child's illness has the following elements:

- physiological processes (recognising that the dying phase has been entered and tapering physical care and symptom management accordingly), identifying that death has

occurred, and care of the body after the child's death
- psychosocial and spiritual elements both for the child and their family and for the carers
- legal and ethical issues.

Knowing how to get 'dying care' right is difficult in a subject area where the lack of research evidence is glaringly obvious. Miller (personal communication, 2005) explains that recognising the terminal stage is one of the challenges, if not *the* challenge, of palliative care.

What are the actual biological processes that occur when someone dies? If these are well understood, then decisions about what should be done (e.g. suction, oxygen, continuing feeds) and what should not be done (e.g. intubation, cardiopulmonary resuscitation) are much more straightforward. What might be considered a grey area (e.g. intravenous fluids, antibiotics, non-invasive ventilation) can also be discussed at the appropriate time.

Similarly, symptom control, especially pain relief, should not be seen as another dilemma. If the nurse who is administering pain relief is anxious that he or she might be seen as giving 'the last dose before the child died', it could be implied that it was the medication that caused death. This type of thinking occurs when the carer does not fully understand the processes involved in the 'dying phase.' On the one hand it clouds the assessment that the child needs the medication, and that the child's eventual death is due to the fact that life has become unsustainable due to terminal shutdown of all the major body systems. On the other hand, it can leave practitioners feeling vulnerable with regard to their own practice. Harrington Jacob[2] has explained the principle of 'double effect', and the reader is encouraged to consult this article. Two important points emerge from it. First, nurses should not hesitate to use full and effective doses of pain medication for the proper management of pain in the dying patient. Secondly, a nurse may believe that by not giving an opioid drug they might cause benefit by avoiding the death of the patient. Yet many people, including children in pain, would argue that more harm than good is done by not giving pain medication, because the patient would be very uncomfortable. Miller (personal communication, 2005) sees the overriding role of clinical staff as ensuring that the child is symptom free. There is no dignity in severe pain. Other aspects of care, such as maintaining autonomy and doing no harm, come second. Harrington Jacob[2] asserts that unease about this practice is to be anticipated, and institutional support in the form of ethics committees can help nurses to navigate these ethical dilemmas.

The setting

The way in which some aspects of care are dealt with also depends to a large degree on the setting in which a terminally ill child receives care. A team that is experienced in 'dying care', whether it is based in a hospital, a hospice or the community, is likely to have a mechanism in place that offers expertise and support within a multi-disciplinary team. Staff in settings where either children are infrequently cared for, or young adults are for the first time receiving care from adult services, can feel very vulnerable during the final pathway of these patients.

The four ACT categories have been used to structure the order in which the scenarios in this book have been presented. In each of these categories (and also within the categories themselves) the needs of the child or young person and their family have differed. Solomon *et al.*[10] point out that hospitals have rarely developed the mechanisms necessary for specifically responding to those needs. The authors state that during their training physicians and nurses are given virtually no opportunities to practise the skills necessary for communicating effectively with dying children and their families. According to these authors, practising healthcare professionals also lack guidance on how best to manage the conflicting goals and values that can arise in difficult circumstances.

END OF LIFE AND BEREAVEMENT

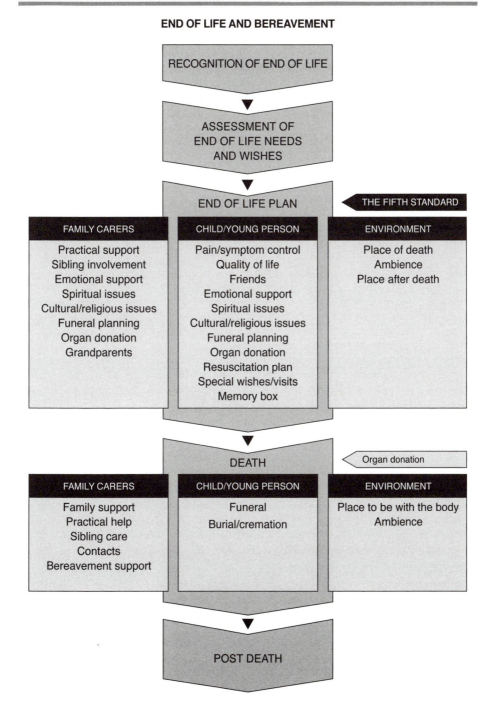

Rushton[8] asserts that a culture of 'cure at all cost' overshadows the obligation to provide dignified, humane and compassionate care. This is often incompatible with 'letting go.'

Hynson *et al.*[6] highlight the fact that the death of a child results in more intense parental grief than is experienced in response to other forms of loss (e.g. the death of a spouse). This is associated with a higher risk of complicated grief reactions and an increased mortality rate in bereaved parents. These authors point out that although siblings are almost universally distressed and might not share their feelings with their already burdened parents, little research has been done on the impact of a child's death on the grandparents.

Davies[11] has studied the need of mothers to be with their dying child, and to be with their child's body after death. The mothers whose child had died in a children's hospice experienced a slow and gentle separation during which it was possible to attend to the child's body while the staff understood and responded to the mothers' need for time, space and privacy.

Cultural needs can be met where such a philosophy can be practised. Davies[11] gives an account of a British-Asian mother whose faith required the baby to be buried within 24 hours of death. She was able to be with her dead baby for several hours, thereby fulfilling her need to hold her child before burial. This contrasted sharply with hospital deaths in the same study, where only a curtain around a bed space separated a child who was having an asthma attack from a family saying their goodbyes to their child. Mothers had limited opportunities to be with their child, because of the need for removal of the body to the hospital mortuary and funeral director. These mothers had limited memories of this time, and those memories were more likely to be a cause of distress: '…the hardest thing I ever had to do is walk away from the hospital.'[11]

Rushton[8] points out that the healthcare organisation and all its members are accountable for the environment in which care is delivered. Within organisations, individuals are responsible for striving to reach the goal of respect and preserving integrity in every encounter and decision.

The journey towards 'letting go'

Knowing that it is going to happen

Rushton[8] examines the concept of 'respect' for parents in relation to helping parents to honour their commitment to their child. It is not a matter of parents proving their commitment to their child, but rather of healthcare professionals challenging their own assumptions, often unverified, about the capacities and intentions of parents. This might lead to a new perspective on working with families. Rushton[8] draws different conclusions about the request that 'everything be done':

> When parents demand that 'everything be done' in the face of a dismal prognosis and overwhelming odds of death, they may not be in denial or misinformed, but rather intent on fulfilling their parental obligations by pursuing every option on their child's behalf…what healthcare professionals may consider denial or a challenge to their competence and judgement may, in fact, be an expression of the parents' need for reassurance that *everything appropriate* has been done.

Fear of the unknown

'Fear of the unknown' is probably the aspect that worries parents the most once it becomes obvious that the point of death is approaching. Very few parents will have seen anyone die, and they might have distressing misconceptions about death. It is vital to explore this with the parents and to give them information in a sensitive way and in general terms as a starting point from which deeper issues, such as fear of not coping or fear of a violent death, can be explored and reassurance given. Not all parents will ask questions, and sometimes it is necessary to anticipate what the parents might need to know (e.g. 'Would you like me to tell you what might happen?', which might include areas such as 'We can ensure that your child is pain free', 'You can hold your child if that is what you want' or 'Are you worried about how you will know that your child has died?'). Similarly, there might be a tendency to hide behind previously observed routines pertaining to the care of the child's body, and parents might not realise that unless the death has become a coroner's case the child's body could be taken home or to a children's hospice. Davies[11] describes the anger of a mother who found out a year after her child's death that this would have been a much wanted option had she only known about it.

Death anxiety among healthcare professionals

The Scottish Partnership Agency for Palliative and Cancer Care[12] states that care delivery with a palliative approach is a core skill that every healthcare professional in every setting should possess if they are dealing with patients with incurable progressive disease. This statement clearly extends across the full range of palliative care. Yet it is the stress associated with death that prompted Boyle and Carter[13] to examine death anxiety among nurses in greater detail and to link it to factors such as personality, life experience, age and religion.

The human experience of death involves confronting the cessation of life and the reality of one's own death-related fears, which according to Boyle and Carter could be said to depict contemporary society's suppressed views of and distaste for death, which are likely to be carried over into the occupational subculture and reflected in the behaviour of healthcare professionals. This may negatively influence attitudes and behaviours towards dying patients and their families, creating obstacles due to fear and anxiety, and leading to responses of avoidance, denial and repression.

Student nurses as well as any member of the multi-disciplinary team who has never seen anyone die also have great concerns about 'dying care', and look for role modelling from more experienced staff. Some 'experienced' staff will have had limited or possibly negative experiences themselves, making them reluctant to engage in this type of conversation. A website accessed through the Liverpool Care Pathway website[14] illustrates just how urgently a pooling of informal evidence is needed. Contributors to a discussion forum discuss 'diagnosing dying', and have noticed a 'pinched-nose' look and other features in dying elderly patients. Although some contributors remembered having heard of this during their nursing training, all of them agree that this observation is not research based. A doctor finally offers the explanation that changes in features are evidence based, and that these features are caused by the profound weakness (including physical fatigue and mental obtundation) and are described in the Liverpool pathway.

The process of death and dying

Copp[15] has examined current theories of death and dying. She discusses Buckman's[16] expansion of the five-stage theory of Kubler-Ross,[17] including aspects such as 'fear of dying, guilt, hope, despair and humour.' Often overlooked is the fact that 'dying' can vary in duration, and may be rapid, slow or plateau, characterised by short-term improvements and relapses, before a final downward plunge.[18] Copp[15] also identifies conflict and tensions in the patient, their family and the medical/nursing staff when an expected death trajectory changes, which disrupts the organisation of work (e.g. when a patient either dies unexpectedly or continues to linger when death is expected). In this context Corr[19] has suggested a model which, like any model, if it is to be of use must contribute to:

- improved understanding
- empowerment
- participation and guidance for helpers to cope with dying.

Copp[15] suggests that clinical practice should take into consideration the following:

- the feelings and responses of individuals to death and dying (e.g. denial, anger, etc.)
- the interactions and interplay between the dying person and other individuals (e.g. mutual pretence, closed awareness, suspicious awareness, etc.)
- the shape, form and duration of the dying process, which affect not only the individual who is dying, but also others around the person
- the nature of the dimensions or tasks of dying – people who are dying normally have to cope with four primary dimensions or tasks of dying, namely physical, psychological, social and spiritual
- the implications of carers – improved understanding, empowerment, participation and guidance are seen as important for helpers in coping with dying.

No cross-referencing of theories has been noted between the paediatric and adult literature. Research with a paediatric focus has been reported by Bluebond-Langner.[20–22]

The biological processes of death

Death encompasses aspects that affect the body, mind and soul of the child or young person who is dying, and also of the family members, for whom the memories of this event will last for ever. Although the biological processes are the focus of this section, it is recognised that emotional and spiritual aspects continue concurrently.

Winston[23] explains that the process of death is not a single quick event, but a slow winding down. It is difficult to say when every cell in the body ceases to have life. Long before we stop breathing the brain may die, our personality lost for ever, but the biology can look cold and distant from the human story.

Literature about the actual process of dying is not easily accessible, although this knowledge is utilised when caring for patients in the terminal stages of their illness. Miller (personal communication, 2005) explains that death occurs when a major organ fails, with the consequences of lack of oxygen supply to other organs, which means that they also fail. Medical management is usually aimed at recognising impending organ failure and then supporting this organ until recovery takes place. Often support of a failing organ requires extraordinary intervention that is invasive and potentially painful, and carries the risk of severe complications.

A terminal stage is reached when the child is unlikely to gain long-term benefit from intervention and there will be no significant improvement in their quality of life.

Miller stresses the subjective phrases in this last sentence – 'terminal stage', 'long-term benefit' and 'quality of life', highlighting the fact that there may be disagreements or different points of view.

He explains that heart, respiratory, liver, kidney or gut failure are all clearly recognised and have clear outcomes if not reversed. However, irreversible 'failure' of the higher cerebral functions is very difficult to diagnose. Failure of the brainstem inevitably leads to death and does have clear guidelines for diagnosis.

In a child with cystic fibrosis the primary problem is lack of oxygen uptake by the lungs, and without oxygen all the other organs fail. Describing events in terms of the laws of thermodynamics, Miller explains that everything deteriorates into chaos (entropy). The state of chaos always increases. Living beings fight to maintain themselves in an attempt to reverse entropy, and require energy to do so. When sufficient energy cannot be generated to maintain an organism, that organism dies.

Pillitary[24] describes how as death draws near, physiological changes such as slowed metabolism, decreased cell oxygenation and cell dysfunction begin to occur.

- The stroke volume of the heart decreases, and ineffective circulation gives the child a mottled and cyanotic appearance. Just before death, blood begins to pool towards dependent body parts, making them appear purple.
- Respiration slows down.
- Muscular function decreases.
- The digestive system slows down.
- The level of consciousness decreases.

Implications for practice

Absorption of a drug from the gastrointestinal tract, a muscle or through the skin via patches becomes virtually impossible. Miller (personal communication, 2005) states that at this point the child is likely to be comatose, and does not have an awareness of their symptoms.

He suggests that a child who is cognate enough to experience discomfort is likely to have sufficient perfusion to absorb medication given enterally if a nasogastric tube or gastrostomy is *in situ*. If absorption is impaired, it is common safe practice to increase the dose until the drug becomes effective. This takes account of the fact that a proportion of the medication will not be absorbed. Intravenous medication is not usually instigated at this point unless the child already has intravenous access (e.g. a portacath). A child dying in hospital who already has intravenous access is likely to be given medication via this route.

Physical care needs to be tapered to this altered situation, and according to Ellershaw and Ward[7] it should include the following.

- Inappropriate interventions, including blood tests and measurement of vital signs, should be discontinued.
- Although the evidence is limited, it suggests that continuing to give artificial fluids to the dying patient is of limited benefit and in most cases should be discontinued.
- Patients who are in the dying phase should not be subjected to attempts at cardiopulmonary resuscitation, as this constitutes a futile and inappropriate medical treatment.
- Regular assessment should be made and adequate symptom control maintained, including control of pain and agitation.
- Attention to mouth care is essential in the dying patient, and the family might wish to provide this care.

Hockenberry *et al.*[25] explain that although there might be wide variation, there is an overall decline in the child's physical condition. This might be interspersed with brief spurts of energy, causing the parents to become exhausted and overwhelmed. The direct results of the child's physiological decline are manifested as follows.

- The child sleeps more.
- Their appetite and thirst will decrease. Eventually the child will have difficulty swallowing and will stop taking food and drink.
- Consequently their urinary output will decrease, and the urine will become more concentrated.
- The child will gradually become less responsive.
- There is loss of the senses. Tactile sensation decreases, and there is increased sensitivity to light.
- Hearing is the last sense to fail.
- There is a change in respiratory pattern to Cheyne–Stokes respiration (waxing and waning of the depth of breathing, with regular periods of apnoea) and the 'death rattle' (noisy chest sounds due to the accumulation of pulmonary and pharyngeal secretions).
- The skin may have a pale, greyish-blue colour and may be cool to the touch.

- The child's eyes may be slightly open, with a fixed gaze.
- Relaxation of the muscles occurs. This may alter the appearance of the individual.[26]

The family needs to be prepared for these changes, so that they can continue with care-giving activities that promote a loving presence for the child.

Although their article was based on adults, Ellershaw and Ward[7] state that a constant source of frustration and anger reported by bereaved relatives was that no one sat down with them and discussed the fact that their loved one was dying. This also influences psychological care as well as spiritual care for both the patient and their relatives.

Although little is known about how children experience death, pooling observations by carers might be a useful starting point for ensuring the emotional safety of the dying child.

Hockenberry et al.[25] describe how some children may experience visions of angels, or of friends or family members whom they had known and who have since died. Children might mention that they are not afraid and that someone is waiting for them. In most cases this appears to provide a comforting and reassuring presence for the child and their family.

Winston[23] explores two phenomena commonly described by adults who have had near-death experiences.

- Bright light at the end of a tunnel. Winston attributes this to the fact that the brain is starved of oxygen. This causes the neurons involved in vision to fire at random, giving a sensation of bright light. There are more neurons at the centre of vision than at the periphery, thus giving the appearance of a tunnel.
- Sensation of euphoria. The brain releases endorphins to relieve the acute distress and pain of terminal events. According to Winston, these may produce hallucinations in the part of the brain that deals with memories and emotions.

When death has occurred

Quested and Rudge[27] offer a discourse analysis of the nursing care of dead bodies. They recognise that death necessitates a reconfiguration of the understanding of the patient. The main points in their article pertaining to the care of children and young people are summarised below.

- These authors argue that death involves a transition during which the individual is reconfigured conceptionally, physically, socially and culturally through the practices of care for the dead body. This transition is mediated by medicine in the defining, pronouncement and procedures of death, and by the nurses in the physical acts of care for the dead body.
- In the living, the presentation of the self is critical, as the validity of the person is often seen to be manifested in the nature of their outer bodies. This means that by removing layers of coverings (and in the case of adult patients by dressing them in a shroud) nurses transform the patient into a corpse, creating new meanings. This transformation occurs before the nurses' eyes and by their actions. (Within paediatrics it has become customary for parents to participate in this process if they wish and feel able to do so. Children and young people are dressed in clothes of either their own or their parents' choice. This has no research basis but is thought to make the process of 'letting go' less traumatic.)
- At the point of this final aspect of care the 'body' challenges the understanding of embodiment, humanity, society, life and death. Embodiment is challenged as the body physically alters, cooling and discolouring. Humanity is challenged as death reminds us that we are all essentially alone while being part of a social group that will outlive the individual. Finally, death is challenged as the body progressively dies, not all at once, but as part of a slow continuum.

Pike[28] reviewed practices with regard to the manual handling of the deceased child in children's hospices. She found that the manual handling guidelines that were in place for living patients were often not adhered to during and after a child's transfer to the 'special bedroom'* and during care (e.g. when changing the child's clothes or bedding, or lifting them into a coffin prior to the funeral). Pike reported that staff found it difficult to move and handle a dead body, as they felt that they were disturbing the child or not leaving them in peace. This may mean that they rush the task and do not use appropriate equipment, such as a hoist or slide sheet, because they feel that it is intrusive. Although the weight of a child will remain the same, the changes to the body that take place after death (including rigor mortis for up to 24 hours after death) may make handling the body particularly difficult. The bed that is used in the 'special bedroom' might not be adjustable in height, or it might not be free-standing to allow access from both sides. Both the emotional stress experienced and the temperature of the room influence the motor performance of the carer. Pike recommends that manual handling training should be adapted to include these issues, and that specific policies need to be in place to enable services to fulfil their manual handling obligations to the staff by providing an environment that reduces any risk to a minimum, while still being true to its philosophy.

Time-of-death arrangements

The ACT family pack[29] has a section on 'planning end-of-life care' which explains aspects such as 'do not resuscitate' orders, organ donation, post-mortem, time-of-death arrangements, and support afterwards.

Miller (personal communication, 2005) states that there is some flexibility with regard to confirming expected deaths. A doctor has to confirm a death, but in the case of an expected death this is not a medical emergency. This means that if a child dies at home and their death was expected, the parents might wish to wait until the following morning before contacting a GP for formal confirmation of death. However, they also might need the reassurance of someone visiting the home to provide emotional support and confirm the death so that they can start the grieving process. A death certificate is issued by a qualified doctor who has seen the child before and is prepared to sign the certificate. If no doctor is willing to sign the certificate, the coroner is informed and a post-mortem will then probably take place.

Post-mortems

Occasionally a post-mortem or a limited post-mortem examination is requested for a child who has died of a life-threatening or life-limiting illness.

If the child's death has become a coroner's case (e.g. after a sudden unexpected death) the post-mortem is a legal requirement, and the parents cannot withhold consent. However, the parents will still need support and information about why the procedure is necessary and may help to explain the child's death.

Many hospitals will have access to a post-mortem coordinator. The paediatric pathologist or the consultant who has been looking after the child will explain the results of the post-mortem to the parents. In some situations parents who allow a post-mortem might feel comforted by the fact that this may have helped another child's treatment.

Following high-profile scandals concerning the failure to obtain informed consent from parents with regard to the retention of organs of deceased children, the

---

* The term 'special bedroom' refers to a room that can be maintained at about 7°C, where a child's body can remain up to the time of the funeral if appropriate, and where families can visit as often as they wish.

Department of Health has put in place stringent guidelines that require detailed information to be given.[30,31]

Post-mortem information is presented sensitively, but is also very detailed. The document is currently adapted by local health authorities and will gradually be replaced. The Paediatric Intensive Care Society[32] offers an excellent description of 'What happens in a post-mortem examination.' It includes an explanation of the fact that although most organs are replaced after they have been inspected and a small section has been taken for microscopic examination, this is not possible with the brain, for which the preparation process takes a week before the organ can be returned to the child's body. The parents may opt to wait for the organs to be returned before the child is buried or cremated. Knowledge of what actually happens is useful and important, and the Paediatric Intensive Care Society suggests that a trained person, namely the bereavement adviser, is involved in this process. They also suggest that a post-mortem should be compared to an operation, and is always performed in a respectful manner and in such a way that it leaves virtually no marks.

Self-reflection

Harrington Jacob[2] offers the following advice which, although sobering, seems a suitable conclusion to this chapter:

> At a minimum, a nurse should be self-reflective when feelings of conflict arise. The nurse should question intent and whose needs are being met. Personal opinion is not sufficient justification for maintaining a particular stance on a topic...and generally results in a disservice to the nurse, patient, family and team.
>
> This is another example of an ethical dilemma that is based on the comparison between harm and benefit. More often than not, the harm in imposing personal opinion outweighs the benefit.

Summary

This chapter has considered the final part of the ACT Care Pathway, namely 'recognising dying.' The setting in which death might take place as well as the emotional journey towards 'letting go' have been discussed. Fear of the unknown and death anxiety among healthcare professionals have been examined, as well as theories of death and dying. The biological processes of dying have been described and implications for practice established. Attitudes towards caring for the body, certification of death and post-mortem examinations have also been discussed.

SWOT

It might be useful to revisit the SWOT analysis at this point in order to determine any further learning needs in relation to this chapter.

Strengths	Weaknesses
Opportunities	Threats

Resources and demands exercise

At this point the reader might wish to examine the resources and demands in their own personal and professional life and to reflect on how their personal coping strategies could be bolstered before determining any further learning needs in relation to this chapter.

Resources	Demands
•	•
•	•
•	•
•	•
•	•
•	•
•	•
•	•

Action plan for further learning

<table>
<tr><td></td></tr>
<tr><td></td></tr>
<tr><td></td></tr>
</table>

References

1. Neuberger J (2003) Commentary: a 'good death' is possible in the NHS. *BMJ.* **326:** 34.
2. Harrington Jacobs H (2005) Ethics in pediatric end-of-life care: a nursing perspective. *J Pediatr Nurs.* **20:** 360–9.
3. Department of Health (2004) *The NHS Knowledge and Skills Framework (NHS KSF) and the Development Review Process.* Department of Health, London.
4. All the documents for the National Service Framework for Children can be accessed via the Department of Health website; www.dh.gov.uk/PublicationsAndStatistics/ Publications/PublicationsPolicyAndGuidance/PublicationsPolicyAndGuidanceArticle/f s/en?CONTENT_ID=4123874&chk=CKADiz
5. Elston S (2004) *Integrated Multi-Agency Care Pathways for Children with Life-Threatening and Life-Limiting Conditions.* ACT, Bristol.
6. Hynson J, Gillis J, Collins J *et al.* (2003) The dying child: how is care different? *Med J Aust.* **179:** S20–2.
7. Ellershaw J and Ward C (2003) Care of the dying patient: the last hours or days of life. *BMJ.* **326:** 30–4.
8. Hylton Rushton C (2005) A framework for integrated paediatric palliative care: being with dying. *J Pediatr Nurs.* **20:** 311–25.
9. Jack B, Gambles M, Murphy D *et al.* (2003) Nurses' perceptions of the Liverpool Care Pathway for the dying patient in the acute hospital setting. *Int J Palliat Nurs.* **9:** 375–81.
10. Solomon M, Dokken D, Fleischman E *et al.* (2002) The Initiative for Pediatric Palliative Care (IPPC): background and goals. Education Development Centre, Inc., Newton, MA; www.ippcweb.org
11. Davies R (2004) New understandings of parental grief: literature review. *J Adv Nurs.* **46:** 506–13.
12. The Scottish Partnership Agency for Palliative and Cancer Care; www. palliativecarescotland.org.uk
13. Boyle M and Carter D (1998) Death anxiety amongst nurses. *Int J Palliat Care.* **4:** 37–43.
14. Palliativedrugs.com; www.palliativedrugs.com/forum/read.php
15. Copp G (1998) A review of current theories of death and dying. *J Adv Nurs.* **28:** 382–90.
16. Buckman R (1993) Communication in palliative care: a practical guide. In: D Doyle, G Hanks and N MacDonald (eds) *Oxford Textbook of Palliative Medicine.* Oxford Medical Publications, Oxford.
17. Kübler-Ross E (1969) *On Death and Dying.* Tavistock Publications, London.
18. Glaser BG and Strauss AL (1968) *Time for Dying.* Aldine, Chicago.
19. Corr C (1992) A task-based approach to coping with dying. *Omega.* **24:** 81–94.
20. Bluebond-Langner M (1978) *The Private World of Dying Children.* Princeton University Press, Princeton, NJ.

21. Bluebond-Langner M (1996) *In the Shadow of Illness: parents and siblings of the chronically ill child*. Princeton University Press, Princeton, NJ.

22. Bluebond-Langner M and DeCicco A (2006) Children's view of death. In: A Goldman, R Hain and S Liben (eds) *The Oxford Textbook of Paediatric Palliative Care*. Oxford University Press, Oxford.

23. Winston R (1997) *The Human Body*. BBC Publications, London.

24. Pillitary A (1999) *Child Health Nursing*. Lippincott, Philadelphia, PA.

25. Hockenberry M, Wilson D, Winkelstein M *et al.* (2003) *Wong's Nursing Care of Infants and Children*. Mosby, St Louis, MO.

26. Woodhouse J (2005) A personal reflection on sitting at the bedside of a dying loved one: the final hours of life. *Int J Palliat Nurs.* **11:** 28–32.

27. Quested B and Rudge T (2003) Nursing care of dead bodies: a discourse analysis of last offices. *J Adv Nurs.* **41:** 553–60.

28. Pike A (2004) Manual handling the deceased child in a children's hospice. *J Child Health Care.* **8:** 198–209.

29. The ACT family pack; www.act.org

30. Department of Health; www.doh.gov.uk/tissue/pmconsentchildhosp.pdf

31. Department of Health; www.doh.gov/pmchildinfo.pdf

32. Paediatric Intensive Care Society (2002) *Standards for Bereavement Care*. Paediatric Intensive Care Society, London.

Conclusion and areas of further research

This book has discussed different situations in which children and young people experience life-limiting or life-threatening illness or a sudden, unforeseen terminal event. An attempt has been made to map the considerations required to give the best possible care against the available evidence as well as the National Service Framework for Children and in particular the ACT Care Pathway. Contemporary issues have been highlighted within each subject area discussed. In each chapter, various clinical governance exercises have allowed the reader to focus on examination of their own practice, feelings, attitudes and learning needs.

Writing this book has been an amazing journey. At the outset I wasn't sure how much evidence I was going to find. In the end I found more than I had expected. Research projects could be identified in virtually every area of palliative care that I examined. Some areas simply excel with regard to the information that is offered for parents, children, young people and even grandparents. The more I searched, the more I found – and it just kept coming!

As a specialty, children's palliative care has come a long way. There has been some pioneering work done in some areas of palliative care for children and young people – for example, on care for young people with degenerative musculoskeletal disease. In the context of the National Service Framework there is now a framework to facilitate this and examine how through effective collaboration the best possible care for children, young people and their families can be achieved.

Many areas within palliative care for children and young people are well on their way to meeting the 10-year target of implementing the National Service Framework. An impressive amount of work has been done, and is ongoing and constantly being refined to identify the needs of families and how these can be met most effectively. This work will also provide the ammunition for funding in an area that relies so heavily on charitable funding.

Despite ongoing research and a significant knowledge base, gaps have been identified in some areas that require further work and sharing of knowledge which might well be out there, but is not readily accessible. The list is not exhaustive, and I expect that the clinical governance exercise at the end of each chapter will uncover further gaps which I hope colleagues will find the confidence to address! Listed below are the areas that I felt warranted further research.

1. Understanding the concept of 'life-limited' – there seem to be huge discrepancies in understanding of the term within the different settings in which some children and young people may find themselves. Sometimes it is difficult to determine whether a reluctance to identify a child or young person as life-limited refers purely to an expectation that they are unlikely to die in the foreseeable future, or whether it has more to do with entitlement to service provision.
2. The extent to which being given the 'label' of 'life-limited' has a negative effect on the child or young person. No published evidence could be identified in this context, but it appears to be recognised now that from the young person's perspective the outcome in terms of quality of life is not so favourable if they have a life-limited label. The outcome is better if there are periods of time when they are free from the label, until the terminal stage of the illness is approaching.

3. Ongoing evaluation of the experience of our service users and their inclusion in the creation of services. Around 25 years ago it could not be anticipated that children with a number of conditions would survive into adulthood, and therefore services prided themselves on remaining alongside families until after the death of a child. We need to know more about when families wish to receive services, and how those services should be set up so that they are acceptable to families, flexible, and can be accessed at short notice if needed, with the families safe in the knowledge that they are still there even if the need doesn't arise for many years to come.

4. Our understanding of the physiological processes of death – so that 'dying care' is based on evidence-based practice and can be tailored to individual needs.

5. Very young parents – are they slipping through the net?

6. Childhood dementia – if we can identify a clear pattern of how children with progressive neurological illness lose their cognitive abilities, might it be possible to help a child to 'make memories' that can help later in the disease process?

7. Complementary therapies – there is a great deal of very informal evidence of how complementary therapies work. Few people would doubt the benefit of therapies such as music therapy, massage, etc., but there is limited evidence, for example, of how these might help to make the environment both physically and emotionally safer for a child who has no concept of danger or who might be experiencing hallucinations.

SWOT

It might be useful to revisit the SWOT analysis one final time (*see* chart on next page) in order to recognise existing expertise and how this can be shared and applied, and also to determine any further learning needs in relation to this book.

Action plan for further learning

Strengths	Weaknesses
• Both as a team and as individuals we do recognise our strengths. • I have found the scenario work easy. • On our unit we have followed through how the care for the young person in the relevant scenario would have worked. • We now have a small working group of staff exploring how we can adapt the ACT Care Pathway for our purposes and improve the care for families in this kind of situation. • This is supported by all relevant members of the multi-disciplinary team.	• I have found some of the material presented in the 'contemporary issues' sections difficult. • I have not previously thought of some of the areas covered as relevant to my field of practice. • I have limited experience with computers, and although I have access to the Internet at work I try to avoid it. • On reflecting on the emotional needs of carers, I have been surprised by the interaction between my personal life and my work.
Opportunities	**Threats**
• During clinical supervision we have agreed that I can go on an in-house IT course. • The working party looking at the implementation of the ACT Care Pathway has also instigated a resource that includes some of the reference material suggested. • We are now looking at staff support and how we can address the balance of resources and demands. • We are making emotional support a distinct feature of clinical supervision.	• It is very difficult to find protected time to follow up the resources that have been suggested. • There is continued pressure on staff due to staff shortages. We are finding it difficult to recruit into some areas due to a lack of expertise.

The key documents

This chapter covers

Content

- The ACT Care Pathway
- Integrated care pathways
- 'Every Child Matters'
- The Children Act 2004
- The Children's Bill
- The National Service Framework for Children, Young People and Maternity Services: standard for hospital services
- The NSF exemplars
- The National Service Framework for Children, Young People and Maternity Services: commissioning children's and young people's palliative care services
- The Knowledge and Skills Framework
- The common core of skills and knowledge for the children's workforce
- The framework for specialist palliative care
- The framework of competencies for basic specialist training in paediatrics
- The Liverpool Care Pathway for the Dying Child
- Keeping up to date

A brief résumé of the main guidance documents applied in this book is given below, as they provide the guiding principles for the evidence-based care that is required for children and young people and their families.

The ACT Care Pathway[1]

The ACT Care Pathway provides the structure that enables healthcare professionals to meaningfully organise care for life-threatened and life-limited children and young people and their families. The pathways are used to critique the care proposed for the families described in the book. Although the scenarios present only a snapshot of the family's journey, a child is unlikely to have one carer throughout. It is envisaged that the reader will consider what has happened to a family before contact with them, and also on the remainder of the journey.

Some of the salient points are summarised below, but the reader is strongly recommended to access the complete text.

Ladyman[2] explains that the ACT Care Pathway represents a pathway for engaging with the needs of the child and their family, which can be used to ensure that all the pieces of the jigsaw are in place, so that the family has access to the appropriate support at the appropriate time.

This document was written to complement the children's National Service Framework (NSF), specifically guidance presented in the NSF Standard 8 on Disabled Children and Young People, and those with complex health needs.

The Care Pathway has three stages:

- Pathway 1: diagnosis or recognition
- Pathway 2: living with a life-threatening illness (LTI) or a life-limiting illness (LLI)
- Pathway 3: end of life.

Five sentinel standards

Each stage begins with a key event of vital significance for the family.

The template sets out five sentinel standards along the pathway that should be developed as a minimum for all families, with the aim of achieving equity for all families wherever they live. The stages identify the weakest points for many families in their pattern of care. Elston[1] identifies them as the points at which there are frequently difficulties with communication and integrated working by professionals, and they are therefore key actions that should be given the highest priority. They include the following:

1. the prognosis – breaking bad news
2. transfer and liaison between hospital and community services
3. multi-disciplinary assessment of needs
4. child and family care plan
5. end-of-life plan.

The template is intended to be a generic one for developing individual care packages, with the primary intention of providing the means for essential components that could underpin more detailed local pathways. Elston[1] emphasises that those at local level will need to develop their own pathway and delivery plans to take account of existing local services, available resources and geographical area. Using the pathways to their full potential might include mapping where on the pathways individuals find themselves at any one time. Browne (personal communication, 2005) states that this can be enlightening, as it is possible that the child, either parent or the professionals involved might not share the same perspective on this. It is therefore suggested that the reader uses the pathways as a working document throughout the text. Browne recommends that the end-of-life plan is drawn up early on in the child's disease trajectory, so that it can be reviewed. This has a dual function. It allows one to touch base and to become matter of fact in a positive way, and it also avoids a feeling of 'giving up on the child' when a child enters the final pathway, as well as regrets along the lines of 'Why didn't we look at this earlier?'

Miller (personal communication, 2005) asserts that in order to achieve ownership of the pathways by families, the pathways should be held by families. 'Parent-held records' such as the 'Red Book' have had mixed success in creating a continuous record including hospital and clinic records for children under the age of 5 years. A number of children's services have attempted to use a type of portfolio for children with complex needs that travels with the child between home, school and hospital to provide continuity.

Integrated care pathways[3]

In a wider context, integrated care pathways (ICPs) according to the Department for Education and Skills and the Department of Health 'are a tool and a concept that embed guidelines, protocols and locally agreed, evidence-based, patient-centred best practice into everyday use for the individual patient.'[3]

An ICP aims to have the right people doing the right things in the right order at the right time in the right place with the right outcome, all with attention to the patient experience.

'Every Child Matters'[4]

'Every Child Matters' provides the legislative backbone to the National Service Framework. It has five key outcomes that need to be kept in mind when making decisions with families, whether for the sick child or young person or the siblings.

- *Being healthy:* enjoying good physical and mental health and living a healthy lifestyle.
- *Staying safe:* being protected from harm and neglect and growing up able to look after themselves.
- *Enjoying and achieving:* getting the most out of life and developing broad skills for adulthood.
- *Making a positive contribution:* to the community and to society and not engaging in antisocial or offending behaviour.
- *Economic well-being:* overcoming socio-economic disadvantages to achieve their full potential in life.

The Children Act 2004[5]

Building on 'Every Child Matters', the Children Act 2004 sets out reforms of children's services, which have been summarised by Joy[6] as including the following:

- Children's Commissioner for England
- local authorities have a duty to promote cooperation between agencies (through Children's Trusts which bring together health, education and social services within a single agency and will enable multi-agency working)
- key agencies have a duty to safeguard children
- local authorities are required to appoint a Director of Children's Services and designated lead members
- integrated inspection framework and joint area review.

The practical application is discussed in Chapter 11 and must be considered both in relation to the child in need of service provision, and also in relation to potential child protection work.

The Children's Bill[7]

This is the first bill to implement measures contained in the 2003 Green Paper, 'Every Child Matters.'

The measures include the following:

- the establishment of new Local Safeguarding Children Boards to focus on child protection
- a power to set up a new database containing basic information about children
- the appointment of a Director of Children's Services who will be accountable for local authority education and children's social services, and a Lead Council Member for Children's Services
- enabling and encouraging local authorities and relevant agencies to form Children's Trusts
- a Children's Commissioner for England, independent of Parliament, to be a voice for all children and young people, especially the most vulnerable. The Commissioner will listen to the views of children and young people and make sure that they are fed into policy making and service delivery, both locally and nationally.

The National Service Framework for Children, Young People and Maternity Services: standard for hospital services[8]

Note: Although the NSF is structured around 'Standards', the ACT standards use the same terminology for a different outcome.

The following is a summary of the core standards[9] taken from the *Executive Summary*.[10]

Standard 1: Promoting health and well-being, identifying needs and intervening early

The health and well-being of all children and young people are promoted and delivered through a coordinated programme of action, including prevention and early intervention wherever possible, to ensure long-term gain, led by the NHS in partnership with local authorities (p.11).

Standard 2: Supporting parents

Parents and carers are enabled to receive the information, services and support which will help them to care for their children and equip them with the skills they need to ensure that their children have optimum life chances and are healthy and safe (p.14).

Standard 3: Child-, young person- and family-centred services

Children and young people and their families receive high-quality services which are co-ordinated around their individual and family needs and take account of their views (p.15).

Standard 4: Growing up into adulthood

All young people have access to age-appropriate services which are responsive to their specific needs as they grow into adulthood (p.16).

Standard 5: Safeguarding and promoting the welfare of young people

All agencies work to prevent children suffering harm and to promote their welfare, and provide them with the services they require to address their identified needs and to safe-guard children who are being or who are likely to be harmed (p.17).

Standard 6: Children and young people who are ill

All children who are ill, or thought to be ill, or injured will have timely access to appro-priate advice and to effective services which address their health, social, educational and emotional needs throughout the period of their illness (p.18).

Standard 7: Children in hospital

Children and young people receive high-quality, evidence-based hospital care, developed through clinical governance and delivered in appropriate settings (p.20).

Standard 8: Disabled young people and those with complex needs

Children and young people who are disabled or who have complex health needs receive coordinated, high-quality child- and family-centred services which are based on assessed needs, which promote social inclusion and, where possible, enable them and their families to live ordinary lives (p.21).

Standard 9: The mental health and psychological well-being of children and young people

All children and young people, from birth to their eighteenth birthday, who have mental health problems and disorders have access to timely, integrated, high-quality multi-disciplinary mental health services to ensure effective assessment, treatment and support for them and their families (p.22).

Standard 10: Medicines for children and young people

Children, young people, their parents and carers, and healthcare professionals in all settings make decisions about medicines based on sound information about risk and benefit. They have access to safe and effective medicines that are prescribed on the basis of the best available evidence (p.24).

Standard 11: Maternity services

Women have access to supportive, high-quality maternity services, designed around their individual needs and those of their babies (p.26).

Evidence[11]

There are further modules available providing evidence that underpins each of these standards.[11] One chapter in the same text highlights gaps in current research evidence, and indeed a couple of chapters in this book put to the test where we are currently on the continuum of the 10-year plan for implementing the NSF.

The NSF exemplars[12]

The Department of Health and the Department for Education and Skills[1] state that the exemplars selected are intended to highlight themes such as responding to the views of children and their parents, involving them in key decisions, providing early identification, diagnosis and intervention, and delivering flexible, child-centred, holistic care. Care is integrated between agencies and over time, and is sensitive to the individual's changing needs. The Department for Education and Skills acknowledges that not every child with the same condition will follow the same journey or have the same type or severity of condition as that illustrated. The exemplars may be useful in a number of different ways.

- They highlight further references which relate to evidence in the NSF and elsewhere, including key clinical guidelines.
- They stimulate local debate and assist multi-agency partners to re-evaluate the way they collaborate on, commission and deliver children's services, for this and other conditions, to the benefit of children and their families.
- They provide an aid to examining and improving local clinical and non-clinical governance.
- They provide a multi-disciplinary training tool for staff working with children and young people to raise awareness of specific issues and stimulate discussion.
- They canvass the views of children and families on specific children's issues.

- They provide a starting point or template for debate prior to the development of new local strategies for managing complex childhood conditions.

Examples of NSF exemplars mentioned in this book include the following:

- complex disability (*see* Chapter 11)
- acquired brain injury (*see* Chapter 10)
- discharge and support of children requiring long-term ventilation in the community (*see* Chapter 10).

The National Service Framework for Children, Young People and Maternity Services: commissioning children's and young people's palliative care services[13]

This supporting document provides national guidance that will help to raise awareness of life-limited or life-threatened children and will provide information for commissioners when planning provision for their needs. The document gives the following policy and legislative context.

- The Children's NSF forms the health and social care developmental standards for services to children and young people by 2014. The child protection element of 'Safeguarding Children' is core, under 'Standards for Better Health.' As part of the commitment to double funding for end-of-life care, it brings implementation of palliative care standards much further forward than 2014. Other related policies impact on the delivery of this commitment.
- Building on the five key outcomes set out in 'Every Child Matters' and the Children's Act 2004, Standard 8 of the Children's NSF expects high-quality palliative care to be available to all children and young people who need it 'to ensure provision takes account of the child's or young person's and their family's physical, emotional, cultural and practical needs in a way that promotes choice, independence, creativity and quality of life.'
- Primary care trusts should take into account the specific requirements under Section 10 of the Children's Act 2004 with regard to their duty to cooperate with local authorities and a number of 'relevant partners' to improve the five outcomes for children in 'Every Child Matters.'

The NSF delivery cycle

The Department for Education and Skills[14] has stated that the basic delivery cycle for the NSF consists of the following:

- assessing the needs of children, young people and pregnant women
- identifying priorities, targets and standards
- planning services
- commissioning services to meet those needs
- managing performance, and assessing and inspecting outcomes.

The Knowledge and Skills Framework[15]

Skills required by staff are mapped against the NHS Knowledge and Skills Framework (NHS KSF).[15] The Department of Health[16] states that the NHS KSF and the development process will enable individuals to:

- be clear about what knowledge and skills they need and how to apply them to meet

the demands of their job
- access appropriate learning and development for their work
- see how their work relates to that of others
- identify the knowledge and skills that they need to learn and develop in order to progress in their careers.

According to the Department of Health,[16] this in turn will enable organisations to audit knowledge and skills within the organisation, to make informed decisions about staff deployment, to identify skills and knowledge gaps and plan how to address those gaps, to organise training and development across staff groups, across the organisation and possibly with other organisations, and to develop effective recruitment processes.

The Department of Health[15] describes six core dimensions, and there are also 30 specific dimensions against which individuals would need to apply their skills. The core dimensions are as follows:

1. communication
2. personal and people development
3. health, safety and security
4. service improvement
5. quality
6. equality and diversity.

There are also specific dimensions that are broken down into health and well-being, estates and facilities, information and knowledge, and a general category. These are non-hierarchical. With these come 'level descriptors' which play a critical part in relating the KSF to actual jobs.

The NHS KSF is a broad generic framework that focuses on the application of knowledge and skills, not on the exact knowledge and skills that individuals need in order to develop.[15] This document is specifically for the NHS and is also the definitive document for 'Agenda for Change' job evaluation. For the purpose of this book solely the KSF is considered, with a proposal that non-NHS settings would do well to put a framework in place to respond to the clinical governance requirements of their organisation.

The common core of skills and knowledge for the children's workforce[17]

Coinciding with the KSF is a further module in the 'Every Child Matters' series, namely a common core of skills and knowledge for the children's workforce that focuses on effective communication and engagement with children, young people, their families and carers, development considerations, safeguarding and promoting child welfare, supporting transitions, multi-agency working and information sharing.

The skills and knowledge are set out in the Common Core prospectus under six main headings as follows:

1. effective communication and engagement with children, young people and families
2. child and young person development
3. safeguarding and promoting the welfare of the child
4. supporting transitions
5. multi-agency working
6. sharing information.

The framework for specialist palliative care[18]

Within palliative care the Royal College of Nursing Hospice Nurse Managers Group has produced a framework for nurses working in specialist palliative care, clearly outlining the competencies required.

The framework of competencies for basic specialist training in paediatrics[19]

The framework of competencies for basic specialist training in paediatrics, produced by the Royal College of Paediatrics and Child Health, has been included in this book because it identifies a range of practical skills, mapping topics and skills that could be immensely helpful to specific roles and client groups.

It should be noted that there is a comparatively short section on palliative care in this document,[19] the requirements for a prospective paediatrician being merely 'awareness', 'being familiar', 'know[ing] the importance' and 'understand[ing].' It focuses on the following topics:

- national and local guidelines on withdrawing and withholding treatment
- management of sudden infant death
- legal and ethical issues relating to withdrawal of life support
- factors that determine when care of a patient becomes palliative
- seeking advice when treatment may not be in the best interest of a child
- therapeutic interventions in symptom control
- ethical issues arising from therapeutic interventions in children with life-limiting conditions
- opportunities for respite care, including hospice availability
- tests for brainstem death
- effects of loss and grief on the health and well-being of children, families and healthcare professionals
- local bereavement and support services
- drawing on the skills and experience of other professionals involved in the care of the dying child for support networks
- the need to respect the wishes of the child or young person, particularly when these are different from those of the family and healthcare professionals.

This framework implies that junior paediatricians have a more senior colleague to role model for them and guide them, and that there is a willingness to work on a multi-disciplinary basis. This is totally in the spirit of the KSF and the NSF.

The Liverpool Care Pathway for the Dying Child[20]

Matthews *et al.*[20] describe a retrospective study of 39 sets of case notes over a 57-month period. The results indicate that although evidence of the delivery of appropriate care to dying children and their families was available in the documentation of the organisations that were reviewed, some lack of consistency resulted in the researchers being unable to draw firm conclusions about the quality of care delivered. Based on the Liverpool Care Pathway for the Dying Patient,[21] which provides guidance on appropriate end-of-life care for the adult population, the Liverpool Care Pathway for the Dying Child is at an early stage. Pending analysis of a pilot study completed in April 2006 and further piloting in a variety of settings, it is envisaged that the Liverpool Care Pathway for the Dying Child will be focusing on the last days of life. Gamble (personal communication, 2006) explains that there will be differences in the detail to make it applicable to children and young people in different situations and settings. There will also be variants built in to allow for difference in care required. It can be anticipated that the Liverpool Care Pathway for the Dying Child will supplement the ACT Care Pathway 3 'End of Life' by providing the detail for care planning.

Keeping up to date

There are currently many complex relevant documents, which in turn refer to other relevant material. A great deal of work has gone into compiling these documents, and new ones continue to be published, making it difficult to keep up to date. As well as knowing that these texts exist (and most of them are easily accessible on the Internet), it is also important to disseminate them automatically to staff in the field in a structured way. This could be done by email alerts through a centralised system, perhaps at the Department of Health.

Each practitioner is professionally accountable for their actions, which should be based on an up-to-date knowledge of the evidence and current developments. This is a key requirement for effective advocacy for children, young people and their families.

However, it is neither easy nor straightforward and, as has been demonstrated in this book, requires not only a sound knowledge of the disease process, psychological needs, current treatments and new developments in treatment, but also a familiarity with and ability to integrate and apply numerous sections of the children's NSF,[8,9] the adult NSF,[22] and in some instances the older people's NSF,[22] the NSF for long-term conditions,[22] the renal NSF,[22] the ACT Care Pathway,[1] the KSF[15] and the various exemplars that are being published for specific conditions (e.g. complex disability,[9] ventilation[9]), as well as companion documents, such as the Barnados publication by Noyes and Lewis,[23] in order to advocate for their patient.

References

1. Elston S (2004) *Integrated Multi-Agency Care Pathways for Children with Life-Threatening and Life-Limiting Conditions.* ACT, Bristol.
2. Ladyman S (2004) Foreword. In: Elston S. *Integrated Multi-Agency Care Pathways for Children with Life-Threatening and Life-Limiting Conditions.* ACT, Bristol.
3. Department for Education and Skills and Department of Health (2005) *Evidence to Inform the National Service Framework for Children, Young People and Maternity Services;* www.dh.gov.uk/PolicyAndGuidance/HealthAndSocialCareTopics/ChildrenServices/ChildrenServicesInformation/ChildrenServicesInformationArticle/fs/en?CONTENT_ID=4089111&chk=U8Ecln
4. 'Every Child Matters'; www.dfes.gov.uk/everychildmatters
5. Children Act 2004; www.opsi.gov.uk/acts/acts2004/20040031.htm
6. Joy I (2005) *Valuing Short Lives: children with terminal conditions.* New Philanthropy Capital, London.
7. Children Bill 2004; www.publications.parliament.uk/pa/pabills.htm
8. Department of Health; www.dh.gov.uk/PublicationsAndStatistics/Publications/PublicationsPolicyAndGuidance/PublicationsPolicyAndGuidanceArticle/fs/en?CONTENT_ID=4006182&chk=oiSEI1
9. All the documents for the National Service Framework for Children can be accessed via the Department of Health website; www.dh.gov.uk/PolicyAndGuidance/HealthAndSocialCareTopics/ChildrenServices/ChildrenServicesInformation/ChildrenServicesInformationArticle/fs/en?CONTENT_ID=4089111&chk=U8Ecln
10. Department for Education and Skills and Department of Health (2004) *Executive Summary.* Department for Education and Skills and Department of Health, London; http://dh.gov.uk/PolicyAndGuidance/fs/en
11. Department of Health and Department for Education and Skills (2005) *National Service Framework for Children, Young People and Maternity Services: evidence to inform the National Service Framework for children, young people and maternity services.* Department of Health, London.
12. Department of Health and Department for Education and Skills (2005) *National Service Framework for Children, Young People and Maternity Services: complex disability;*

www.dh.gov.uk/policyAndGuidance/HealthAnd SocialCareTopics/ChildrenServices/fs/en

13. Department of Health and Department for Education and Skills (2005) *National Service Framework for Children, Young People and Maternity Services: commissioning children's and young people's palliative care services. A practical guide for the NHS Commissioners;* www.dh.gov.uk/PublicationsAndStatistics/Publications/PublicationsPolicyAndGuidance /PublicationsPolicyAndGuidanceArticle/fs/en?CONTENT ID=4123874&chk=CKADiz

14. *National Service Framework for Children, Young People and Maternity Services;* www.dh.gov.uk/PublicationsAndStatistics/Publications/PublicationsPolicyAndGuidanc e/PublicationsPolicyAndGuidanceArticle/fs/en?CONTENT ID=4123874&chk=CKADiz

15. Department of Health (2004) *The NHS Knowledge and Skills Framework (NHS KSF) and the Development Review Process.* Department of Health, London.

16. Department of Health (2003) *The NHS Knowledge and Skills Framework and Related Development Review (Working Draft).* Department of Health, London.

17. Department for Education and Skills (2005) *Common Core of Skills and Knowledge for the Children's Workforce;* www.everychildmatters.gov.uk

18. Royal College of Nursing Hospice Nurse Managers Group (2002) *A Framework for Nurses Working in Specialist Palliative Care: competencies project.* Royal College of Nursing, London.

19. Royal College of Paediatrics and Child Health (RCPCH) (2004) *A Framework of Competences for Basic Specialist Training in Paediatrics.* RCPCH, London.

20. Matthews K, Gambles M, Ellershaw J *et al.* (2006) Developing the Liverpool Care Pathway for the dying child. *Paediatr Nurs.* **18:** 18–21.

21. Ellershaw J and Wilkinson S (eds) (2003) *Care of the Dying: a pathway to excellence.* Oxford University Press, Oxford.

22. Link to National Service Frameworks mentioned in this section: www.dh.gov.uk/AdvancedSearch/SearchResults/fs/en?NP=1&PO1=C&PI1=W&PF1= A&PG=1&RP=20&PT1=national+service+framework&SC= dh site&Z=1

23. Noyes J and Lewis M (2005) *From Hospital to Home: guidance on discharge management and community support needs of children using long-term ventilation.* Barnados, Ilford; www.longtermventilation.nhs.uk

Some things don't turn out as planned
As I give you to our father's hand
I want you to remember that we laughed.

We Laughed, **by Billy Bragg and**
Maxine Edgington
From the CD *Rosetta Requiem* **(2005)**
produced by Rosetta Life, London.

Index